# Functional Electrical Stimulation in Neurorehabilitation

Thomas Schick

Editor

# Functional Electrical Stimulation in Neurorehabilitation

## Synergy Effects of Technology and Therapy

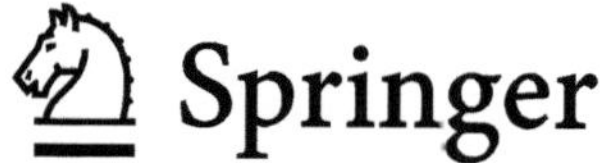 Springer

*Editor*
Thomas Schick
Department Neurorehabilitation STIWELL
MED-EL
Innsbruck, Tirol, Austria

ISBN 978-3-030-90125-7      ISBN 978-3-030-90123-3   (eBook)
https://doi.org/10.1007/978-3-030-90123-3



This Springer imprint is published by the registered company Springer Nature Switzerland AG
The registered company address is: Gewerbestrasse 11, 6330 Cham, Switzerland

# Preface

Within the treatment of neurological diseases, neurorehabilitation is still a young special discipline. No other medical field aims for a need of such close cooperation between the disciplines and players. For this reason, this book addresses large parts of the neurological rehabilitation network.

Neurorehabilitation has changed significantly over the past 30 years as a result of a steady increase in knowledge in the areas of motor learning, neuroplasticity, and the efficacy of therapeutic procedures. Significant research activity, particularly in the last two decades, has challenged existing treatment approaches and introduced new ones. One of these modern therapeutic approaches, Functional Electrical Stimulation (FES), is presented comprehensively in this book with its many possible applications in a wide variety of diseases. These range from the treatment of sensorimotor disorders to forms of therapy in the neck area for improving swallowing and speech. Neuro-urological application areas are also discussed.

This book reveals therapeutic possibilities to the professional audience on how various neurological diseases can be treated in a target-oriented, evident way. The importance of FES is underlined by a steadily growing body of evidence.

This fascinating therapeutic progress has been made possible by global research activity in this field. The further development of medical technology for user-friendly electrical stimulation devices tailored to patient needs has also led to an improved range of products. The added value of this development can be seen particularly in individualizable and adaptable multichannel therapy devices for electrical stimulation which in many cases also enable patient-directed movement triggering.

In their contributions, the authors expressly refrain from naming and describing commercially available medical devices for functional electrical stimulation. Instead, they describe the therapeutic requirements for the patient and thus the requirements that are placed on the medical devices to be adequately used for the respective applications.

The aim of the book is to provide the reader with therapeutic instructions for treatment as well as relevant background information on the mode of action of FES. It is not intended to be another book on electrotherapy, but a first comprehensive standard work on FES and its great importance in the context of therapy in neurorehabilitation.

All authors contributing to this book are scientifically active and clinical experts in the field of neurorehabilitation, FES, or electromedical engineering.

We have deliberately focused on the treatment of structural, functional, and activity deficits in upper and lower motor neuron damage, improving mobility, sensitivity, and perception, as well as facial expression, swallowing, and oral function.

I hope this book contributes to many inspiring insights into FES with its wide range of applications in neurological patients.

Innsbruck, Austria                                              Thomas Schick

# Acknowledgments

A book project of this kind requires many active supporters until it is successfully produced, who, in addition to the authors, have a significant influence on the success of the book. At this point, I would like to express my gratitude to these persons. In particular, I would like to thank all authors for their very carefully prepared and consistent high-quality contributions.

My appreciations and thanks go to Ms. Anja Fuchs, who has tirelessly contributed with great creativity and extraordinary skills to the successful design and implementation of the countless graphics, tables, photographs, and video sequences in all chapters as well as Ms. Andrea Weiler, (MA) and Ms. Mag. Ursula Lehner-Mayrhofer for their great commitment and many hours of translating and proofreading of various chapters.

I would also like to express my special thanks to Ms. Patricia Meier (MSc) and Ms. Maria Steinmetz (BA) for the intensive and very constructive discussions in the early and late phases of the preparation of the book concept and for proofreading my contributions.

We would like to thank our photo models Ms. Carla Greier, Ms. Franziska Lauerwald (BSc), Ms. Vera Sprenzinger (BSc), Ms. Sabrina Falgschlunger, Mr. Oliver Hinzmann, and Mr. Stefan Ossanna for their great commitment and patience as well as the therapy department of the private clinic "Sanatorium Kettenbrücke" in Innsbruck, Austria, where we created the visual content and especially their therapy director Mr. Manuel Krug. He supported us in a very cooperative and uncomplicated way by officially providing us with the therapy rooms and materials for the two photo shoots to create the countless photographs and video sequences.

Furthermore, I would like to thank the company MED-EL, department of Neurorehabilitation STIWELL in Innsbruck, for the electrical stimulation devices and the necessary accessories they provided. This support enabled the vivid and illustrative design of the whole project.

My thoughts also go to university professor DI Dr. med. Stefan Golaszewski who passed away unexpectedly while this book was in preparation. He was a passionate advocate of various forms of electrical stimulation. He made a very large contribution to the establishment of these forms of therapy through his intensive research activities and as a dedicated physician. We will miss him and are pleased, however, that we are able to preserve and convey a part of his extensive knowledge and experience to the interested professional community through his exciting book contribution, supporting also his spirit.

Innsbruck                                                            Thomas Schick
April 2022

# Contents

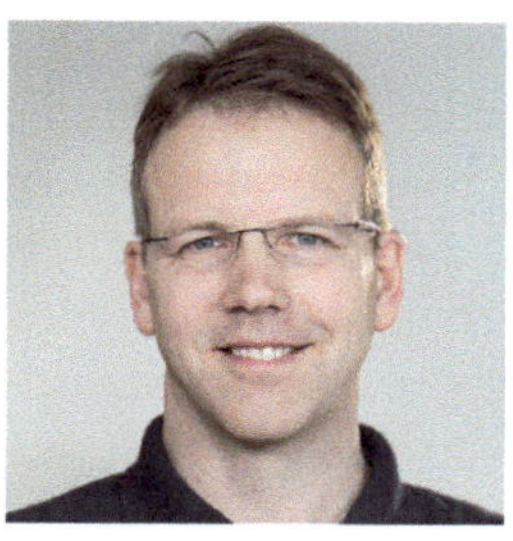

**Thomas Schick, MSc** gained extensive experience as a physiotherapist since 1993 and has led several rehabilitation teams at German clinics for neurorehabilitation. He also graduated as a specialist in social and health care. For more than 20 years, he has been a lecturer for various rehabilitation procedures in neurology. Among other things, he regularly teaches at the master's degree programs in neurorehabilitation and occupational therapy at the Center for Neurorehabilitation at the Danube University Krems, Austria. The main focus of his work is to convey and deepen the knowledge of FES and in particular EMG-triggered multichannel electrical stimulation. After completing his studies in neurorehabilitation with a master's degree in 2015, He joined Neurorehabilitation STIWELL, which is a department of the international company MED-EL, based in Innsbruck, Austria. Here, he is working on the development of medical products from a medical-therapeutic point of view, the implementation of training events and scientific work in the field of FES. He is member of the IFESS and published several articles in professional journals and a German-language therapeutic textbook about "Functional electrical stimulation in Neurorehabilitation" previously.

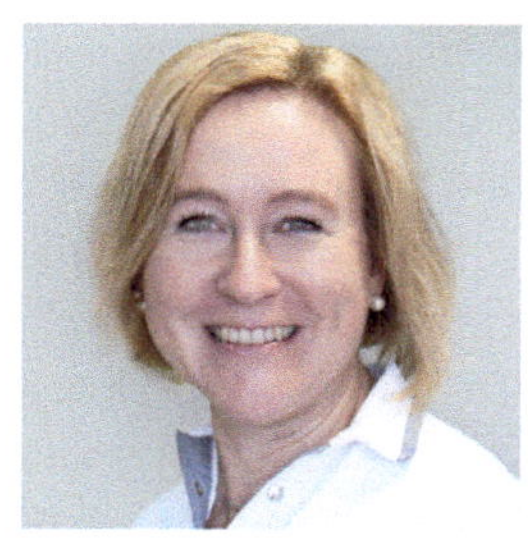

**Ines Bersch-Porada, MSc, PhD** is working at the Swiss Paraplegic Centre since 1991 and has been Head of the International FES Centre® since 2018. Her work is focusing on functional electrical stimulation (FES) and its implementation in the rehabilitation of people suffering from paraplegia and neuromusculoskeletal disorders.

Additionally, she teaches at the Universities of Applied Sciences in Bern and Basel. In 2012, the author obtained a Master of Science in

Neurorehabilitation Research and her PhD in Clinical Sciences at the University of Gothenburg. Her topic was focusing on upper and lower motoneuron lesions in tetraplegia—diagnostic and therapeutic implications of electrical stimulation. Apart from her clinical work, she gives lectures and organizes workshops. As a clinician, scientist, lecturer, and active member of the IFESS, she implements FES in clinical practice based on clinical study results and new technologies.

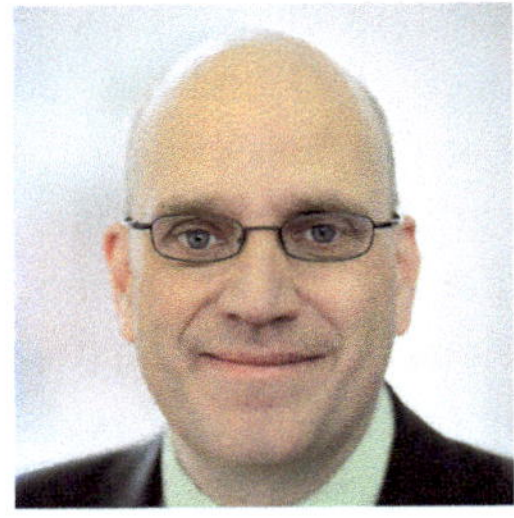

**Christian Dohle, MD, MPhil** is physicist, neurologist, and rehabilitation physician. Currently, he is leader of the P.A.N. Center for Post-Acute Neurorehabilitation and Head of research, both at the Fürst Donnersmarck Foundation in Berlin. Besides, he is teaching at different academic institutions, including the Charité—University Medicine Berlin and vice president of the German Society for Neurorehabilitation. His main scientific focus lies on evidence-based motor rehabilitation procedures, especially with visual stimulation (mirror therapy, virtual reality). Besides, he is working on determining factors of quality in neurorehabilitation.

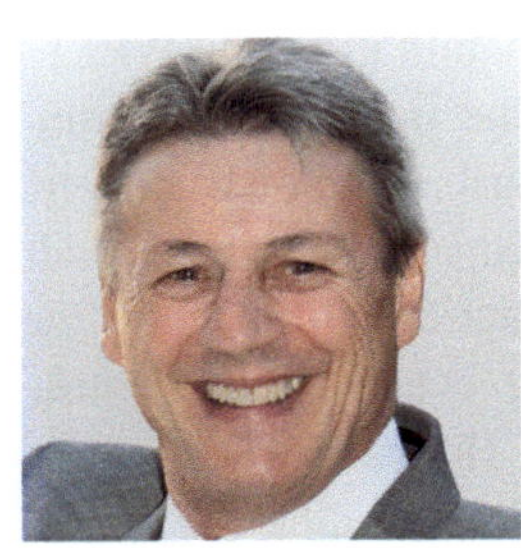

**Klemens Fheodoroff, MD** specialist in neurology/psychiatry who achieved his diploma in Manual Medicine and Psychotherapeutic Medicine (ÖÄK). He is teaching the university course for medical managers in Graz. He is working as a senior physician in Neurorehabilitation at the Gailtal Klinik in Hermagor since 1994. Moreover, he is teaching at the Carinthia University of Applied Sciences and the Danube University Krems. Additionally, he is a member of the Scientific Advisory Board/Austrian Society for Neurological Rehabilitation (OeGNR) and the World Forum Neurorehabilitation (WFNR), especially in the special interest groups on MAC and robotics. He organized the Neurorehabilitation-Curriculum OeGNR between 2006 and 2018 and is a member of the BoNT Certification Committee of the Austrian Dystonia and Botulinum Toxin Working Group (ÖDBAG). Over 40 publications on spasticity and

BoNT, goals, ICF, and HRQoL were published including his expertise.

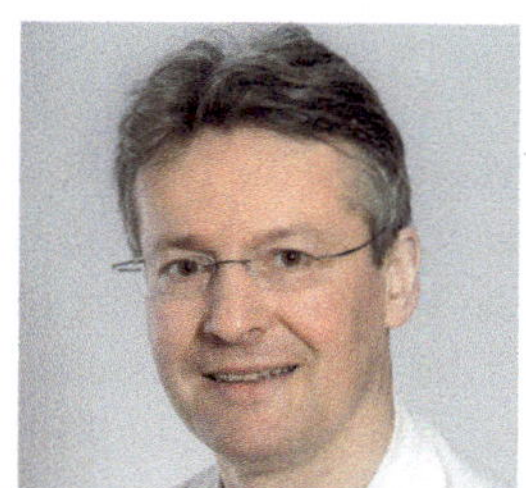

**Stefan M. Golaszewski, MD** was born in Vienna in 1964 and died unexpectedly at the end of 2020. He studied technical physics and medicine in Vienna. Between 1995 and 2001 he was working as a resident in neurology at the MR Institute of the University Hospital Innsbruck with a focus on scientific research in clinical applications for fMRI. He continued his residency in neurology from 2001 to 2002 at the Neurology Department at the Medical University of Graz and completed it between 2002 and 2004 at the Alfred Krupp Hospital in Essen and at the Department of Neurology, St. Mauritius Therapy Clinic near Düsseldorf. After that, he started working at the University Clinic of Neurology at the Paracelsus Medical University (PMU) Salzburg, where he habilitated in neurology in 2006.

From 2010, Prof. Golaszewski was medical director at the Neuroscience Institute of the PMU, where he was appointed associate university professor in 2019. Prof. Golaszewski has published a total of 150 articles in international peer-reviewed journals.

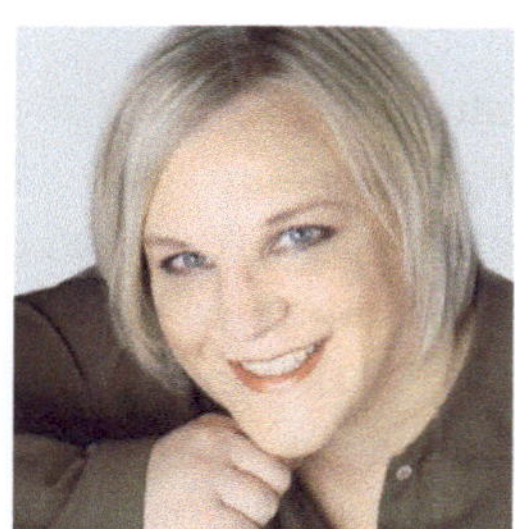

**Kerstin Schwenker** works in the field of Neurorehabilitation, Neuroscience, and Paraplegia Research (SCI-TReCS, Spinal Cord Injury and Tissue Regeneration Center Salzburg) at the Department of Neurology at the University Hospital Salzburg, at the Paracelsus Medical University Sazburg and at the Karl Landsteiner Institute for Neurorehabilitation and Space Neurology, Salzburg, Austria. At the Medical University of Graz, Austria, she completed the university course Clinical Trial Specialist with distinction. Until the sudden death of Dr. of medicine Stefan M. Golaszewski, university professor and engineer, in November 2020, she had been his assistant for many years. She is currently completing her extra-occupational master's degree in Study Management at the Medical University of Vienna, Austria, as well as studying human medicine at the Paracelsus

Medical University of Salzburg, Austria. In addition to her clinical and scientific work, she is also active in teaching and in the organization of congresses and workshops.

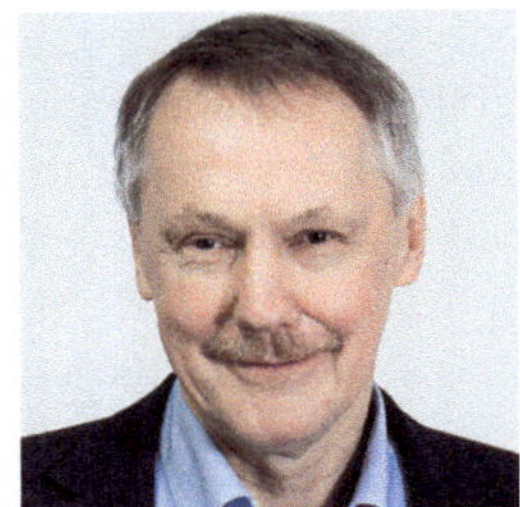

**Winfried Mayr** has worked at the Medical University in Vienna after he completed his studies in electrical engineering at the Vienna University of Technology in 1983. In 1992, he wrote his dissertation on "Reactivation of paralyzed muscles by FES with implants." Subsequently, he worked on noninvasive FES applications in paraplegic rehabilitation, in space and for the elderly. He coordinated the EU project RISE with 20 partner groups, which resulted in a novel clinical method including a market-ready stimulator for denervated muscles. His current focus is on spinal cord stimulation after injury. Between 2009 and 2017, he was president of the Austrian Society for Biomedical Engineering (ÖGBMT), since then vice president and board member of the European umbrella organization EAMBES (European Alliance for Medical and Biological Engineering and Science). He is one of the founders and board member of the International FES Society (IFESS) and a section editor for FES at the Journals Artificial Organs and Frontiers in Neuroscience.

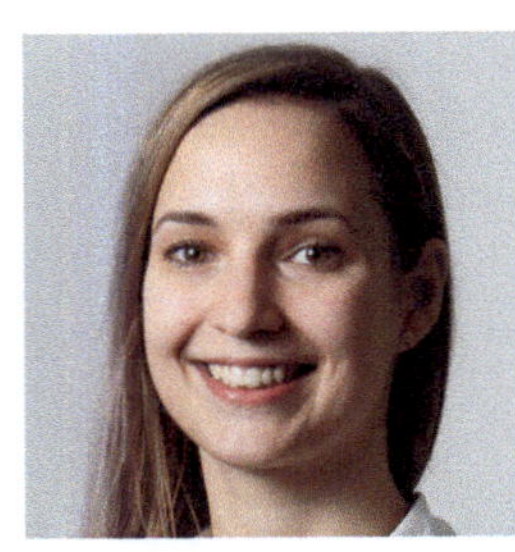

**Patricia Meier, MSc, PhD student** graduated as a physiotherapist in 2010 from the University of Applied Sciences for Health, Innsbruck, Austria. She continued her further qualification at the Danube University Krems, where she finished her master's degree in neurorehabilitation with distinction in 2018. Since 2019, she is studying part-time in the PhD program for neuroscience at the Medical University of Innsbruck. She is working at the Medical University of Innsbruck, Department of Neurology, since 2011 and as a research associate (MED-EL Medical Electronics, VASCage GmbH) since 2018, focusing intensively on motor learning and rehabilitation processes and their effects on cortical reorganization. Moreover, she has been a lecturer in the field of neurorehabilitation for several years at the University of Applied Sciences for Health, Innsbruck. Within her professional career, she has been involved in the planning and implementation of several studies and the development of guidelines (treatment pathway stroke). Apart from that she has given lectures at international congresses.

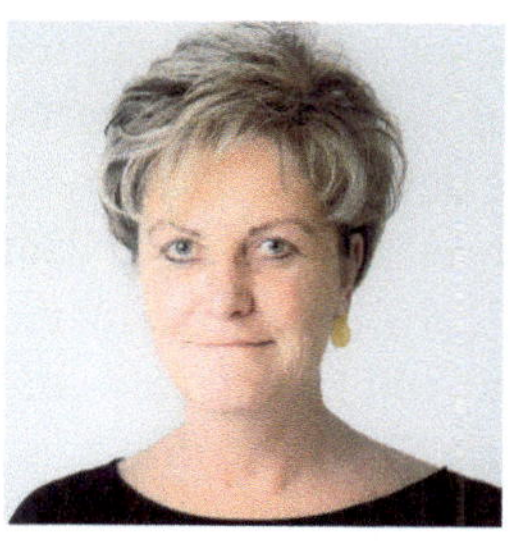

**Michaela M. Pinter, MD, MAS** is Full Professor for Neurorehabilitation Research at Danube University Krems, Austria, and Head of the Department of Clinical Neurosciences and Preventive Medicine as well as Head of the Center for Neurorehabilitation.

Her scientific focus is on neuromodulation as well as on restoration of neuronal functions. She actively conducts clinical studies on the modification of muscle tone and restoration of motor functions.

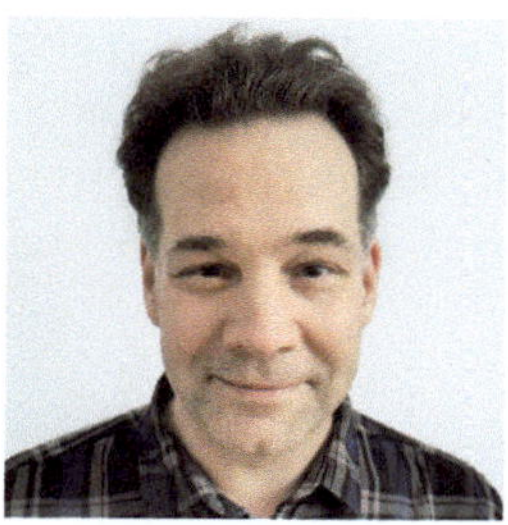

**Carsten Kroker** is a television technician and became a speech therapist in 1999. He is currently Head of Speech Therapy at the Clinic Saarbrücken (neurological acute clinic incl. stroke unit) and has his own practice in Saarbrücken, Germany. He has published various articles in professional journals and two monographs (including Aphasie—Schnell Test). He is a lecturer at several institutions, including the "interkantonale Hochschule für Heilpädagogik" (HfH) in Zürich, Switzerland. Since 2004, he has dedicated himself to electrical therapy and was co-developer of the FES treatment program for dysarthria "Dys-SAAR-thrie Therapie."

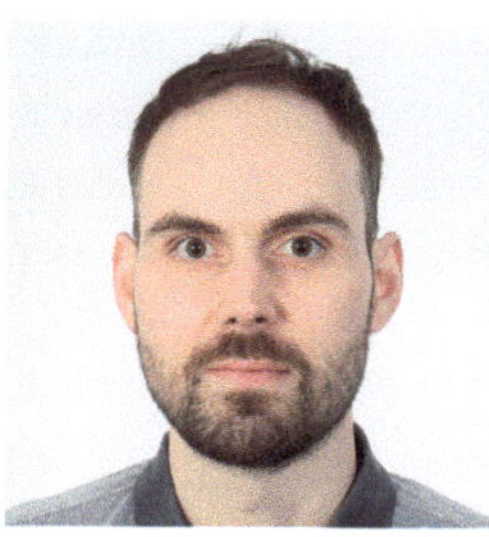

**Jan Faust, B of Health** graduated in 2011 with a degree in Speech and Language Therapy (Logopedics) from HAN University of Applied Sciences in Nijmegen, the Netherlands. Since then, he has practiced as a speech therapist with a clinical focus on neurorehabilitation and holds certifications on fiberoptic endoscopic evaluation of swallowing (FEES). Since 2016, he has been practicing at Helios Hospital Krefeld, Germany, which has the status of Academic Hospital of RWTH Aachen University. The author lectures on FES in speech, voice, and swallowing disorders for health care professionals through various educating and training institutes. Since 2020, he has been studying the MSc program in Teaching and Research Logopedics at RWTH Aachen University.

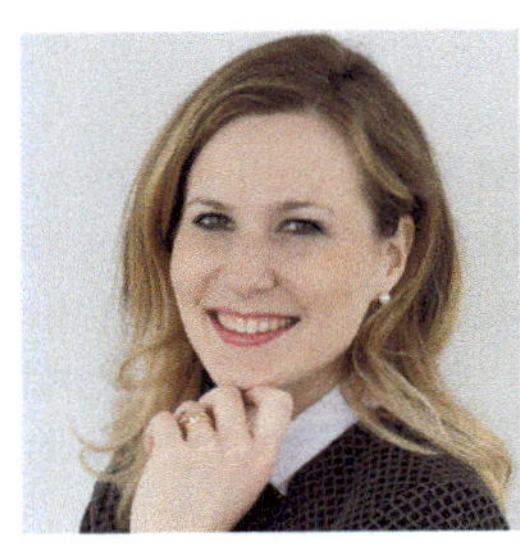

**Christina A. Repitsch, BSc, MSc** graduated from the Carinthia University of Applied Sciences, Austria, in 2012 with a bachelor's degree in speech therapy. Since then, she has worked as a speech therapist at the Department of Speech Therapy at the Hospital Klagenfurt as well as in independent practice. Between 2015 and 2018, she studied at the Danube University Krems and completed the course "Neurorehabilitation." She specialized her work in the treatment of facial paresis. In 2016, she founded the Facial Outpatient Clinic in cooperation with the Department of Plastic, Aesthetic and Reconstructive Surgery at the Klagenfurt Hospital. Here, the focus is on the therapeutic treatment of pre- or postoperative patients with facial nerve paresis. FES is also part of this therapeutic treatment concept. Furthermore, the author is hosting seminars on rehabilitation of facial paresis for therapists.

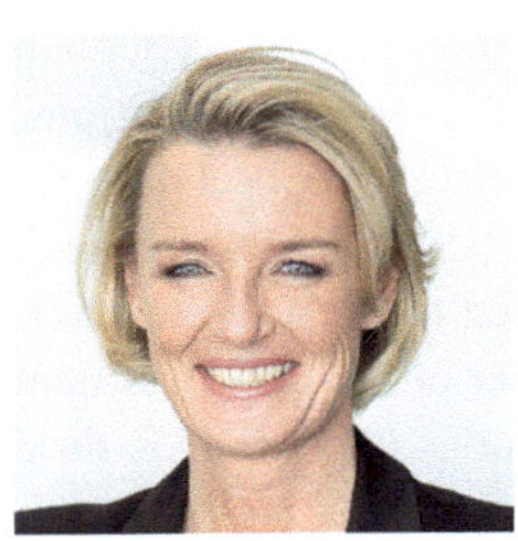

**Berit Schneider-Stickler** is otolaryngologist, phoniatrician, and singer. She is Deputy Head of the Division of Phoniatrics-Logopedics of the Medical University Vienna.

Her clinical focus and her research interests have been focused on voice diagnostics and voice therapy for more than two decades. She is particularly interested in neurological voice disorders like vocal fold paralysis, spasmodic dysphonia, and voice tremor. Her activities significantly contribute to the establishment of neurolaryngology in Austria.

She is co-founder of the working group "Austrian Neurolaryngology" of the Austrian Society for Ear, Nose and Throat Disorders.

She is author and coauthor of many scientific papers and co-editor of two textbooks.

Since 2014, Berit Schneider-Stickler is president of the Austrian Society of Logopedics, Phoniatrics, and Pedaudiology.

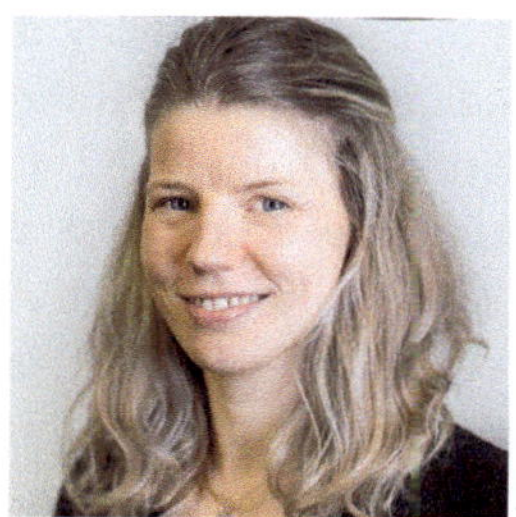

**Birgit Tevnan, MSc** is working as an occupational therapist since 2012. She studied at the University of Applied Sciences for Health Professions in Upper Austria and is working at the Neuromed Campus, Linz, in the Department of Neurological Acute Aftercare since 2013. In 2017, she achieved her master's degree at the University of Applied Sciences Vienna for Health Assisting Engineering. Her research was focusing on the review and evaluation of user-friendliness of FES medical devices in home therapy. Since 2018, the author has additionally been working as a freelancer, specializing in neurological follow-up of patients after stroke in the home-setting. In 2019, she joined the start-up Rewellio as a part-time clinical expert for the development of a therapy app for the neurological follow-up of patients with neurological disorders after stroke.

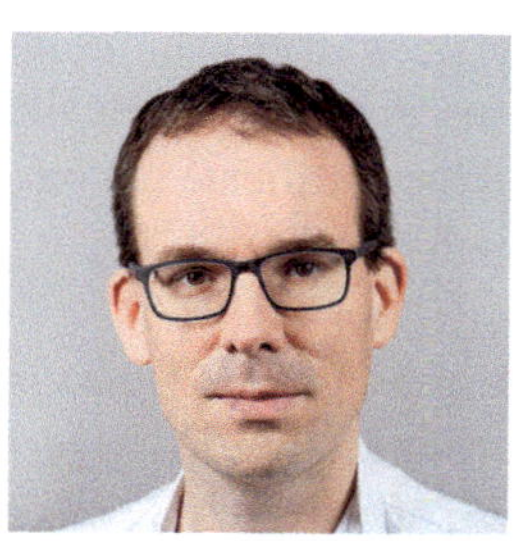

**Gerd F. Volk, MD** is working as a physician in the Department of Otorhinolaryngology at the Jena University Hospital since 2006. Since 2012, he is Head of the interdisciplinary Facial Nerve Center Jena, Germany, a cooperation of the departments of psychology, neurology, physiotherapy, radiology, and ENT. In addition to the interdisciplinarity, the special feature is a two-week biofeedback training for patients with peripheral facial nerve palsy with defect healing. In addition to surface EMG, constrained induced movement techniques known from "deaf training" are used for biofeedback. Already during his medical studies in Münster, Volk was working in the research group of Solon Thanos, specializing on quantification and improvement of nerve regeneration. His clinical interests are electrophysiological and imaging techniques for the assessment and visualization of the muscles and nerves of the face and larynx, the application of botulinum toxin in the head and neck region, and the functional diagnosis and therapy of peripheral nerve lesions. His scientific focus is on the development of new methods for reconstruction and rehabilitation of facial and laryngeal nerve lesions, electrical stimulation as a diagnostic and therapeutic tool, central nervous changes after cranial nerve lesions, especially of the facial and vestibular nerves, and mechanisms for their compensation.

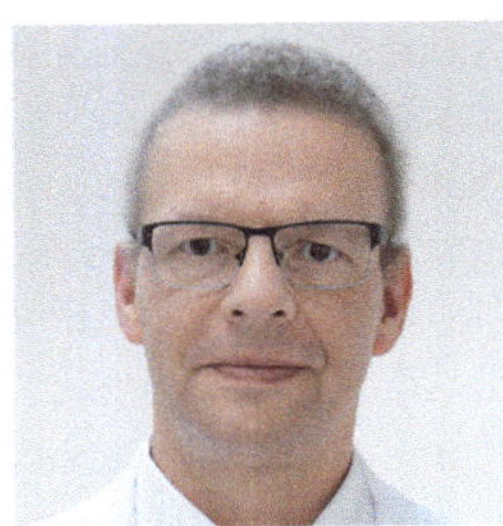

**Jürgen Pannek, MD** born in Essen, Germany in 1963, studied human medicine at the Ruhr-University in Bochum, Germany from 1982 to 1888. He completed his training as a urologist at the university hospitals of Bochum and Essen. A research stay at the Johns Hopkins Hospital in Baltimore, USA, from 1996 to 1997 led to his habilitation at the Ruhr-University Bochum, Germany in 1999, where he received the extraordinary professorship for urology in 2005. From 2003 to 2007 he was Head of the Neuro-urology Department at the University of Bochum, Germany. Since 2007, he has been Head of the Neuro-urology Department at the Swiss Paraplegic Centre in Nottwil, Switzerland; therefore, in 2011 he was rehabilitated and appointed titular professor at the University of Bern, Switzerland.

In addition to additional urological qualifications (focus titles for special urological surgery, neuro-urology, and urology of women), he completed the training to become a "Certified Health Care Manager" and acquired the certificate of competence in classical homeopathy.

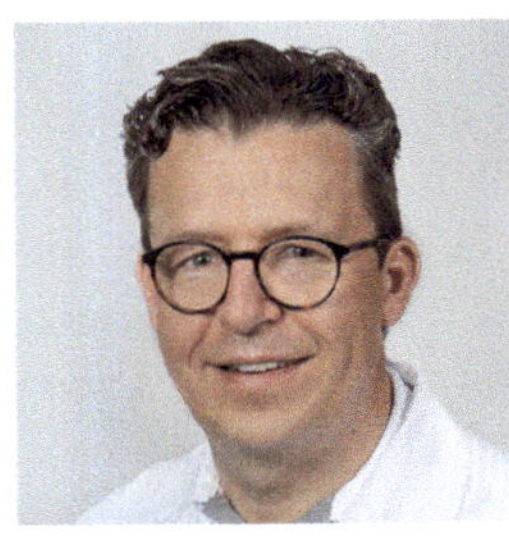

**Jens Wöllner, MD, EMBA** is Senior physician in the Department of Neuro-urology in Swiss Paraplegic Centre, Nottwil, Switzerland since 2013. In 2020, he gets his "Venia legend" at the medical school of the University of Mainz in Germany and a master's degree in Master of Business Administration in Medical Management (EMBA), PHW Bern, Switzerland. He is medical doctor (MD) since 2008 and specialist in urology since 2009. The primary education ended in 2003 at medical school university of Mainz, Germany.

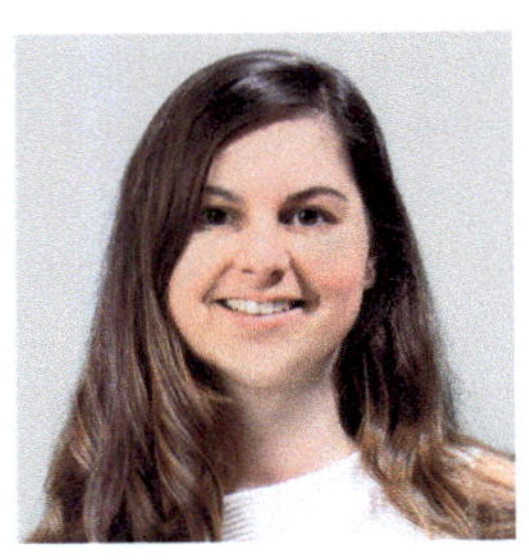

**Anja Fuchs** graduated in graphic and communication design from the HTL 1—Construction and Arts in Linz, Austria and now working as a multimedia designer in Innsbruck, Austria. In close cooperation with the authors and the editor, she created the photo and video content including the selection and edit of these extensive recordings. Her professional and descriptive graphic preparation of the figures and tables resulted in a uniform and clear design that runs through the entire book. She was also the responsible graphic designer for the German edition of *Functional electrical stimulation in neurorehabilitation* in the publication year 2020.

# Contributors

**Ines Bersch-Porada** International FES Centre®, Swiss Paraplegic Centre, Nottwil, Switzerland

**Christian Dohle** P.A.N. Center for Post-Acute Neurorehabilitation, Fürst-Donnersmarck-Stiftung, Berlin and Center for Stroke Research, Charité—University Medicine Berlin, Berlin, Germany

**Jan Faust** Helios Klinikum Krefeld, Department of Otolaryngology, Krefeld, Germany

**Klemens Fheodoroff** Gailtal Klinik Hermagor, Hermagor, Austria

**Anja Fuchs** MED-EL, Department Neurorehabilitation STIWELL, Innsbruck, Austria

**Stefan M. Golaszewski** Salzburg, Austria

**Carsten Kroker** Praxis für Logopädie, Saarbrücken, Germany

**Winfried Mayr** Medical University of Vienna, Vienna, Austria

**Patricia Meier** Medical University of Innsbruck, Department of Neurology, Innsbruck, Austria

VASCage GmbH, Research Centre on Vascular Ageing and Stroke, Innsbruck, Austria

**Jürgen Pannek** Swiss Paraplegic Center, Department Neuro-Urology, Nottwil, Switzerland

**Michaela M. Pinter** Danube-University Krems, Department for Clinical Neuroscience and Prevention, Krems, Austria

**Christina A. Repitsch** Klinikum Klagenfurt am Wörthersee, ENT Department, Klagenfurt, Austria

**Thomas Schick** MED-EL, Department Neurorehabilitation STIWELL, Innsbruck, Austria

**Berit Schneider-Stickler** Medical University of Vienna, Division of Phoniatrics-Logopedics, Department of Otorhinolaryngology, Vienna, Austria

**Kerstin Schwenker** University Hospital Salzburg, Department of Neurology, Spinal Cord Injury and Tissue Regeneration Center Salzburg, Paracelsus Medical University, Salzburg, Austria

**Birgit Tevnan** Kepler University Hospital, Neuromed Campus, Linz, Austria

**Gerd F. Volk** Friedrich-Schiller-University Hospital, ENT Department, Jena, Germany

**Jens Wöllner** Swiss Paraplegic Center, Department Neuro-Urology, Nottwil, Switzerland

# Introduction and History of Functional Electrical Stimulation

**Thomas Schick**

**1**

Persons interested in neurorehabilitation are confronted with a wealth of technical information and scientific findings. Filtering out the most important and current information for one's own professional field from this wide range of information would require regular study of scientific literature. Also, the decision for the appropriate therapy method – depending on the problem constellation of the patient – such as functional electrical stimulation (FES), can be a challenge. This book is intended to provide valuable assistance for searching specific and therapy-relevant approaches. This makes it easier to achieve the goal of patient-centered, high-quality therapy. The main focus of this book is FES and its wide range of applications in neurological patients with various symptoms. The special nature of modern FES with its importance in the context of motor learning and its strongly task-oriented approach compared to classic methods is discussed intensively. It is not uncommon for initial difficulties to arise in the search for current literature due to the internationally very variable use of FES terms. In this chapter, the reader gets a basic overview of the numerous technical terms and their meaning.

T. Schick (✉)
MED-EL, Department Neurorehabilitation
STIWELL, Innsbruck, Austria
e-mail: schick@neuro-reha.info

## 1.1 Introduction and Explanation of Terms

It is intended to provide a useful classification of the inconsistent terminology and reflects the opinion of the author. The most frequently used terms are described. Fig. 1.1 illustrates the terms and their predominant use for the therapeutic field in the context of electrical stimulation (ES).

Figure 1.1 is based on extensive literature research and experience of the most common usage and does not claim to represent the language choice of all actors in electrical stimulation in a universally valid way. This list is to be understood as a contribution to the improved comparability of studies and clinical applications. The classification and division of the forms of therapy is based on the structure and function level as well as the activity level of the ICF (International Classification of Functioning, Disability and Health).

In this book, the authors use the umbrella term *FES*. This was coined by the scientists Moe and Post in 1962 [1]. The older term *Functional Electrotherapy (FET)* [2] has not gained acceptance among experts (Fig. 1.2) and is now used only occasionally [3]. The term FES is probably the most commonly used term in literature [4]. Electrical stimulation is called functional if the contractions triggered by the stimulation are coordinated in a way that they compensate for a restricted or absent support function.

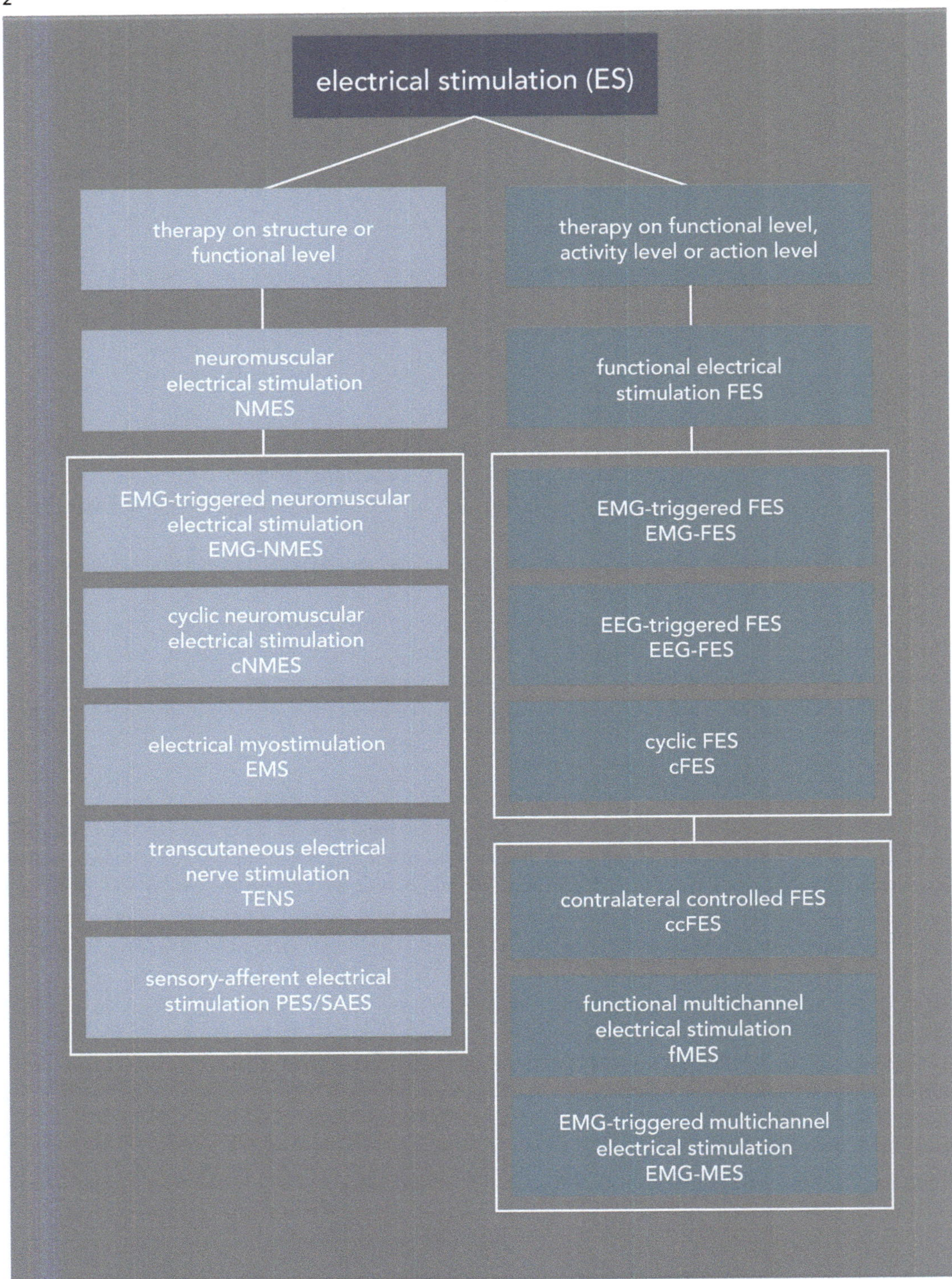



**Fig. 1.1** Comparison of functional electrical stimulation (FES) and neuromuscular electrical stimulation (NMES) and their further development

Thus, FES in the proper sense does not denote muscle stimulation that triggers contractions of muscle groups or a single muscle by means of an electrical stimulus [5]. According to another logical definition, the FES is an electrical stimulation during the execution of a voluntary movement.

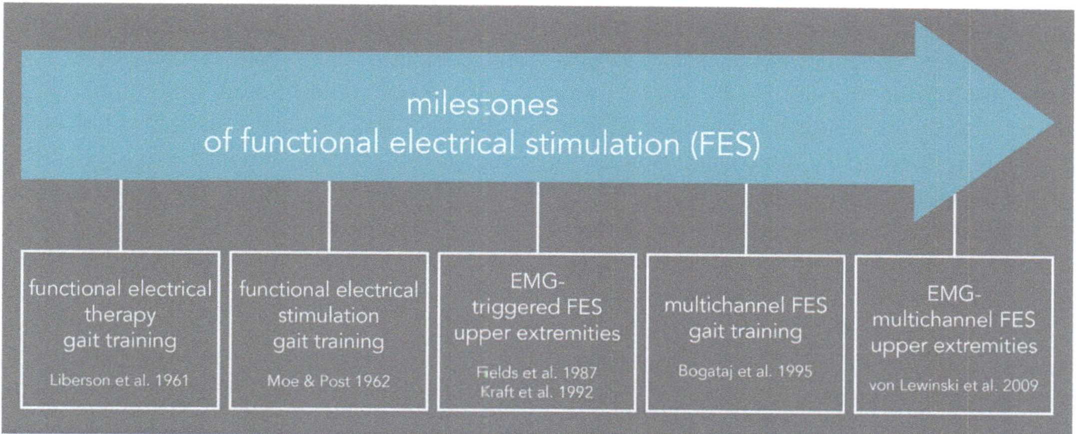


**Fig. 1.2** Milestones in functional electrical stimulation

This means that every time a person wants to perform a movement, he or she receives electrical assistance from the electrical stimulation device [3]. This distinguishes FES from passive neuromuscular electrical stimulation (NMES), which is not designed for active, functional, or task-oriented patient cooperation. Some authors consider FES a sub-area of NMES [6]. The author of the contribution does not agree with this classification. NMES has a rather passive treatment approach which focuses mainly on structural and functional deficits. It is used for atrophy prophylaxis, muscle strengthening, toning or detonation of muscles, for certain forms of spasm treatment, to promote blood circulation, or to improve sensory perception. This represents a significant difference from the above-mentioned definitions.

If the stimulations are given by an electrical stimulation device at defined, temporally repeating intervals, this is referred to as cyclic neuromuscular electrical stimulation (cNMES).

Early work further specifies FES as Electromyography (EMG)-triggered FES (EMG-FES), in which impulses are triggered when a certain threshold is reached according to EMG measurement [7, 8]. EMG-triggered stimulations are mostly described in the literature as EMG-triggered neuromuscular electrical stimulation (EMG-NMES) [9]. The emphasis of the therapy with EMG-NMES is based on a cyclic movement electrically supported by the stimulation device, which is actively initiated by the patient. The conscious initiation of movement and muscular activity of a stroke patient is the main focus of EMG-NMES. EMG-triggered stimulation devices with only one stimulation channel are usually used in these cases [10]. This form of therapy focuses on the repetitive aspect similar to cyclic stimulation. This distinguishes the EMG-NMES from EMG-triggered multichannel electrical stimulation (EMG-MES; see below), in which a task-oriented, active therapy approach is explicitly required. Switch-triggered neuromuscular electrical stimulation (sNMES) [11] is another option. This technique is used to assist stroke patients or paraplegic patients while walking, again mainly using the term FES [3]. Transcutaneous electrical nerve stimulation (TENS) is used not only in pain treatment, but also in electrical myostimulation (EMS), for example in postoperative functional paresis, in sports, but also occasionally in stroke therapy [9]. In the case of TENS, which is also designed to be passive, the minimization of muscle atrophy rather than functionality is usually the first priority apart from pain treatment. Muscle contractions in this case are amplitude-dependent, since one cannot only stimulate in the sensory-threshold area but in the motor-threshold area via neuromuscular excitation at the motor end plate [12].

Also, the term EMS is misleading since the muscle itself is not directly stimulated, but always the upstream nerve based on the corresponding stimulation parameters. Only a few studies on muscle stimulation after nerve damage in animal experiments use EMS in the study description [13]. In sports therapy, EMS is used for additional non-specific recruitment of muscles under forced activity. However, this approach significantly differs from the functional approaches required and used in neurorehabilitation.

In neurorehabilitation, peripheral or sensory-afferent electrical stimulation PES/SAES has developed further in recent years as a subform of TENS, which is characterized by the stimulation of sensitive nerve fibers aiming for a change in sensorimotor functions [14]. Both TENS and PES/SAES, as well as EMS, can be considered subsets of NMES. However, SAES can also be actively used in therapy in a task-oriented manner and with the aim of improving functionality, and can thus be assigned to FES (Chap. 9).

In electrical stimulation of denervated muscles in lower motor neuron syndrome (LMNS), FES has been established to support reinnervation even in partial denervation. Electrical stimulation is performed directly on the denervated muscle since stimulation via upstream nerves is no longer possible. Here, the term EMS would actually make sense in the early phase, but this does not correspond to the common use and indication of EMS. Also, EMS stimulation devices are not regularly designed for the treatment of denervated muscles due to their technical equipment.

Examples of the treatment of neurological patients with LMNS are described in detail below (Chap. 8). The therapeutic treatment approach of the FES considerably differs from the forms of stimulation used for damage to the first motor neuron or upper motor neuron syndrome (UMNS) in the selection of the necessary current parameters, e.g., pulse widths, frequencies, and current shapes. This treatment approach also focuses on the therapeutic goal of improving functionality and requires the active cooperation of the patient according to his possibilities, and thus justifies the name FES.

A clinically relevant form of FES in the context of motor learning in patients with UMN impairment is patient-initiated FES or EMG-FES. However, many available electrical stimulation devices have only one stimulation channel, which considerably reduces the possibilities for functional and action-oriented therapy.

For modern products with four or more stimulation channels, another specification for multichannel FES (MFES) for the treatment of UMNS is EMG-triggered multichannel electrical stimulation (EMG-MES) [15–17]. The special possibilities of using this modern method are described in detail and illustrated with practical examples in Chap. 6.

As could be seen in the previous section, it is usually difficult to identify a uniform term for electrical stimulation. The following example will illustrate this. The American Stroke Association (ASA) guideline on post-stroke care [18] recommends, among other things, the use of NMES in stroke patients with minimal functions and shoulder subluxations. According to the authors, these recommendations are based on several randomized control trials (RCTs) primarily on FES in stroke patients [19, 20]. Also, there is no uniform use of terms. This shows the urgent need to agree on international uniform definitions of the different forms of stimulation.

To simplify and improve clarity and for reasons of plausibility, the authors of this book predominantly use the designations FES, EMG-triggered electrical stimulation (EMG-ES), and EMG-triggered multichannel electrical stimulation (EMG-MES). The reason for this is mainly the emphasis on the manifold possibilities especially of EMG-MES in the context of task-oriented practice and the expected positive effects on plastic changes and synaptic reorganization in the context of motor learning.

The classical electrotherapy procedures are not described in this book, as the activity-enhancing FES therapies are preferred in neurorehabilitation.

**Summary**

Electrical stimulation is said to be functional if the contractions triggered by the stimulation are coordinated in a way that they support a restricted or absent function.

## 1.2 History of Functional Electrical Stimulation

It was a long way of acquiring knowledge and experience in the field of electrical engineering as well as human physiology and pathophysiology until the FES emerged in its differentiated form as it is available to the user in neurorehabilitation today. Records of the use of electrical shocks by citterrays or electric eels date back to the 4th millennium BC [21]. In antiquity, the Greek natural philosopher Thales first described the electrostatic charging of amber (Gr.: ἤλεκτρον/ Electron), which still shapes the name of electrical therapy today [22].

Targeted attempts at electrical stimulation in humans only became public with the discovery and invention of the "Leiden bottle" by von Kleist in 1745. A kind capacitor enabled the application of electricity [23]. Early written documentation of experiments and hypotheses of effects on humans can be found in the book of the French mathematician and philosopher Louis Jallabert who, as an experimental physicist in Geneva in the middle of the eighteenth century, described the first observations of the effects of electricity on humans [24]. In the same book, interesting experimental observations in stroke patients are described by Professor de Sauvages from Montpellier in the form of a missive to his colleague Doctor Bruhier. Therein, he reports on systematic, daily electrical stimulation of patients who, following the treatment series, regained functions of the hand and arm and improved their walking and stair climbing.

In 1770, the German Johann Friedrich Hartmann published an extensive work with a detailed set of rules for electrical stimulation in various diseases. One of his focal points was the treatment of neurological patients with paralysis using electricity [25]. Only 6 years later, the German physician Gottlieb Schäffer published a book on the effects of electricity on paralyzed limbs [26]. The next milestone was set by the Italian anatomist Luigi Galvani who became the founder of electrophysiology. In 1780, he randomly discovered the simultaneous twitching of a prepared frog's leg while a spark was being passed through a nearby "electrifying machine." Galvani suspected electrical energy directly in the muscle. These observations and countless follow-up experiments with various electrical conductors as well as comprehensive records were the basis for the Italian physicist Alessandro Volta to develop his own energy source in the form of a battery at the beginning of the nineteenth century. He was the founder of the theory of electricity [27].

In the same century, the French physiologist and neurologist Guillaume-Benjamin Duchenne developed muscle stimulation; he is still considered the father of electrotherapy. Among other things, he made numerous experiments on the stimulation of facial muscles [28]. During this time, the neurologist Robert Remark from Berlin described the first specific paralysis treatments of the hand where he defined the muscle stimulation points [12].

In 1831, Michael Faraday developed the electromagnetic machine, a precursor of today's electrical therapy devices which generated alternating current by means of a rotating metal coil. The term "faradic current" has evolved at this time [29]. Since that time, the application of current in the body was also used for diagnostics. It was clinically observed that paralyzed musculature reacts only to galvanic (direct current), but not to faradic current (alternating current).

The French neuroscientist Louis Lapicque shaped the beginning of the twentieth century with the term *rheobase* as a measure of the membrane potential. Thus, the excitation threshold could be determined. The rheobase describes the current intensity at which excitation was just achieved for an infinitely long stimulus time [30]. Another parameter was the Determination of the *chronaxy* which is the shortest current flow duration for tissue excitation at double rheobase. The determined parameters were now also used for the diagnostic assessment of nerve damage. Adrian [31] produced the first curves for the assessment of healthy and damaged human muscles.

From the 1950s, portable, battery-powered electrical stimulation devices were available. The invention of the transistor in 1948 enabled the development of such portable electrical stimulation devices. A few years later, Vladimir Liberson emphasized on the term "electrical stimulation" for the first time.

*Functional electro-therapy (FET)* for percussive patients with foot dorsiflexion weakness is a current-assisted functional alternative to conventional orthoses. He documented improved functional outcomes after electrical stimulation [2]. A short time later, the term was changed to *Functional Electrical Stimulation (FES)* [1] which has endured to this day. Despite encouraging reports over more than two and a half centuries, functional electrical stimulation (FES) did not become established in the rehabilitation of neurological patients until the twenty-first century. Until the turn of the millennium, it was still rarely used in patients with central paralysis, although significant studies on EMG-triggered FES in stroke patients [7, 8] and first papers on multichannel electrical stimulation to improve walking [32] had already been published in the 1980s and 1990s. Vogedes wrote in the Year 2000 "...still the treatment of central paralysis with electrical therapy is rarely performed in Germany. For many physicians and therapists, the treatment of central paralysis is still an absolute contraindication for the entire spectrum of electrical therapy" [33]. However, the same author referred to new therapeutic possibilities of EMG-triggered electrical stimulation. In 2004, Wenk writes justifying "*...the treatment of central paresis is still met with skepticism today. (...) Critics must be told in no uncertain terms that this electrical therapeutic method is only ever used in combination with recognized methods such as Bobath, Vojta or PNF. Electrical therapy can only provide a positive basis in the sense of inhibition and facilitation primarily at the spinal cord level*" [34].

This aforementioned skepticism and criticism are now outdated and overcome. Chapter 3 provides modern approaches to clarify the actual mode of FES. Bossert writes in 2014 about EMG-ES: "*...even in central paresis, the 1st motor neuron should be activated and thus movement reinitiated*" [12]. Fortunately, FES is becoming increasingly established in neurorehabilitation, due to an increase in research activities in the field of FES, but also in motor learning [35], and neuroplasticity [36] (Chap. 2). This process has been supported by the development of modern electrical stimulation devices, which no longer control impulse triggering in a purely device-driven manner, but in a patient-initiated manner, e.g., by EMG or sensor triggering.

In recent years, technological progress has provided additional impetus: User-friendly modern electrical stimulation devices with more than one stimulation channel have been developed, described, and investigated [15, 16, 32, 37, 38]. These can be used to target stimulation not only of individual muscle groups but also of entire movement sequences in patients with UMNS [4].

Functional, activity-enhancing and action-oriented electrical stimulation has thus arrived in modern neurorehabilitation and is becoming increasingly established. The many therapeutic options of FES for increasing the function and activity of a neurological patient are summarized in detail in this book. Well-founded, up-to-date knowledge from science and extensive clinical empiricism are intended to provide users, as well as criticists, with an understanding of the current data situation and the rehabilitative application possibilities. Fig. 1.2 shows the significant publications from the early FET and FES in single-channel application to the first FES with EMG triggering, MFES, and later of EMG-MES in stroke patients.

**Summary**

The term FES was first mentioned in the literature in 1962 and is still predominantly used today.

## References

1. Moe J, Post H. Functional electrical stimulation for ambulation in hemiplegia. J Lancet. 1962;82:285–8.
2. Liberson W, Holmquest H, Scot D, Dow M. Functional electrotherapy: stimulation of the peroneal nerve synchronized with the swing phase of the gait of hemiplegic patients. Arch Phys Med Rehabil. 1961; 42:101–5.

3. Popovic M, Masani K, Micera S. Neurorehabilitation technology, 2. Aufl. Springer Science, s.l.; 2016

4. Doucet B, Lam A, Griffin L. Neuromuscular electrical stimulation for skeletal muscle function. Yale J Biol Med. 2012;85:201–15.

5. van Kerkhof P. Das Elektrotherapieskript. Muskelstimulation wwwPhysiosupportorg 12 October; 2013:S1–260.

6. Eraifej J, et al. Effectiveness of upper limb functional electrical stimulation after stroke for the improvement of activities of daily living and motor function: a systematic review and meta-analysis. Syst Rev. 2017;6(1):40.

7. Fields R, et al. Electromyographically triggered electric muscle stimulation for chronic hemiplegia. Arch Phys Med Rehabil. 1987;68:407–14.

8. Kraft G, Fitts S, Hammond M. Techniques to improve function of the arm and hand in chronic hemiplegia. Arch Phys Med Rehabil. 1992;73(3): 220–7.

9. Iruthayarajah J, et al. Evidence-based review of stroke rehabilitation. London: Evidence-Based Review of Stroke Rehabilitation; 2018.

10. Monte-Silva K, et al. Electromyogram-related neuromuscular electrical stimulation for restoring wrist and hand movement in poststroke hemiplegia: a systematic review and meta-analysis. Neurorehabil Neural Repair. 2019;33(2):96–111.

11. Coscia M, et al. Neurotechnology-aided interventions for upper limb motor rehabilitation in severe chronic stroke. Brain. 2019;142:2182–97.

12. Bossert F-P, Vogedes K. Elektrotherapie, Licht- und Strahlentherapie, 3. Aufl: Elsevier GmbH, Urban & Fischer, München; 2014.

13. Willand M, et al. Electrical muscle stimulation elevates intramuscular BDNF and GDNF mRNA following peripheral nerve injury and repair in rats. Neuroscience. 2016;15(334):93–104.

14. Golaszewski S, Frey V. Neuromodulation in der Neurorehabilitation nach Schlaganfall. Jatros Neurol Psychiartrie. 2019;3:12–8.

15. von Lewinski F, et al. Efficacy of EMG-triggered electrical arm stimulation in chronic hemiparetic stroke patients. Restor Neurol Neurosci. 2009;27(3): 189–97.

16. Kapadia N, et al. Functional electrical stimulation therapy for grasping in traumatic incomplete spinal cord injury: randomized control trial. Artif Organs. 2011;35:212–6.

17. Schick T, et al. Synergy effects of combined multichannel EMG-triggered electrical stimulation and mirror therapy in subacute stroke patients with severe or very severe arm/hand paresis. Restor Neurol Neurosci. 2017;35(3):319–32.

18. Winstein C, et al. Guidelines for adult stroke rehabilitation and recovery: a guideline for healthcare professionals from the American Heart Association/American Stroke Association. Stroke. 2016;47(6):e98–e169.

19. Alon G, Levitt A, McCarthy P. Functional electrical stimulation (FES) may modify the poor prognosis of stroke survivors with severe motor loss of the upper extremity: a preliminary study. Am J Phys Med Rehabil. 2008;87(8):627–36.

20. Hara Y, Ogawa S, Tsujiuchi K, Muraoka Y. A home-based rehabilitation program for the hemiplegic upper extremity by power-assisted functional electrical stimulation. Disabil Rehabil. 2008;30(4):296–304.

21. Moller P. Review: electric fish. Bioscience. 1991;41(11):794–6.

22. Hackmann W. Electrostatic machine. In: Bud R, editor. An historical encyclopedia. Instruments of science. New York: Garland; 1998. p. S221–4.

23. Lommel E. Ewald Georg von Kleist, Allgemeine Deutsche Biographie. Allgemeine Deutsche Biographie. 1882;16:112–3.

24. Jallabert L. Experimenta electrica usibus medicis applicata. J. R. im Hof, 312 S. Pappband der Zeit, Basel; 1750

25. Hartmann JF. Die angewandte Elektrizität bei Krankheiten des menschlichen Körpers. s.n., Hannover; 1770

26. Schäffer JG. Die Elektrische Medicin oder die Kraft und Wirkung der Elektricität in dem menschlichen Körper und dessen Krankheiten besonders bei gelähmten Gliedern aus Vernunftgründen erläutert und durch Erfahrungen bestätigt, 2. Aufl. Johann Leopold Montag, s.l. 1766

27. von Oettingen A, Galvani A, Volta A (Hrsg). Abhandlung über die Kräfte der Elektricität bei der Muskelbewegung: (Comm. Bonon. Sc. et Art. Inst. et Acad. T. 7); (1791)/von Aloisius Galvani. Untersuchungen über den Galvanismus: (1796–1800)/von Alessandro Volta, 2. Aufl. Bolognia (Hrsg), Thun/Frankfurt am Main; 1996

28. Duchenne G-B. Mécanisme de la physionomie humaine ou analyse électro-physiologique de l'expression des passions. Deuxième édition ed. Paris: Librairie J.-B. Bailliere et Fils; 1876.

29. Baker L, Bowman B, Waters R, Benton L. Funktionelle Elektrostimulation. Geschichte der Elektrostimulation. Darmstadt: Dr. Dietrich Steinkopff Verlag Gmbh & Co. KG; 1983.

30. Lapicque L. Définition experimentale de l'excitabilité. 24 Juillet. Comptes Rendus Acad Sci. 1909;67: S280.

31. Adrian E. The response of human sensory nerves to currents of short duration. J Physiol. 1919;53: 70–85.

32. Bogataj U, et al. The rehabilitation of gait in patients with hemiplegia: a comparison between conventional therapy and multichannel functional electrical stimulation therapy. Phys Ther. 1995;75(6):490–502.

33. Vogedes K. Treatment of central paralysis with electrotherapy. Z Elektrostim Elektrother. 2000; 2:24–8.

34. Wenk W. Elektrotherapie. ISSN 2627–3179. 1 Auflage. Berlin Heidelberg: Springer-Verlag; 2004.

35. Hardwick R, Rottschy C, Miall R, Eickhoff S. A quantitative meta-analysis and review of motor learning in the human brain. J Neuro-Oncol. 2013;67:283–97.

36. Taub E, et al. Technique to improve chronic motor deficit after stroke. Arch Phys Med Rehabil. 1993;74(4):347–54.

37. Tan Z, et al. The effectiveness of functional electrical stimulation based on a normal gait pattern on sub- jects with early stroke: RCT. Biomed Res Int. 2014;2014:545408. https://doi.org/10.1155/2014/545408.

38. Teasell R, Bhogal S, Foley N, Speechley M. Gait retraining post stroke. Top Stroke Rehabil. 2003;10(2):34–65.

# Plasticity and Motor Learning

**2**

Patricia Meier

For a long time, treatment concepts in neurorehabilitation were based on the assumption that recovery of motor function is determined exclusively by sensory input. This hypothesis was the basis of many traditional treatment methods, such as the Bobath or the Vojta concept. However, none of these therapeutic methods could achieve reasonable results in scientific studies [1].

Technological advancements, particularly in diagnostic imaging, and the growing knowledge of brain function helped to change this belief. The knowledge about neuronal plasticity and the evidence of changes on a structural and functional level led to a rethinking of therapeutic interventions in neurorehabilitation.

Modern treatment approaches have evolved from the more restrictive to exercise-dominant treatment methods that follow the principles of Motor Learning [2]. The comparison of these "Motor relearning programs"with the traditional concepts confirms the usefulness of this rethinking especially in terms of effectiveness and regarding the quality of the movement [3].


P. Meier (✉)
Medical University of Innsbruck,
Department of Neurology, Innsbruck, Austria

VASCage GmbH, Research Centre on Vascular
Ageing and Stroke, Innsbruck, Austria


## 2.1 Plasticity

Plasticity or neuroplasticity describes the ability of the nervous system to adapt its structure or function in response to internal or external conditions. This can manifest through a transformation of cortical areas or an increase in synaptic efficiency [4].

Neural plasticity can be based on a wide variety of neuroanatomical and neurophysiological processes, so that we speak of either structural or functional plasticity in each case:

- Structural or anatomical plasticity describes changes on a structural level. Structural adaptations are, for example, an increase in dendritic branches and synapses or the sprouting of axons.
- Functional or chemical plasticity encompasses all changes on a functional level. Functional changes are pre- or postsynaptic adaptations, such as increased neurotransmitter release or increased receptor density at the postsynaptic membrane [5].


**Summary**
Depending on the underlying mechanisms of neuroplasticity we speak of:

- Structural or anatomical plasticity.
- Functional or chemical plasticity.

Therefore, the nervous system is not a rigid structure but can change due to external or internal influences such as an increased use of an extremity or a traumatic event, like a stroke.

After neurological damage, a reorganization of the brain happens based on these plastic changes. This process is referred to as injury-induced neuronal plasticity. Injury-induced plastic changes occur primarily in the first weeks and months after an acute event [6].

Brain damage initiates sprouting of axons as well as unmasking of neural pathways and synapses. Unmasking means that usually unused, inactive synaptic connections are stimulated into activity [5]. In stroke, the decrease of the edema around the infarct area additionally leads to functional improvement, as non-destroyed areas can become active again.

However, as described, neuronal plasticity does not only take place initiated by damage, but also by an increased use of the (affected) extremities in the sense of a Motor Learning process. This type of plasticity plays an important role in rehabilitation and is referred to as training-induced neuronal plasticity [7]. Even in healthy individuals, a change in cortical structures is observed owing to increased use. For example, frequent practice with a guitar can increase cortical representation of the fingers in the homunculus. Until now various imaging techniques made it possible to observe pronounced plastic changes in the brain during several physiotherapeutic interventions. The restructuring of the neuronal system subsequently leads to an improvement in motor function, whereby various mechanisms at the neuroanatomical, neurochemical, and neurophysiological levels may be responsible for the recovery of function [4].

The basic mechanism of these plastic processes is long-term potentiation (LTP). LTP means that repeated activation in rapid succession improves synaptic efficiency and thus the transmission of excitation [8]. Subsequently, the persistence of increased synaptic connectivity can lead to structural changes such as synapse assembly or synaptic remodeling.

▶ Long-term potentiation (LTP) is the basic mechanism for plastic processes during Motor Learning.

Because of LTP, cells that are active together link together. This process, which is important for training-induced plasticity, is often described with the words "what fires together – wires together" and is known as Hebbian plasticity [9]. This synchronization of neuronal activity promotes not only synaptic efficiency but also axonal growth [10] or the sprouting of dendritic branches with the aim of forming new synapses for the corresponding connection.

Therefore, it is crucial that the therapist knows his responsibility to design functionally relevant tasks to effectively link the cells. In neurorehabilitation, this principle is known as "practice makes perfect".

**Summary**
Depending on the cause of appearance of neuroplastic changes we distinguish between:

- Injury-induced neuronal plasticity.
- Training-induced neuronal plasticity.

The recovery of functions, especially after a central lesion or a tumor, is thus largely dependent on compensatory mechanisms of the brain [11], like cortical restructuring. Induced through injury and training of motor functions increased activation in associated brain regions near or far from the lesion can be shown [7] as well as increased neuronal activity in cortical areas where the trained body part is represented.

Therefore, various brain mechanisms can lead to functional improvement: On the one hand, surrounding cortex regions can at least partially take over or support the function of the damaged brain area. On the other hand, intraregional changes take place, changes within the affected area of the (motor) cortex, defined as map expansion. Also, activation of the same region of the contralesionally (unaffected) hemisphere supports reorganization [7] and recovery of motor functions [12].

Conversely, in the absence of a stimulus, i.e., when individual functions are no longer needed, the corresponding cortical representation can be reduced. This follows the well-known principle of "use it or lose it" [13, 14].

Functional improvement after cortical lesions can also be achieved through compensatory mechanisms of voluntary motor function. This is described by the principle of motor equivalence. It means that even years after a brain damage function can increase despite motor and neurological deficits [15].

Neuronal plasticity is a continuous and dynamic process, meaning that it does not only take place in case of a spontaneous healing process of the nervous system, but it can also be achieved by any Motor Learning process through consistent training.

## 2.2 Motor Learning

Motor Learning represents a relatively permanent improvement in a person's capability to perform a motor skill and describes the process of acquiring motor skills and complex actions through training. The learning process is based on the same principles both in patients with damage to the (central) nervous system and in healthy individuals. The neuroplastic changes that occur because of the learning process differ though.

### 2.2.1 Stages of Motor Learning

Every Motor Learning process can be seen in stages [16]. Transitions from stage to stage are fluid, so it is not always clear in which phase the learner is. Roughly, however, three phases can be distinguished:

- In the initial stage of Motor Learning, the cognitive stage, different strategies are tried to master a certain motor task. The therapist's support, either in the form of manual assistance or verbal feedback, is most needed. Verbal feedback can also be given during performance and should therefore be short, clear, and reduced to essential hints. For the same feedback, the same wording should be used [12]. The patient needs to be focused and aware of the task to be able to perform it, yet some errors take place in this stage [17].
- In the associative stage motor pathways of the task to be learned are already better consolidated, meaning the task is performed with less

and less variability until the optimal strategy is finally found [17]. From this point on, the therapist should refrain from manual support, but targeted feedback is still important. However, this feedback should be given with latency to the task to avoid overlapping with the intrinsic feedback for movement control [18]. Once the movement strategy has been established, exercises can be varied slightly.
- In the autonomous stage of Motor Learning the movement program of the task to be learned is already automated. This means that the movement can be performed almost optimally without requiring greater attention or concentration [17]. At this stage, it is possible to focus more precisely on individual components of the movement to economize them. Variation of the exercises as well as the incorporation of difficulties is now necessary to maintain the patient's motivation [12].

**Summary**
Stages of Motor Learning:

1. Cognitive stage: The patient needs to be focused and aware of the task, yet some errors take place in this stage. The goal is to develop an overall understanding of the skill.
2. Associative stage: The patient demonstrates a more refined skill at the end of this stage with almost no errors during the movement.
3. Autonomous stage: The motor skill becomes mostly automatic. The task should be varied until it can be done in every environmental condition.

### 2.2.2 Principles of Motor Learning

When acquiring a new task, certain principles must be followed for an efficient Motor Learning process.

A central requirement is frequent repetition [19–21]. This is particularly plausible because, as already described in Sect. 2.1, cortical reorganization only occurs with repeated stimulation

(LTP). It is not possible to give an exact figure for the number of repetitions because of the numerous factors influencing the learning process. However, it is certain that an immense number of repetitions at regular intervals is required to stimulate neuroplastic changes [22].

In the associative and autonomous stages of learning, however, the movements must not always be repeated identically, but should be variable [23]. The variation of the movement may only be given by small changes and must be done systematically. For example, in grasping exercises, the object to be grasped could be exchanged or placed on a different position. This guiding principle of Motor Learning is known as "repetition without repetition"[17].

Another fundamental principle is shaping. Shaping means that the exercise to be learned should be adapted to the patient's performance limit. Adjustments can be made either through increasing or decreasing the degree of complexity [12]. The "shaping to the performance limit"can be done in a variety of ways:

- From single-joint to multi-joint movements.
- Isolated practice with one limb to complex actions (involving the whole body).
- From slow to fast movements.
- From static to dynamic exercises (regarding trunk or balance training).
- From closed to open kinematic chains.
- From simple to difficult body position (lying, sitting, standing, etc.)
- From undivided to divided attention.
- None, one, several objects (for movements of the upper extremity).
- None, one, several obstacles (for movements of the lower extremity).

Shaping of the affected limb (also in combination with restriction of the unaffected side) serves to promote the inclusion of the limb in everyday activities. When this principle is not taken into account, the negative movement experience with the affected side and the positive experience with the healthy side can develop into "learned non-use"of the affected limb [24].

Exercises in physical therapy should also be close to everyday life and action-oriented [21], since biomechanical and neuromotor mecha-

nisms are organized during activity. Therefore, the more the exercise situation corresponds to reality, the easier it is to transfer what has been learned to everyday life [22]. Yet, it is not enough to work through standard exercises that are generally close to everyday life. The exercises should be individual and thus relevant to the patient, so that the learner can muster the necessary attention and motivation. Therefore, a detailed assessment of the patient's condition and a joint formulation of goals is very helpful [17].

▶ When practicing situations of everyday life with the patient, also think about external factors of everyday life (fellow human beings, street noise, etc.) and try to include them in therapy.

If the patient lacks the physical prerequisites, for example, strength or range of motion, to master a task, it can also be useful to split the task into different components. In this case, the learner must be made aware of the complex end goal of the exercise to understand its meaning [25].

Task- and problem-specific training should take place five times per week for 30 to 45 minutes in order to achieve an improvement in motor skills [26]. Additional independent home training and attendance at group physical training are recommended to consolidate what has been learned [17]. For this very reason, it is advantageous for patients to find themselves in an enriched environment at home or in rehabilitation [22]. The stimulus for physical activity and social interaction (enriched environment) has a positive effect on the reorganization of the brain and thus on the rehabilitation process.

**Summary**
Principles of Motor Learning:

- Repetitive training.
- Variable practice.
- Shaping.
- Restriction (of the unaffected side).
- Action-oriented and task-specific training.
- Goal-oriented training.
- Frequent training (dosage/duration).
- Enriched environment.

### 2.2.3 Factors Affecting the Motor Learning Process

Every learning process can be positively or negatively influenced by a wide variety of factors. In Motor Learning, motivation, but also the correct use of manual guidance and feedback play an important role in the various learning stages.

Motivation is the central aspect of Motor Learning [17]. Motivation can be intrinsic, driven by internal rewards, or extrinsic, led by external factors:

- The patient's intrinsic motivation depends strongly on the movement experience and on successes made in physical therapy. It can therefore be promoted by the therapist through adequate exercise design (Sect. 2.2.2).
- The extrinsic motivation can be enhanced through an adequate therapy-goal (external factor) that should be defined in collaboration with the patient.

Positive reinforcement plays a central role in promoting motivation. Feeling successful to provide a positive experience in the brain of a learner can be achieved by the therapist giving positive feedback (explicit feedback). The principle of giving positive feedback on a "successful" movement is already known from Edward Taub when reporting about learned non-use [27] and is also applied in Motor Learning.

Feedback should be adapted to the learning stage and should therefore be given either during the exercise in the cognitive stage or with latency in the associative and autonomic stage [1]. Feedback can either be given about the result of the movement (knowledge of results/KR) or about the performance (knowledge of performance/KP) but should primarily be positive. To be able to give positive feedback on the execution of movements, the degree of difficulty of the exercises must always be adapted to the patient's performance level (shaping) (Sect. 2.2.2). Complexity of the exercises should just be

manageable and only be increased when patients improve. Conversely, complexity should be reduced in case of repeated failure [12]. If the patient is always in a situation in which he can perform an activity or develop a motor strategy, this in turn creates a positive movement experience, which promotes the patient's intrinsic motivation.

If demands are too high, stress and anxiety can occur and negatively influence the learning process [28]. Consequently, the therapist has to adjust the exercises, give the patient more breaks or, if necessary, seek a conversation to find out about the cause or other factors that may trigger stress and overload [17].

Movement learning is not only influenced by augmented feedback from the therapist, but also by intrinsic feedback of movement perception [12]. Modern treatment approaches, however, reduce the internal focus, e.g., "Stretch your elbow!", as the superiority of practicing with an external focus has been shown in studies [29]. In grasping exercises, an external focus can be a glass, for example. The therapist's instruction would follow this focus by saying "Grasp the glass!". The results in favor for an external focus in practice are not surprising, since no one is likely to think about what position their joints are in when stirring their tea, but only whether the tea and sugar are mixing well. External focus can be provided not only by visual cueing, but also by tactile or auditory cueing (in terms of rhythm).

Another factor influencing the Motor Learning process is manual guidance provided by the therapist. In the initial learning stage, when an effective movement strategy is developed, manual guidance ("hands on") can be beneficial for the learning process [17]. In the later learning stages, in which the exercise is nearly errorless and the transfer of the movement into different situations is most important, working without manual support ("hands off") is more effective. Hence, it can be said that "hands on" and "hands off" can have a positive and negative influence, depending on the learning stage in which they are used [1].

**Summary**
The process of Motor Learning is influenced by:

- Intrinsic/extrinsic motivation.
- Reinforcement.
- Intrinsic/augmented (KP/KR) feedback.
- Focus of attention (internal/external).
- Cueing.
- Manual guidance: "hands-on"/ „hands-off".

## 2.3 Motor Learning and FES

Therapy with FES after neurological damage focuses on the restoration of movement skills. There is no concept that must be followed, but the principles and influencing factors of Motor Learning should be considered. In fact, these principles can be easily taken into account in therapy, since FES coincides in many aspects with the approaches in Motor Learning (see Table 2.1).

**Summary**
The following aspects are of great relevance in Motor Learning and can be ideally implemented in therapy with FES:

- High repetition.
- Active training.
- Motivation.
- Reinforcement (positive reward-prediction error).
- Task-specific and goal-oriented training.
- Shaping.
- Variable practice.
- External focus of attention.
- Feedback.
- Frequent training (dosage/duration).

First and foremost, targeted, reproducible functions should be practiced with frequent repetition. The FES device's request for stimulation triggering (in the case of EMG-triggered stimula-

tion) particularly motivates increased repetition. The triggering function works like a recurring request to move and therefore facilitates extrinsic motivation.

Since an active training should be preferred, EMG-triggered FES is to be aimed for even in more severely affected patients [21]. When using an EMG trigger, the patient must cross an individual preset activity-threshold with one of the muscles to be stimulated. This activity threshold can be set very low, as most devices have a sensitive EMG measurement. As the patient starts the movement, this weak impulse is then amplified by the electrical stimulation device and starts the stimulation of all channels with the set parameters of contraction and release time. Consequently, the FES enables an active training even in patients with severe paresis. Without the support of stimulation, it is often difficult to execute adequate functional training due to a low residual function, and only partial components that can be trained.

However, the FES not only promotes increased repetition and an active training, but also a constant reproducibility of a movement by supporting and guiding the movement. This provides relief to the learner, especially in the cognitive phase. The enabling of a reproducible movement helps to gain positive movement experiences (reinforcement through a positive reward-prediction error), which encourages the patient's intrinsic motivation. Furthermore, the support provided by electrical stimulation gives the feeling of a certain ease of exercise (positive feedback), even though patients exercising with FES train on their limit of performance.

▶ Observe patients' positive emotions when FES assists them while carrying out a movement as well as their satisfaction when they are able to perform a task for the first time again due to the support of the stimulation.

With a multichannel system technology, FES also enables complex movements and thus actions related to everyday life. Since the relevance of an exercise for everyday living (also consider an adequate goal setting) is particularly

**Table 2.1** FES and the Motor Learning process

| motor learning | FES support factor for motor learning | rehabilitation phases (R) & learning stages (L) where the FES support factor can be beneficial |
|---|---|---|
| high repetition | - repetitive EMG-trigger<br>- support of muscle strength/contraction<br>- acoustic signal at the start of the movement | R: all phases<br><br>L: all stages |
| active training | - EMG-trigger<br>- support of muscle strength/contraction<br>- adaptation of frequency and pulse widths | R: all phases: advantage in acute care when active training is not yet possible due to a severe paresis<br><br>L: all stages |
| motivation | - repetitive EMG-trigger<br>- support of muscle strength/contraction<br>- constant reproducibility of a movement | R: all phases<br><br>L: all stages |
| task-specific and goal-orientated training | - multichannel system technology<br>- individual plateau-pause settings for each channel<br>- adjustable rise time and fall time settings | R: all phases: especially important when activities of daily living and back-to-work activities are focused<br><br>L: all stages |
| shaping | - multichannel system technology<br>- individual plateau-pause settings for each channel<br>- adjustable rise time and fall time settings<br>- adaptation of frequency and pulse widths | R: all phases<br><br>L: especially helpful in cognitive stage when the level of difficulty has just been increased |
| variable practise | - multichannel system technology<br>- possibility to alter channels/stimulated muscles<br>- individual plateau-pause settings for each channel<br>- adjustable rise time and fall time settings | R: all phases<br><br>L: especially helpful in later learning stages, as the combination of therapy and FES allows more gradations of variation |
| external focus of attention | - tactile cueing: initiation of the movement through the increase of the current<br>- auditory cueing by an acoustic signal at the beginning of the movement<br>- the constant rhythm of movements generated by plateau-pause times makes it easier for the patient to concentrate on an external visual focus | R: all phases<br><br>L: cueing strategies through FES particularly facilitate the cognitive stage |
| feedback | - proprioceptive feedback through the electrical stimulation<br>- visual feedback of the successful movement through the support of the FES | R: all phases<br><br>L: all stages |
| frequent training | - unsupervised training possible; increases the necessary therapy dosage/ duration/ frequency<br>- individual therapy through individual programs (set by the therapist) | R: especially important in later phases when supervised therapies take place less often (e.g. only twice a week)<br><br>L: all stages |

important for the Motor Learning process, a multichannel system should be preferred in any case. Task-oriented training is easy to implement because of the individually adjustable channels. Phases of stimulation (plateau) and pauses (contraction and relaxation time of the muscles) can be adjusted like the rise and fall times (rise and fall of the current) for each muscle involved in a movement. This helps to mimic a physiological movement as accurate as possible and supports the learning of any everyday activity.

▶ For complex movements, the therapist must be more skilled in using the FES to recognize the activation patterns of the actual movement and to adequately adjust the various parameters and plateau-pause times.

When exercising with FES, it is as important as in training without stimulation, to adapt the exercises to the patient's performance level. Shaping can be done even more precise, because of additional parameters to adjust on the stimulation device, like force (stimulation frequency) or movement velocity (contraction-, release-, rise-, and fall time).

▶ If you want to adjust an exercise, do not change all channels at the same time, but change one channel (one joint or movement component) first, then two channels, and so on to make the transitions smoother.

FES eases the shaping process, when increasing the complexity of a task, for example, when the limb to be trained should be incorporated into an action like grasping and moving an object or when several body parts should get involved. The FES supports the patient in the cognitive phase because the affected limb is kept in the usual movement sequence that was already trained with the preset stimulation program. Thus, more concentration remains for the actual task, the objects or the steps of execution, which additionally helps to shift to an external focus.

▶ If grasping in sitting already succeeds without problems and even with variation (object size and position), the stimulation protocol can be maintained and the context can be changed, for example, by moving the glasses from the countertop to the cupboard in a standing position.

Variability in the exercise situation can be obtained with FES from two sides:

– On the one hand, you can, as usual, vary the objects or the environment with which or in which you work. For this purpose, the stimulated muscles and the plateau-pause times do usually not need to be changed, since the movement merely takes place in a different context.
– On the other hand, you can change the patient's starting position (ASTE), which slightly alters the movement. In this case, it is recommended to additionally adjust the plateau-pause times to the new movement.

▶ When you start working with FES, don't give up if it seems difficult or takes a little longer to change program settings on the device. After some tries, you will be faster than you think – it is very intuitive!

The constant rhythm of movements generated by electrical stimulation (preset plateau-pause times) has proven to be particularly beneficial for Motor Learning, as this corresponds to tactile cueing. The cueing of the movement rhythm takes place through the increase of the current (external stimulus) at a certain point in time, depending on the preset stimulation protocol. The support of the timing of the movement makes the task easier for the patients because they are less focused on coordinating the sequence of movements in the task-solving process. Accordingly, there is facilitation in the cognitive stage and thus acceleration of the onset of the associative stage of Motor Learning. Training with an external focus, in the sense of visual cueing, is supported by the guiding of the movement (plateau-pause times), as the learner can focus more on the target. Auditory cueing also takes place in FES to a certain extend. An acoustic signal from the device reports back to the patient when the pause is over, and the movement should be started again.

Cueing strategies through FES do not only serve to initiate or ease movement, but also support augmented feedback of the movement (KP) and feedback on movement success or failure (KR).

To gain motor function or maintain what was learned, regular individual training is necessary, but often problematic when patients leave acute care facilities, due to various reasons. These can either be a lack of facilities nearby, a lack of time (appointments), or a lack of financial support of the insurance companies. However, the recommended therapy frequency of five times per week for 30-45 minutes [26] can be easily achieved with FES therapy, that can be done in an unsupervised setting after some training sessions. Especially in an outpatient setting, where therapy often takes place only twice a week, FES is particularly beneficial for supporting independent practice (Chap. 17).

▶ Consider using FES to support independent practice at home if you think your patient can benefit from it.

# References


1. Freivogel S. Grundkonzepte der Physiotherapie. In: Dettmers C, Stephan KM, editors. Motorische Therapie nach Schlaganfall, 1 Aufl. Bad Honnef: Hippocampus; 2011. p. 106–18.
2. Shepherd R, Carr J. Scientific basis of neurological physiotherapy: bridging the gap between science and practice. In: Dettmers C, Weiler C, editors. Update neurologische rehabilitation, 1. Aufl. Bad Honnef: Hippocampus; 2005. p. 61–71.
3. Langhammer B, Stanghelle JK. Can Physiotherapy after stroke based on the Bobath concept result in im- proved quality of movement compared to the motor relearning programme. Physiother Res Int. 2011;16(2):69–80.
4. Sterr A, Conforto AB. Plasticity of adult sensorimotor system in severe brain infarcts: challenges and opportunities. Neural Plast. 2012;970136:1–10.
5. Ende-Henningsen B, Henningsen H. Neurobiologische Grundlagen der Plastizität des Nervensystems. In: Frommelt P, Lösslein H, editors. Neurorehabilitation, 1. Aufl. Berlin/Heidelberg: Springer; 2010. p. 67–79.
6. Krakauer JW. Motor learning: its relevance to stroke recovery and neurorehabilitation. Curr Opin Neurol. 2006;19:84–90.
7. Scheidtmann K. Nutzen der neuronalen Plastizität. In: Hüter-Becker A, Dölken M, editors. Physiotherapie in der Neurologie, 3. Aufl. Stuttgart: Georg Thieme; 2010. p. 7–8.
8. Bliss TV, Lomo T. Long-lasting potentiation of synaptic transmission in the dentate area of the anaesthetized rabbit following stimulation of the perforant path. J Physiol. 1973;232(2):331–56.
9. Hebb DO. Drives and the C.N.S. (conceptual nervous system). Psychol Rev. 1955;62(4):243–54.
10. Carmichael TS, Chesselet M-F. Synchronous neuronal activity is a signal for axonal sprouting after cortical lesions in the adult. J Neurosci. 2002;22(14):6062–70.
11. Cramer SC. Repairing the human brain after stroke: 1. Mechanisms of spontaneous recovery. Ann Neurol. 2008;63:272–87.
12. Freivogel S, Fries W. Motorische rehabilitation. In: Frommelt P, Lösslein H, editors. Neuro-rehabilitation, 1. Aufl. Berlin/Heidelberg: Springer; 2010. p. 225–66.
13. Nudo RJ, Milliken GW. Reorganization of movement representations in primary motor cortex following focal ischemic infarcts in adult squirrel monkeys. J Neurophysiol. 1996;75(5):2144–9.
14. Elbert T, Rockstroh B. Reorganization of human cerebral cortex: the range of changes following use and injury. Neuroscientist. 2004;10(2):129–41.
15. Lashley KS. The accuracy of movement in the absence of excitation from the moving organ. Am J Phys. 1917;43:169–94.
16. Fitts PM, Posner MI. Human performance. Belmont: Brooks/Cole Publishing Company; 1967.
17. Wulf D. Motorists Lernen. In: Hüter-Becker A, Dölken M, editors. Physiotherapie in der Neurologie, 3. Aufl. Aufl. Stuttgart: Georg Thieme; 2010. p. 41–72.
18. Majsak MJ. Application of motor learning principles to the stroke population. Top Stroke Rehabil. 1996;3(2):37–59.
19. Lang CE, MacDonald JR, Gnip C. Counting repetitions: an observational study of outpatient therapy for people with hemiparesis post-stroke. J Neurol Phys Ther. 2007;31(1):3–10.
20. Lang CE, MacDonald JR, Reisman DS, Boyd L, Kimber-Ley TJ, Schindler-Ivens SM, et al. Observation of amounts of movement practice provided during stroke rehabilitation. Arch Phys Med Rehabil. 2009;90(10):1692–8.
21. Hauptmann B, Müller C. Motorisches Lernen und repetitives Training. In: Nowak D, editor. Handfunktionsstörungen in der Neurologie. Berlin/Heidelberg: Springer; 2011. p. 214–23.
22. Mehrholz J. Frühphase Schlaganfall, 1. Aufl. Stuttgart: Georg Thieme; 2008.
23. Mulder T. Das adaptive Gehirn. Stuttgart: Georg Thieme; 2007.

24. Taub E, Crago JE, Burgio LD, Groomes TE, Cook EW III, DeLuca SC, Miller NE. An operant approach to rehabilitation medicine: overcoming learned nonuse by shaping. J Exp Anal Behav. 1994;61(2):281–93.

25. Horst R. Motorisches Strategietraining und PNF, 1. Aufl. Stuttgart: Georg Thieme; 2005.

26. Freivogel S, Hummelsheim H. Qualitätskriterien und Leitlinie für die motorische Rehabilitation von Patienten mit Hemiparesen. Aktuelle Neurol. 2003;30(8):401–6.

27. Taub E, Miller NE, Novack TA, Cook EW 3rd, Fleming WC, Nepomuceno CS. Technique to improve chronic motor deficit after stroke. Arch Phys Med Rehabil. 1993;74(4):347–54.

28. Singer RN. Motor learning and human performance: an application to motor skills and movement behaviors. New York: Macmillan; 1980.

29. Wulf G. Bewegungen erlernen und automatisieren: Worauf ist die Aufmerksamkeit zu richten? neuroreha. 2011;3(01):18–23.

Patricia Meier

**Summary**
A clinical improvement is associated with cortical reorganization [1–3] since the motor learning process always causes a change in neuronal structures. This knowledge is often sufficient for everyday practice, but for those interested it can be exciting to understand the various neuroplastic mechanisms that are initiated through practice with FES more precisely.

## 3.1 Why Does Neuroplasticity Take Place when Practicing with FES?

When practicing with FES training-induced neuronal plasticity occurs, as in any other exercise-based therapeutic intervention, since FES follows an action-oriented and task-specific approach. FES training covers various aspects that are responsible for changes on different neuronal levels.

► Training-induced plasticity describes changes on a molecular and structural level through practice, for example, through the increased use of a limb. The basic mechanism of these neuroplastic processes is long-term potentiation (LTP, Sect. 2.1). LTP leads to a transformation of synapses, implying structural more stable connections through increased formation of synapses and dendrites as well as increased incorporation of receptors or increased release of neurotransmitters (increase in synaptic efficiency) [4].

FES utilizes the principle of long-term potentiation (LTP), which is fundamental to plasticity, through its exercise design with increased repetition supported by the repeated electrical stimulation. This repeated stimulation in an action-oriented context enhances cortical reorganization [5]. In the sense of the phrase "what fires together – wires together" ( [6]; Sect. 2.1), cells that are active together, for example, through specific movement sequences supported by FES, link together. Increased connectivity affects all synapses involved in this particular movement.

The electrical impulses stimulate the motor nerve fibers antidromically from the periphery, meaning against their physiological "firing direction" (orthodromic). The retrograde impulses depolarize the anterior horn cell. Together with the voluntary initiated activity, i.e., an activation of the corticospinal pathways, it can be assumed that the coupling of the synapses is promoted in the sense of a Hebbian plasticity [7].

Even though you are working in a motor-threshold range with FES, not only motor but

P. Meier (✉)
Medical University of Innsbruck,
Department of Neurology, Innsbruck, Austria

VASCage GmbH, Research Centre on Vascular
Ageing and Stroke, Innsbruck, Austria


T. Schick (ed.), *Functional Electrical Stimulation in Neurorehabilitation*,
https://doi.org/10.1007/978-3-030-90123-3_3

also sensory nerve fibers are stimulated. The stimulation of afferent (sensory) fibers by FES thereby arises not merely from tactile input through cutaneous sensation, but also from increased proprioceptive information from joint receptors, Golgi tendon organs, and muscle spindles. The enhanced multifactorial afferent impulse of the functional stimulation also leads to cortical changes [8–10], increased sensorimotor cortex excitability (SMC), and changes in motor cortical network activity [11, 12]. Thus, increased connectivity results from the various afferent input through the task-oriented focus of FES. Consequently, sensory stimulation leads to increased intracortical excitability of the motor cortex mainly through a functional context [13].

FES also supports muscle recruitment, which further results in a bigger movement [14]. Thus patients can perform movements actively and goal-oriented through the support of electrical stimulation and the reinforcement of muscle strength [15]. Therefore, another advantage of FES compared with other active treatment methods is that movements can be executed mostly without compensatory mechanisms or co-contractions. Consequently, effective linkages can occur from the very beginning of the rehabilitation process even in patients with severe paresis.

Since training with FES includes several factors that positively influence the motor learning process, there is also an accelerated structural reorganization at the neural level. In addition, the visual perception of the amplified movement enhances motivation, enjoyment, and thus motor learning [16].

## 3.2 What Kind of Neuroplastic Changes Are Induced by FES?

Functional electrical stimulation results in plastic changes of neuronal structures, like increased activation of individual primary sensory and motor areas [17], as well as in an accelerated axonal growth and in enhanced myelination of peripheral nerves through changes on a neuromolecular level [18]. Based on current literature the following sections describe neuroplastic changes in motor and sensory cortex, corticospinal tract, and peripheral nerves in detail and discuss initial hypotheses about effects on spinal cord structures.

Most studies investigating these neuroplastic effects of FES chose a very simple setting. That is, in most cases, a functional stimulation of only one or two muscle groups. Most commonly, wrist extensors were stimulated for upper extremity studies and plantar flexors, or dorsal extensors were stimulated in studies involving the lower extremity.

### 3.2.1 Effects of FES on Motor and Sensory Cortex

The effects of FES on cortical structures were first studied in healthy subjects, as it is generally the case in new therapy approaches. In these healthy participants, functional magnetic resonance imaging (fMRI) showed an increased activation of the contralateral primary sensorimotor cortex (SMC) and of the supplementary motor area (SMA) due to electrical stimulation [19]. Another fMRI study demonstrated changes in activation of movement-relevant cortical regions as well. Functional stimulation resulted in an increased activation of the contralateral primary motor cortex (M1), the primary somatosensory cortex (S1), and the premotor cortex (PMC) as well as a bilateral activation of SMA and secondary sensory areas (S2) [11] (Fig. 3.1).

Similar findings were obtained in hemiplegic patients as well. Using fMRI, functional stimulation increased bilateral activation of the somatosensory cortex, which remained consistent over time [9]. The more the exercise set-up corresponded to functional training (EMG-triggered stimulation), the more changes in cortical activation patterns shifted from ipsilateral (contralesional) to contralateral (ipsilesional) SMC [20].

▶ Functional improvement may be due to different cortical mechanisms. Commonly a shift to the ipsilesional side is referred to as

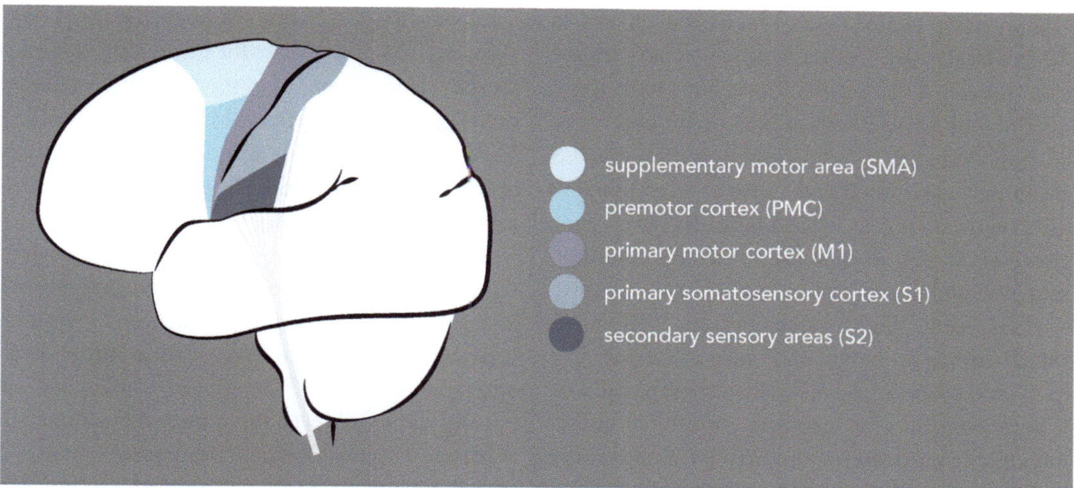


**Fig. 3.1** Motor (M1, PMC, SMA) and sensory (S1, S2) cortex areas with increased activation through training with FES

objective improvement, whereas increased activation of contralesional structures is referred to as compensation.

A study by Shin et al. [20] showed the presence of a cortical shift to the ipsilesional side in association with a significant improvement in all clinical tests after EMG triggered neuromuscular stimulation of the wrist extensors. However, as we know from rehabilitation, this shift is rather rare in patients with large lesions and severe paresis [21]. This was also confirmed for training with FES. Severely affected patients tended to have an increased activation of the contralesional side, whereas activation of ipsilesional regions could only be shown in less severely affected patients [22].

In order to visualize plastic changes in the motor and sensory cortex, different imaging techniques can be used. In addition to fMRI and BOLD-fMRI (blood oxygenation level-dependent, BOLD), which focuses on the blood flow in individual areas (higher spatial resolution), single-photon emission computed tomography (SPECT) or positron emission tomography (PET) can be used (temporal resolution). These two imaging techniques are associated with radiation exposure (albeit low) to the patient and are therefore rarely performed in studies unless they are absolutely necessary.

Unfortunately, there appear to be difficulties in performing imaging while doing an FES training with either of the abovementioned imaging techniques. Apparently, the magnetic field makes it difficult to bring the stimulation device into the area of the tomograph and it is unclear if the magnetic field alters the sensation of current or if the electrical stimulation influences the imaging results [18]. Although there have been studies that have attempted to demonstrate that electrical stimulation during such imaging techniques does not cause any problems [11], most studies preferably conduct fMRI or BOLD-fMRI imaging not during, but rather before and after FES treatment.

However, near-infrared spectroscopy (NIRS) can be performed during FES training without any problems, as there are no interactions with the stimulation device. Another major advantage of NIRS is that patients can be in a sitting or standing position during imaging. The basic principle of NIRS is the detection of differences in oxygenated and deoxygenated hemoglobin depending on the absorption of infrared light. The change in oxygenation correlates with the cerebral blood flow [23], which in turn provides information about cortical activation. Thus, Hara et al. [14] were able to demonstrate by using NIRS that cortical blood flow is increased in ipsilesional SMC already during EMG-triggered FES in moderately affected patients. Further studies using NIRS showed increased activity in S2 bilaterally [8]. Consequently, we can observe that these study results correlate with those obtained by fMRI imaging post-treatment.

Improvement in motor function through FES is not only associated with cortical activation, but also with changes in synaptic activity, gene expression, and an increase in neurotransmitter, receptor, and neurotrophin levels [24].

This seems highly plausible, as FES maximized sensory input and motor output. An increased proprioceptive feedback combined with a high frequency of repetitive movement stimulates pre- and postsynaptic activity along motor and sensory pathways. This mechanism, following the principle of Hebbian plasticity, is known to enhance synaptic and neuronal functioning and causes training-induced plasticity [18, 25].

The knowledge of neuroplastic changes along the sensorimotor system through FES gives a good explanation for the superior functional outcomes in EMG-triggered FES approaches. EMG-triggered FES enhances the connection of central activation, i.e., the intention to perform a movement, and peripheral activation through electrical stimulation. Thus, this form of FES corresponds more to the complexity of a motor learning process. This hypothesis has already been supported by studies showing that volitionally initiated (EMG-triggered) functional stimulation has significantly greater effects on motor evoked potentials (MEP) [26] and on activation of the ipsilesional cortex [14] than non-EMG-triggered stimulation or active movement alone. These changes in cortical excitation also correlated with an enhanced improvement of function [14].

Since, as described, the involvement of volitional initiation and prior movement planning plays an essential role in the motor learning process, it becomes understandable why Mental Imagery combined with EMG-triggered FES showed better results than FES alone. Hong et al. showed a significant change in metabolic processes in the cortex (contralesional SMC), accompanied by a significant improvement in the Fugl-Meyer test [27].

Since optimal timing of these two inputs (cortical and peripheral) is critical [28], EEG (electroencephalography)-derived motor imagery was used as a trigger for the electrical stimulation. This form of "motor imagery-based brain-computer interface (MI- BCI) controlling FES" was successfully conducted to induce an optimal temporal match, in terms of a "physiological" arousal [29, 30].

Achieving these physiological excitation patterns is not only important for the central, but also for the peripheral nervous system. Consequently, the movement that is "mimicked" and supported by FES should correspond as closely as possible to the actual movement. To achieve a physiological movement, multiple stimulation channels should be used. Studies that have investigated the use of different numbers of channels have shown that 4-channel stimulation significantly improved motor function and cortical plasticity compared to 2-channel stimulation in stroke patients (5).

▶ Depending on the type of stimulation, effects on the cortex are different. The closer the FES training gets to a physiological movement planning/execution process, the more likely cortical reorganization occurs. Thus, multichannel EMG-triggered FES with a task-oriented approach should be preferred in any case (provided it is adequate for the patient's motor level).

**Summary**

Effects of *FES* on:

- Primary somatosensory cortex and secondary sensory areas (S1, S2).
- Premotor cortex (PMC).
- Primary motor cortex (M1).
- Supplementary motor area (SMA).

### 3.2.2 Effects of FES on the Corticospinal Tract

Even after 2 weeks of functional electrical stimulation of the finger extensors healthy subjects showed an increased activation of the corticospinal tract (CST), which correlated with an improvement in function on the perdue pegboard test (PPT) [31]. In addition to the focal effects at the target muscle, Mang et al. were also able to find global effects on corticospinal excitability in healthy subjects, as demonstrated by MEP (motor evoked potentials) using transcranial magnetic stimulation (TMS) [32]. Although no imaging was performed here, at least a meaningful statement about the functional outcome can be made with the help of TMS [33].

Wei et al. [34] investigated the effects of FES training in subacute stroke patients and showed an improvement in motor function and a change in FA (fractional anisotropy) values of CST in the internal capsule region in diffusion tensor imaging (DTI). This effect has also been demonstrated in other studies investigating the effects of FES on CST [35].

Regarding neuroplastic changes of the CST a multichannel stimulation is also superior. Four-channel FES inducing a cycling movement of the lower extremities based on a gait pattern showed an increase in fibers and an enlargement of fiber bundles in the ipsilateral CST (Fig. 3.2) in tractography using DTI (fMRI) and may therefore be even more effective in promoting motor recovery and plastic changes compared with a two-channel stimulation [5].

Since effects of FES are shown on a cortical level and in the CST, the question arises, if there are effects of FES training even on a spinal cord level. This question will be addressed in Sect. 3.2.3.

**Summary**
Effects of *FES* on:

– Activation of CST.
– Number of fibers in CST.

### 3.2.3 Effects of FES on Spinal Cord Structures

In clinical practice, we see that FES has a positive effect on spasticity. Electrical stimulation leads to a reduction in muscle tone and improved mobility and function [36, 37]. Also in the case of spasticity the superiority of functional stimulation (FES) over conventional electrical stimulation (NMES) is clearly apparent [38]. Thus, it must be assumed that FES intervenes in the mechanism of spasticity and induces changes in spinal neural circuits. Different hypotheses have been put forward in this regard.

Based on the suppositions that spasticity, increased tendon reflexes and the increased mus-

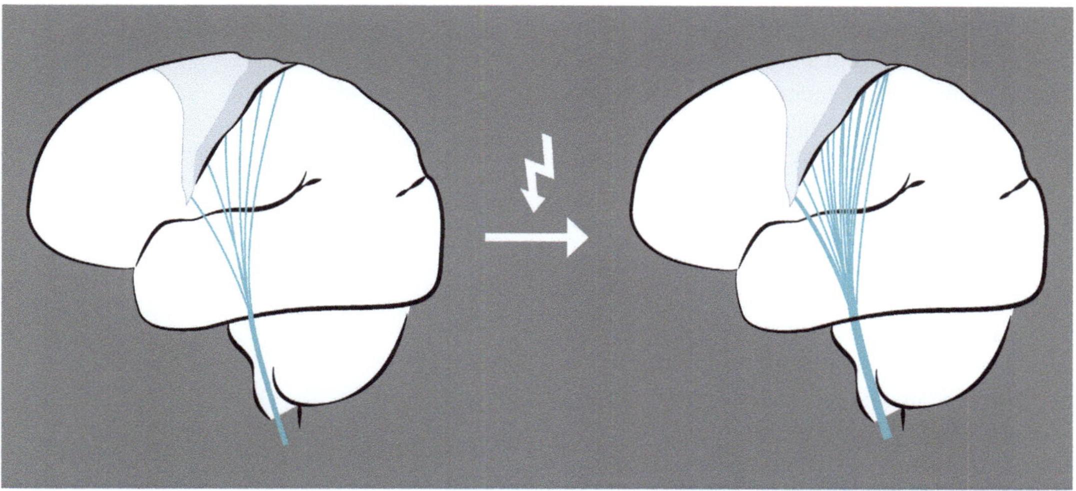

**Fig. 3.2** FES training shows an increased activation and proliferation of fibers of the CST

cle tone result from a reduced cortical input with simultaneous increased occupation of the anterior horn cell by sensitive afferent fibers (especially Ia fibers) of the same segment [39], Rushton [7] seems to have put forward a good hypothesis:

If therapy with FES results in increased cortical activation (Sects. 3.2.1 and 3.2.2), the alpha motor neuron in the anterior horn is again increasingly "needed" by efferent (cortical) pathways, which re-establishes segmental cortico-spinal connections in the sense of a physiological restructuring. In combination with an antidromic excitation of the alpha motor neuron, which is induced by electrical stimulation (Sect. 3.1), motor pathways can be functionally reconnected (Fig. 3.3). This theory seems quite plausible considering that the anterior horn cell responds like a "Hebb synapse" to LTP [40].

However, a clinical change in spasticity could also be induced by other mechanisms since FES influences several structures of the spinal cord and its afferent pathways. Depending on the stimulation frequency and the stimulation protocol (to be investigated), FES could lead to a promotion of reciprocal inhibition (Ia afferent) and/or autogenic inhibition (Ib afferent) by the increased sensory afferent input (muscle spindle, Golgi tendon organ). FES could as well influence a restoration of the recurrent inhibition (Renshaw cell) by antidromic excitation of the alpha motor neuron (Fig. 3.4) and thus cause a reduction of spasticity [41].

Unfortunately, there are yet not so many studies concerning the influence of FES on the underlying neuroplastic changes in the spinal cord, probably because the development of spasticity is a multifactorial and yet not fully understood process and peripheral measurements are more complicated than cortical imaging. Most studies are still conducted in rats and mice, and until now, there are only a few papers published where humans were examined [42].

However, Stowe et al. [43] were able to show a change in the H-reflex after neuromuscular electrical stimulation of the upper extremity in stroke patients. The measurement was made via an EMG signal, whereby an increase of the

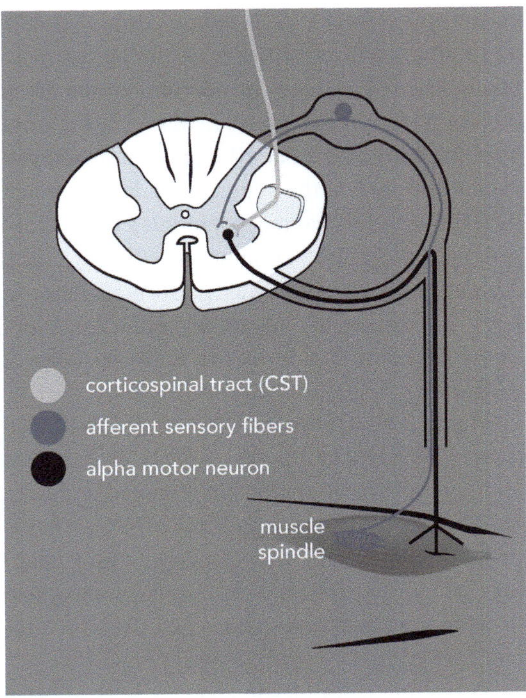


**Fig. 3.3** Hypothesis of FES effects on a spinal cord level: FES promotes the restoration of physiological connectivity of cortical pathways (upper motor neurons) with alpha motor neurons in the anterior horn [7]

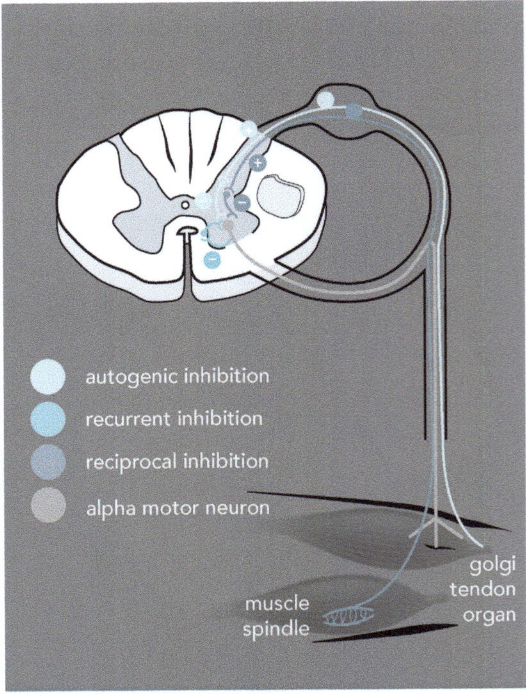


**Fig. 3.4** Hypothesis on neuronal influences of FES at spinal cord level: FES influences spasticity by modulating segmental inhibition of the alpha motor neuron [41]

H-reflex in the paretic wrist extensors and no increase of the H-reflex in the spastic flexors was observed due to electrical stimulation, whereas in the control group the values of the extensors increased less and those of the flexors more. The change in H-reflex due to electrical stimulation even correlated with improved motor function of the upper extremity in the box-and-block test (BBT) [43].

Because of the small study population, the interpretation of the results must be made with caution, but it is a first confirmation of the established hypotheses [41].

▶ The H-reflex (named after the physiologist Paul Hoffmann) corresponds to a muscles intrinsic reflex. It is defined as a reflectory contraction of a muscle due to excitation of the spindle afferents, when a motor or mixed nerve is electrically stimulated [44]. Excitation of Ia fibers (spindle afferents) leads to an activation of alpha motor neurons of the same muscle and its synergists, and to an inhibition of alpha motor neurons of antagonistic muscles via Ia inhibitory interneurons.

Although the process of restructuring neuronal circuits and thus the modulation of spasticity due to FES has not yet been clearly elucidated, having demonstrated plastic changes in the brain and CST and functional changes in spastic skeletal muscles, plasticity on a spinal cord level (alpha motor neuron and its synaptic connections) definitely seems plausible [41].

However, although neuronal effects on spasticity from FES are likely, not all studies can show functional improvement of movement or a change in spasticity [45]. This is probably because the development of spasticity is multifactorial, and the progression of spasticity affects movements and bodily structures on different levels. If spasticity is present, not only the muscle properties and neuronal circuits change, but also stiffness and joint contractures occur [22], which are often more difficult to influence therapeutically, particularly when they persist for a longer period of time.

**Summary**
The effect of *FES* on the following structures should be further investigated:

– Alpha motor neuron.
– Ia afferents.
– Ib afferents.
– Renshaw cell.

### 3.2.4 Effects of FES on Peripheral Nerves

With regard to peripheral nerves, FES plays an important role especially before and after surgery or after peripheral nerve injury. Most studies are currently conducted in animals, primarily rats. After surgical transection of the nerve, accelerated axonal growth was shown, especially by low-frequency stimulation. In humans, similar results were shown by electrical stimulation after damage of sensory and mixed nerves and after peripheral nerve surgery. Electrical stimulation led to an accelerated and increased axonal growth, which resulted in earlier innervation of the target muscles in both humans and animals [42, 46, 47].

Patients with median nerve compression in the carpal tunnel underwent carpel tunnel release surgery (CTRS) followed by electrical stimulation of the median nerve. Even though the stimulation had no functional context and was performed directly on the nerve, once, immediately after surgery, brief low-frequency electrical stimulation showed enhanced axonal regeneration 6–8 months after CTRS. In comparison to the control group motor units increased significantly and sensory nerve conduction values improved [42].

Wong et al. [47] demonstrated enhanced axonal growth and sensory reinnervation as well as accelerated functional recovery by electrical stimulation even in patients who sustained complete digital nerve transection. Daily electrical stimulation after peroneal repair was as well associated with accelerated reinnervation of the denervated muscle, but so far only in animal experiments [48].

The mechanism of electrical stimulation on peripheral nerves is supposed to occur by influencing the cell body. Stimulation results in an increased calcium ion ($Ca^{2+}$) influx, leading to an increase in cyclic adenosine monophosphate (cAMP), which can promote regeneration by increasing the amount of neurotrophic factors [49]. Consequently, nerve regeneration occurs depending on retrograde transmission of action potentials to the cell body [50].

The cause of accelerated axonal regeneration induced by electrical stimulation is therefore an increased release of BDNF (brain-derived neurotrophic factor) or an enhanced expression of mRNA (messenger ribonucleic acid) for BDNF and its receptor trkB (tropomyosin receptor kinase) [51, 52] in sensory and motor nerves (Fig. 3.5).

Electrical stimulation of Schwann cells also caused an increase in BDNF as well as NGF (nerve growth factor), GDNF (glial cell line-derived neurotrophic factor), and myelin protein 22 at both the mRNA and protein levels. The increase of neurotrophic factors in the cell, induced by electrical stimulation, thus leads to increased axonal growth, which could already be demonstrated in vivo, in rats [53]. Similar stimulation protocols were also able to show effects on myelination mediated via enhanced BDNF signals, indicating an accelerated remyelination of Schwann cells as a result of electrical stimulation [54].

In any case, further studies are needed to explain the underlying processes of FES in peripheral nerves in detail.

**Summary**

Effects of *FES* on:

– Neurotrophic factors and its receptors.
– Axonal growth.
– Schwann cell myelination.
– Reinnervation of denervated muscles.

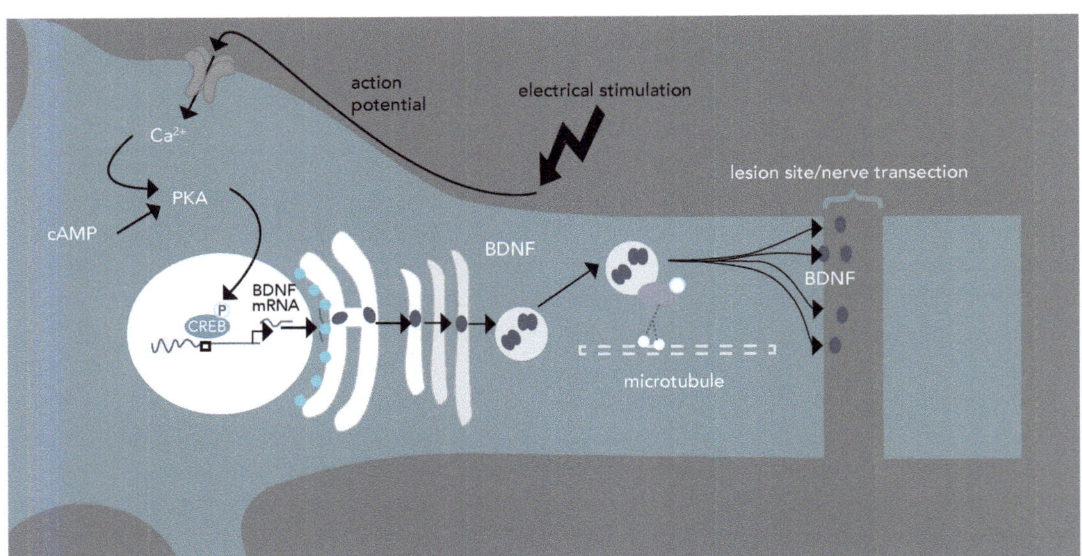


**Fig. 3.5** Explanatory model for the accelerated axonal growth due to electrical stimulation: retrograde transmission of action potentials to the cell body result in the opening of voltage-dependent calcium ion channels. The influx of calcium ions ($Ca^{2+}$) leads, through an increase of cAMP and thus through an activation of protein kinase A (PKA), to the phosphorylation (P) of the transcription factor CREB (cAMP response element-binding protein), thereby starting the process to produce neurotrophic factors (e.g., brain-derived neurotrophic factor, BDNF)

## References


1. Carey JR, Kimberley TJ, Lewis SM, Auerbach EJ, Dorsey L, Rundquist P, et al. Analysis of fMRI and finger tracking training in subjects with chronic stroke. Brain. 2002;125(Pt 4):773–88.
2. Liepert J, Bauder H, Wolfgang HR, Miltner WH, Taub E, Weiller C. Treatment-induced cortical reorganization after stroke in humans. Stroke. 2000;31(6):1210–6.
3. Platz T, van Kaick S, Möller L, Freund S, Winter T, Kim IH. Impairment-oriented training and adaptive motor cortex reorganisation after stroke: a fTMS study. J Neurol. 2005;252(11):1363–71.
4. Frommelt P, Lösslein H. Neuro-rehabilitation. 1st ed. Berlin/Heidelberg: Springer; 2010.
5. Zheng X, Chen D, Yan T, Jin D, Zhuang Z, Tan Z, et al. A randomized clinical trial of a functional electrical stimulation mimic to gait promotes motor recovery and brain remodeling in acute stroke. Behav Neurol. 2018;2018:8923520.
6. Hebb DO. Drives and the C.N.S. (conceptual nervous system). Psychol Rev. 1955;62(4):243–54.
7. Rushton DN. Functional electrical stimulation and rehabilitation—an hypothesis. Med Eng Phys. 2003;25(1):75–8.
8. Lo CC, Lin PY, Hoe ZY, Chen JJ. Near infrared spectroscopy study of cortical excitability during electrical stimulation-assisted cycling for neurorehabilitation of stroke patients. IEEE Trans Neural Syst Rehabil Eng. 2018;26(6):1292–300.
9. Sasaki K, Matsunaga T, Tomite T, Yoshikawa T, Shimada Y. Effect of electrical stimulation therapy on upper extremity functional recovery and cerebral cortical changes in patients with chronic hemiplegia. Biomed Res. 2012;33(2):89–96.
10. Wardman DL, Gandevia SC, Colebatch JG. Cerebral, subcortical, and cerebellar activation evoked by selective stimulation of muscle and cutaneous afferents: an fMRI study. Physiol Rep. 2014;2(4):e00270.
11. Blickenstorfer A, Kleiser R, Keller T, Keisker B, Meyer M, Riener R, et al. Cortical and subcortical correlates of functional electrical stimulation of wrist extensor and flexor muscles revealed by fMRI. Hum Brain Mapp. 2009;30(3):963–75.
12. Ridding MC, Brouwer B, Miles TS, Pitcher JB, Thompson PD. Changes in muscle responses to stimulation of the motor cortex induced by peripheral nerve stimulation in human subjects. Exp Brain Res. 2000;131(1):135–43.
13. Liu H, Au-Yeung SSY. Corticomotor excitability effects of peripheral nerve electrical stimulation to the paretic arm in stroke. Am J Phys Med Rehabil. 2017;96(10):687–93.
14. Hara Y, Obayashi S, Tsujiuchi K, Muraoka Y. The effects of electromyography-controlled functional electrical stimulation on upper extremity function and cortical perfusion in stroke patients. Clin Neurophysiol. 2013;124(10):2008–15.
15. Lotze M, Braun C, Birbaumer N, Anders S, Cohen LG. Motor learning elicited by voluntary drive. Brain. 2003;126(Pt 4):866–72.
16. Rizzolatti G, Craighero L. The mirror-neuron system. Annu Rev Neurosci. 2004;27:169–92.
17. Carson RG, Buick AR. Neuromuscular electrical stimulation-promoted plasticity of the human brain. J Physiol. 2021;599(9):2375–99.
18. Hara Y. Brain plasticity and rehabilitation in stroke patients. J Nippon Med Sch. 2015;82(1):4–13.
19. Han BS, Jang SH, Chang Y, Byun WM, Lim SK, Kang DS. Functional magnetic resonance image finding of cortical activation by neuromuscular electrical stimulation on wrist extensor muscles. Am J Phys Med Rehabil. 2003;82(1):17–20.
20. Shin HK, Cho SH, Jeon HS, Lee YH, Song JC, Jang SH, et al. Cortical effect and functional recovery by the electromyography-triggered neuromuscular stimulation in chronic stroke patients. Neurosci Lett. 2008;442(3):174–9.
21. Rehme AK, Eickhoff SB, Rottschy C, Fink GR, Grefkes C. Activation likelihood estimation meta-analysis of motor-related neural activity after stroke. NeuroImage. 2012;59(3):2771–82.
22. Quandt F, Hummel FC. The influence of functional electrical stimulation on hand motor recovery in stroke patients: a review. Exp Transl Stroke Med. 2014;6:9.
23. Toronov V, Webb A, Choi JH, Wolf M, Michalos A, Gratton E, et al. Investigation of human brain hemodynamics by simultaneous near-infrared spectroscopy and functional magnetic resonance imaging. Med Phys. 2001;28(4):521–7.
24. Dimyan MA, Cohen LG. Neuroplasticity in the context of motor rehabilitation after stroke. Nat Rev Neurol. 2011;7(2):76–85.
25. Cecatto RB, Maximino JR, Chadi G. Motor recovery and cortical plasticity after functional electrical stimulation in a rat model of focal stroke. Am J Phys Med Rehabil. 2014;93(9):791–800.
26. Barsi GI, Popovic DB, Tarkka IM, Sinkjaer T, Grey MJ. Cortical excitability changes following grasping exercise augmented with electrical stimulation. Exp Brain Res. 2008;191(1):57–66.
27. Hong IK, Choi JB, Lee JH. Cortical changes after mental imagery training combined with electromyography-triggered electrical stimulation in patients with chronic stroke. Stroke. 2012;43(9):2506–9.
28. Mrachacz-Kersting N, Kristensen SR, Niazi IK, Farina D. Precise temporal association between cortical potentials evoked by motor imagination and afference induces cortical plasticity. J Physiol. 2012;590(7):1669–82.
29. Reynolds C, Osuagwu BA, Vuckovic A. Influence of motor imagination on cortical activation during functional electrical stimulation. Clin Neurophysiol. 2015;126(7):1360–9.
30. Wang Z, Chen L, Yi W, Gu B, Liu S, An X, et al. Enhancement of cortical activation for motor imagery

during BCI-FES training. Annu Int Conf IEEE Eng Med Biol Soc. 2018;2018:2527–30.

31. Jang SH, Seo YS. Effect of neuromuscular electrical stimulation training on the finger extensor muscles for the contralateral corticospinal tract in Normal subjects: a diffusion tensor tractography study. Front Hum Neurosci. 2018;12:432.

32. Mang CS, Clair JM, Collins DF. Neuromuscular electrical stimulation has a global effect on corticospinal excitability for leg muscles and a focused effect for hand muscles. Exp Brain Res. 2011;209(3):355–63.

33. Koski L, Mernar TJ, Dobkin BH. Immediate and long-term changes in corticomotor output in response to rehabilitation: correlation with functional improvements in chronic stroke. Neurorehabil Neural Repair. 2004;18(4):230–49.

34. Wei W, Bai L, Wang J, Dai R, Tong RK, Zhang Y, et al. A longitudinal study of hand motor recovery after sub-acute stroke: a study combined FMRI with diffusion tensor imaging. PLoS One. 2013;8(5):e64154.

35. Chen D, Yan T, Li G, Li F, Liang Q. Functional electrical stimulation based on a working pattern influences function of lower extremity in subjects with early stroke and effects on diffusion tensor imaging: a randomized controlled trial. Zhonghua Yi Xue Za Zhi. 2014;94(37):2886–92.

36. Sabut SK, Sikdar C, Kumar R, Mahadevappa M. Functional electrical stimulation of dorsiflexor muscle: effects on dorsiflexor strength, plantarflexor spasticity, and motor recovery in stroke patients. NeuroRehabilitation. 2011;29(4):393–400.

37. Yang YR, Mi PL, Huang SF, Chiu SL, Liu YC, Wang RY. Effects of neuromuscular electrical stimulation on gait performance in chronic stroke with inadequate ankle control - a randomized controlled trial. PLoS One. 2018;13(12):e0208609.

38. Sharif F, Ghulam S, Malik AN, Saeed Q. Effectiveness of functional electrical stimulation (FES) versus conventional electrical stimulation in gait rehabilitation of patients with stroke. J Coll Physicians Surg Pak. 2017;27(11):703–6.

39. Benecke R, Berthold A, Conrad B. Denervation activity in the EMG of patients with upper motor neuron lesions: time course, local distribution and pathogenetic aspects. J Neurol. 1983;230(3):143–51.

40. Pockett S, Figurov A. Long-term potentiation and depression in the ventral horn of rat spinal cord in vitro. Neuroreport. 1993;4(1):97–9.

41. Motta-Oishi AA, Magalhães FH, Mícolis de Azevedo F. Neuromuscular electrical stimulation for stroke rehabilitation: is spinal plasticity a possible mechanism associated with diminished spasticity? Med Hypotheses. 2013;81(5):784–8.

42. Gordon T, Amirjani N, Edwards DC, Chan KM. Brief post-surgical electrical stimulation accelerates axon regeneration and muscle reinnervation without affecting the functional measures in carpal tunnel syndrome patients. Exp Neurol. 2010;223(1):192–202.

43. Stowe AM, Hughes-Zahner L, Barnes VK, Herbelin LL, Schindler-Ivens SM, Quaney BM. A pilot study to measure upper extremity H-reflexes following neuromuscular electrical stimulation therapy after stroke. Neurosci Lett. 2013;535:1–6.

44. Bischoff C, Dengler R, Hopf H. EMG, NLG: electromyography, nerve conduction studies. 2nd ed. Stuttgart: Georg Thieme; 2008.

45. Mangold S, Schuster C, Keller T, Zimmermann-Schlatter A, Ettlin T. Motor training of upper extremity with functional electrical stimulation in early stroke rehabilitation. Neurorehabil Neural Repair. 2009;23(2):184–90.

46. Ahlborn P, Schachner M, Irintchev A. One hour electrical stimulation accelerates functional recovery after femoral nerve repair. Exp Neurol. 2007;208(1):137–44.

47. Wong JN, Olson JL, Morhart MJ, Chan KM. Electrical stimulation enhances sensory recovery: a randomized controlled trial. Ann Neurol. 2015;77(6):996–1006.

48. Willand MP, Holmes M, Bain JR, de Bruin H, Fahnestock M. Sensory nerve cross-anastomosis and electrical muscle stimulation synergistically enhance functional recovery of chronically denervated muscle. Plast Reconstr Surg. 2014;134(5):736e–45e.

49. Balog BM, Deng K, Labhasetwar V, Jones KJ, Damaser MS. Electrical stimulation for neuroregeneration in urology: a new therapeutic paradigm. Curr Opin Urol. 2019;29(4):458–65.

50. Al-Majed AA, Neumann CM, Brushart TM, Gordon T. Brief electrical stimulation promotes the speed and accuracy of motor axonal regeneration. J Neurosci. 2000;20(7):2602–8.

51. Al-Majed AA, Brushart TM, Gordon T. Electrical stimulation accelerates and increases expression of BDNF and trkB mRNA in regenerating rat femoral motoneurons. Eur J Neurosci. 2000;12(12):4381–90.

52. Geremia NM, Gordon T, Brushart TM, Al-Majed AA, Verge VM. Electrical stimulation promotes sensory neuron regeneration and growth-associated gene expression. Exp Neurol. 2007;205(2):347–59.

53. Kim IS, Song YM, Cho TH, Pan H, Lee TH, Kim SJ, et al. Biphasic electrical targeting plays a significant role in Schwann cell activation. Tissue Eng Part A. 2011;17(9–10):1327–40.

54. Wan L, Xia R, Ding W. Short-term low-frequency electrical stimulation enhanced remyelination of injured peripheral nerves by inducing the promyelination effect of brain-derived neurotrophic factor on Schwann cell polarization. J Neurosci Res. 2010;88(12):2578–87.

# Role of Electrical Parameters in Functional Electrical Stimulation

**4**

Winfried Mayr

## 4.1 Introduction

Functional electrical stimulation (FES) is a powerful tool in the hands of capable therapists, but by far underrepresented in clinical use yet, far beneath exploiting the evident opportunities. On the one hand the necessary technical and physiological basic education is not considered enough in curricula for neurorehabilitation professionals, which would be crucial for building up confidence for safe and effective application. On the other hand, the vast multiplicity of positive, negative and sometimes contradictory application reports in scientific literature, public media and even in manufacturers' documents can provoke uncertainty and doubts, or else, exaggerated expectations and disappointment. A main goal of this chapter is to support a low-threshold entry in the use of stimulation equipment and guide towards qualified selection and alignment of electrical parameters for useful, effective and safe therapeutic intervention.

▶ Functional electrical stimulation (FES) is a powerful and versatile tool for rehabilitation, provided that adequate basic understanding of physiological mechanisms, capabilities and limits, as well as principles of application safety are given.

W. Mayr (✉)
Medical University of Vienna, Vienna, Austria
e-mail: winfried.mayr@meduniwien.ac.at

### 4.1.1 Selection and Evaluation of Stimulators

Stimulators are available in numerous variations and in vastly different cost segments. Stimulators offered as certified medical products are usually more expensive as they undergo strict and complex approval procedures, and need to comply with mandatory quality management processes in production and sales, which are associated with increased internal costs and fee-based monitoring by governmental authorities. These are the tools of choice for clinical practice for ensuring best possible patient safety and scientifically validated efficacy. Unfortunately, costs are often an impregnable obstacle for availability for patients, in case health insurance refuses to cover costs and devices are not affordable for purchase at their own expense.

The market segment "sports and fitness" offers rather similar devices with comparable technical specifications but for substantially lower prices, due to sparing costs for requirements of medical product regulations. Regarding applicability, a distinction is often difficult. FES-supported neuromuscular training is a topic of interest in neurorehabilitation as well as in sports. Finally, therapeutic responsibility and legal standards are to be weighted as decisive factors for the choice of appropriate devices. Additionally, there is a third, hardly controllable source for stimulators: internet shops. Unvalidated promises and low prices can appear attractive, but product and documentation quality can turn out to be questionable, unfiltered recommendations and unverified technical properties can even get health-endangering. Anyhow, stimulation technology should only be applied under competent medical advice to ensure safe and effective conditions.

### 4.1.2 What Really Matters

Despite all diversity of offered devices, stimulators remain pulse sources that interact with an organism via various electrode configurations, generally non-invasive with electrodes attached to the intact skin surface, in special applications invasive via implanted electrodes.

## 4.2 Monophasic/Biphasic Pulses/DC Component

Even though the marked offers stimulators with alternative voltage or current output waveforms, the vast majority relies on monophasic or biphasic rectangular pulses delivered in various pulse trains via bipolar electrode configurations. Therefore, we focus on such pulse forms and discuss how they interact with the organism. Further, we will discuss, how we can systematically influence this interaction, what limits we face and how far safety-relevant aspects need to be considered.

▶ Essential requirement: charge balance!

For the classical monophasic rectangular pulses there are three basic parameters that can be varied: pulse amplitude, pulse width and pulse frequency respectively the associated period between the leading edges of subsequent pulses. In the meantime, the majority of stimulators relies on biphasic rectangular pulses, where immediately after a monophasic pulse (first phase) an equal pulse of opposite polarity (second phase) follows. Adjustable parameters are the same, only pulse width becomes a pulse phase width, which is to be defined for positive

and negative phase. Usually, both pulse phases are equal, but occasionally there are reasons for using asymmetric ones (Fig. 4.1).

### 4.2.1 Monophasic and Biphasic Pulse Forms and Parameter Definitions for Nerve and Muscle Stimulation

It is a matter of decisive relevance to—except for a few special applications, which have to be handled with great care—avoid DC components in stimulation wave forms. This can be ensured by appropriate design of the output stage of the stimulator electronics and is usually considered by the device manufacturers. Still, we can find even certified medical devices on the market, that have a potentially critical DC component in their output pattern. Therefore, it remains important to carefully check for this feature whenever purchase, recommendations or prescriptions are undertaken. Charge balance without DC component is reliably ensured, if each stimulus, shifting a certain amount of electrical charge across the electrode contact into an organism, is followed by a recharge pulse of opposite polarity with a compensatory backflow of an equal amount of charge. A simple, safe and cost-effective solution is insertion of a capacitor in the output lead between stimulator output stage and electrode connector. A capacitor is a passive component that blocks DC and forces continuous charge balance of traversing alternating currents, even if the shape is complex like in variable sequences of stimuli.

In symmetric biphasic rectangular stimuli, the two subsequently delivered pulse phases of opposite polarity directly compensate residual charge to zero. The influence of an inserted coupling capacitor on pulse shape is minimal. In case of monophasic stimuli capacitive coupling leads to a strong deformation of the wave form, as every pulse is followed by an asymmetric forced recharge phase, usually a spike with exponential decay with dependence on the given electrode tissue impedance—safe in the application, but with some disadvantages regarding control characteristics and efficiency of stimulation, in com-

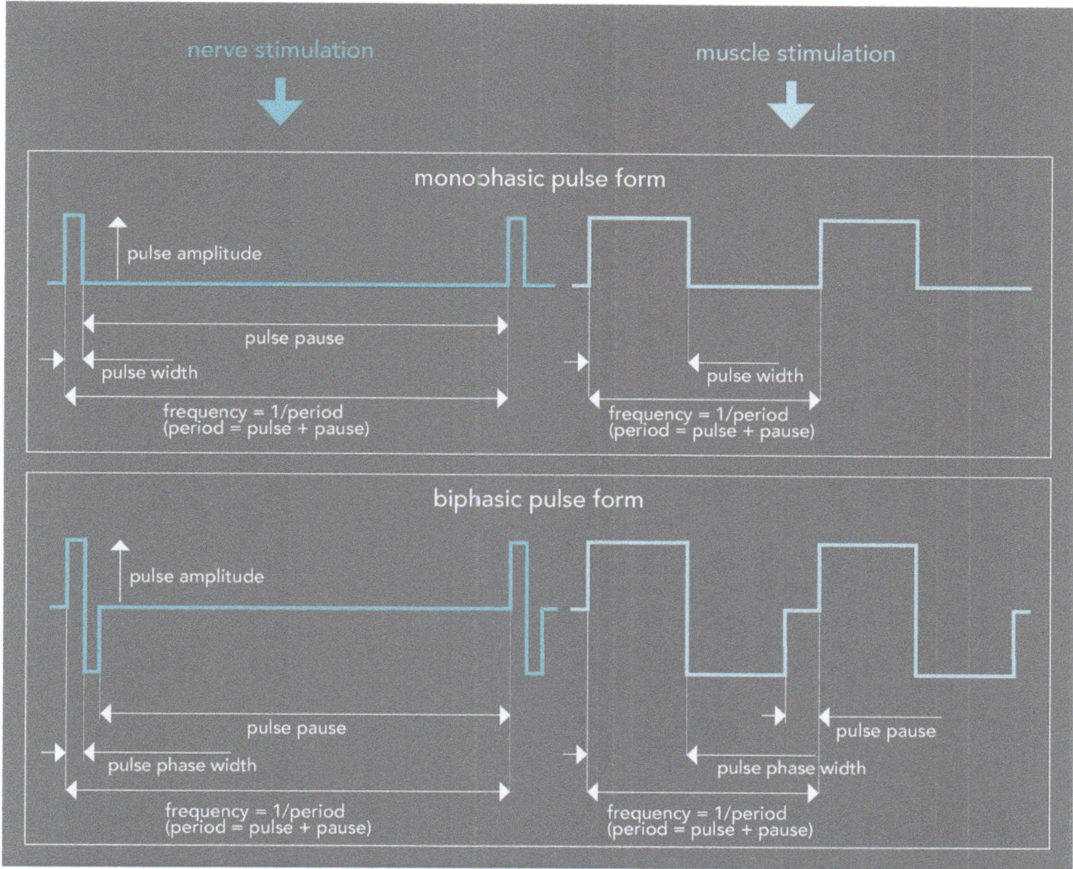


**Fig. 4.1** Monophasic and biphasic pulse forms and parameter definitions for nerve and muscle stimulation

parison to symmetric biphasic stimuli. As DC-decoupled monophasic stimuli are often named "biphasic" in the technical device specifications it is important to specially scrutinize this essential feature, to judge on suitability of an electrical stimulator.

▶ **Note** Caution: DC or "hidden" DC component in a pulse pattern!

An alternative to forced DC-decoupling with capacitors is active control of flow and backflow of electrical charge within a biphasic stimulus via electronic provisions for continuously maintaining charge balance. Monophasic stimuli delivered without DC-decoupling are always associated with a DC-component which varies with adjustment of pulse parameters (Fig. 4.2.).

## 4.3   Monopolar/Bipolar Electrode Configurations

A potential source of misunderstanding is the difference between application of "mono- or biphasic stimuli" and "mono- or bipolar stimulation." The latter relates to an electrode configuration, which is the first to be optimized for an application setup. The decision on the suitable pulse form and allocation of anode and cathode are of high importance.

A bipolar electrode configuration of two identical electrodes, placed over an anatomical target area, is the classical and most common approach. The locally concentrated electrical impulse field elicits action potentials in sensory and motor neurons as soon as the specific threshold intensity is exceeded. In case of peripheral denerva-

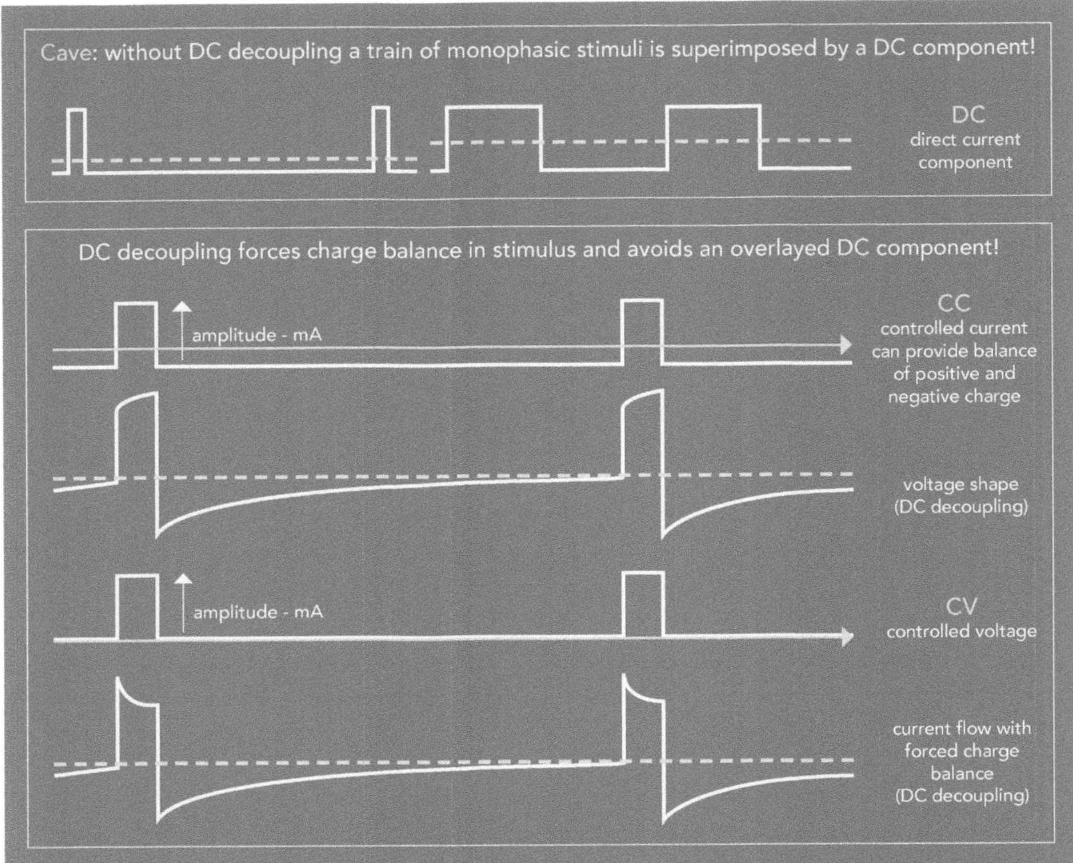


**Fig. 4.2** Monophasic pulse forms undergo some deformation, when delivered through safety-relevant DC-decoupling means, usually capacitors in the output lines, differently for controlled current (CC) or controlled voltage (CV) modes. DC-decoupling respectively charge balance is given, if the area below the trace of the positive pulse phase is exactly counterbalanced by the one enclosed by the negative phase, in relation to the zero line

tion, and only in this condition, appropriate stimuli can also elicit action potentials directly on muscle fibres. Usually this is the arrangement of choice for smooth and efficient activation of neurons or muscle fibres under and in-between the electrodes.

For application of monophasic stimuli, we observe a significantly lower threshold for neural structures close to the cathodic electrode in comparison to the anodic one. If biphasic stimuli are applied, we have the lowest threshold in neurons close to the anode of the first pulse phase ("anode first" polarity).

> **Note** For monophasic stimuli nerve structures close to the cathode respond at a significantly lower threshold than structures near the anode.
>
> For biphasic stimuli this polarity rule reverses with reference to the first pulse phase: the lower threshold appears near the anodic electrode ("anode first").

For selective activation of a locally restricted area a monopolar electrode arrangement can be the best choice. This can be necessary for diagnostic tests as well as for therapeutic intervention, when small target areas should be activated without co-activating anatomically adjacent structures. Examples are local denervation with intact sensory-motor nerve structures around, local hypersensitivity, selective activation of agonist and antagonistic in the treatment of muscles imbalances, or for avoiding electrical field induction in implants or wounds close to therapeutic targets. Preferential electrode arrangements rely on a smaller active cathode in combination with a larger anodic reference. A pronounced depth effect can be accomplished, when the reference electrode is placed anatomically opposite to the active cathode, e.g., when placing electrodes at the trunk or the extremities. Regarding polarity the same rules apply as for bipolar electrode arrangements.

> **Conclusion**
> The best possible selectivity in activating nerve structures can be accomplished using a small size active electrode, which is chosen as cathode for monopolar stimuli or as anode of the first phase of a biphasic stimulus.

## 4.4 Controlled Current (CC)/Controlled Voltage (CV) Stimulus Delivery

A further important device-related question is the electronic control mode of the stimulation output. It can either be based on controlled current (CC) or controlled voltage (CV) . CC means that the desired pulse shape is exactly followed by the current flow, whereas the voltage appears deformed under influence of the electrical resistance properties at the electrode/tissue interfaces and the traversed tissue in the current path (load impedance). CV delivers an exact voltage shape, whereas the current is adapting to the generally non-linear impedance properties (Fig. 4.2).

Basically, the effect of both operation modes is equal if the transverse resistance of the electrode to skin interface and the anatomical contour in the application area remain unaltered during stimulus delivery.

But there is an important safety aspect to be considered, when long-duration pulses with high charge transfer per pulse are applied for direct stimulation of denervated muscles, or in nerve stimulation with very small electrodes: especially in CC a locally excessive current density may occur, which, in a worst case, can lead to irreversible electrochemical processes in the electrode-skin interface with some risk of tissue damage.

In case the load impedance of a stimulator output varies during stimulus delivery, CC mode forces unchanged current flow in the default shape by continuous re-adjustment of the driving voltage source. This provides the advantage that the induced electrical field in the tissue interaction with nerves and muscles remains more or less unaltered. At the same time a risk emerges if worsening of the electrode to skin resistance properties occurs, for example, by partial contact loss of self-adhesive hydrogel electrodes or drying out of contact media between conductive rubber electrodes and skin surface. In such case CC mode ensures unaltered current delivery and forces flow of the entire current through an eventually significantly reduced contact area, with the consequence of a potential risk of electrochemical skin damage. Also, excessive local current density can occur at spots of locally increased mechanical contact pressure like at electrode edges under tension of elastic fixation means. This needs special attention in particular in conjunction with direct stimulation of denervated muscles.

Similar changes of contact properties are far less critical in CV mode, as an increase of load impedance results in concurrent reduction of current. The user notices a decline in stimulation response, but risks of skin damage are neglectable.

Most, but not all the commercially available stimulators rely on CC mode. Preference for choosing CC or CV finally depends on application scenarios and a critical assessment of functional expectations versus tolerable risks.

## 4.5    Role of the Parameter's Amplitude and Pulse Width

Most stimulators offer possibilities for pre-adjustment of pulse width and frequency within a certain range, whereas variation of amplitude is freely variable for intensity adjustments in test procedures and therapeutic application. Occasionally, devices rely on constant pre-adjusted amplitude and modulation of pulse width for control of intensity. For nerve respectively neuromuscular stimulation useful amplitude ranges cover 0–120 mA or 0–120 V, a pulse width range between 100 µs and 1 ms, both related to a pulse phase, and a frequency range between 1 and 120 Hz.

The role of intensity adjustment is a variation of recruitment of neurons, usually situated in bundled form in a neural structure. Regardless of using amplitude or pulse width for recruitment modulation there is always a low-intensity range without any neuron activation, meaning that no action potentials are elicited. Gradual increase first results in reaching a sensory threshold, at least if sensory perception is intact, and with further increase a motor threshold with first signs of muscle activation. With further growing intensity increasing sensory perception and enforced muscle contraction are induced. High intensity saturates the responses and can even lead to blocking phenomena that suppress propagation of action potentials in neurons (Fig. 4.3).

If and at what intensity an action potential is elicited in a neuron depends on the distance to the electrodes respectively the electrical field configuration acting on the neuron, and the diameter of the neuron. The larger a neuron is, the lower is the threshold for an action potential. This has multiple implications for the impact electrical stimulation can have on neural functions.

The largest neurons, with diameters up to 20 µm, are "proprioceptive afferents," which are responsible for feedback on body image, muscle lengths and joint angles. So-called "cutaneous afferents," associated with skin sensor information, have a size spectrum from approximately 14 µm down to 5 µm. Further there is a pool of even smaller fibres in the size range around 1 µm which are mainly related to deep pain feedback.

These afferent sensory neurons proceed in bundles, together with efferent motor fibres, with their diameter range between 18 and 8 µm. Larger

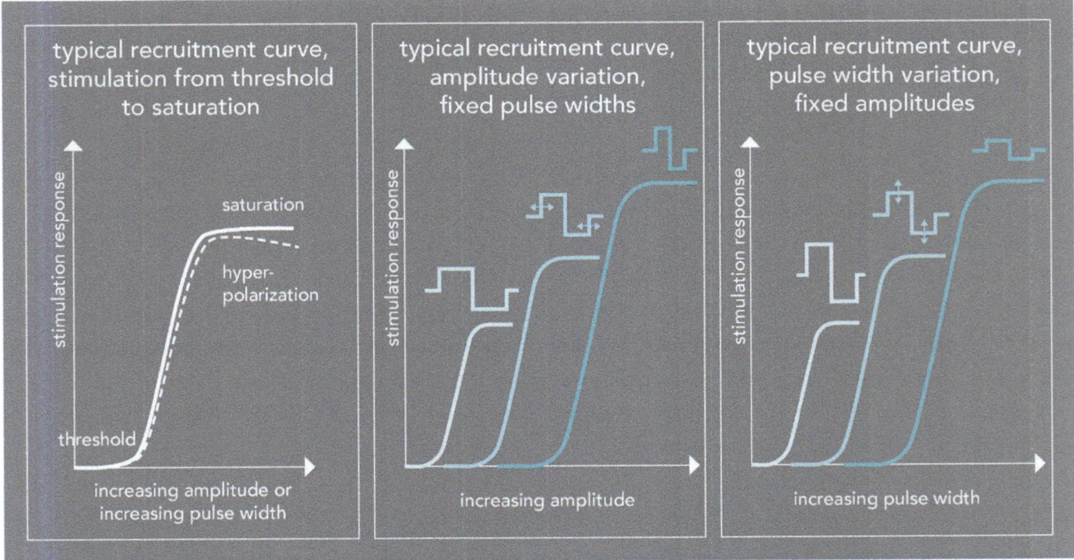


**Fig. 4.3** An increase of stimulation intensity, beginning with "0" leads first to reaching of a threshold, followed by a linear increase of recruitment of nerve or muscle fibres until a saturation plateau is reached and most sensitive fibres can even get hyperpolarised with block of propagation of action potentials. Recruitment can be controlled by either modulating amplitude or pulse width

motor neurons control groups of fast and strong contracting, but fast fatiguing muscle fibres (Type 2, glycolytic metabolism), smaller ones activate fatigue resistent but slower and weaker muscle fibres (Type 1, aerobic metabolism). The combination of a motor neuron cell, situated as integral part in spinal interneuron networks, the associated peripheral motor neuron, its peripheral branching and all connected muscle fibres are called a "motor unit" (MU). In relation to conduction speed, contraction speed and endurance MUs are often classified as "fast" versus "fatigue resistant." Physiological recruitment of MUs relies predominantly on fatigue-resistant ones and co-recruits fast ones only for special demands in force and movement speed (Henneman principle, natural recruitment).

In the size spectrum of neurons, we also find smaller efferent neurons, which interact with muscle spindles, and finally, with diameters below 1 µm, neurons related to the autonomous nerve system and reacting only to electrical stimuli of very high intensity.

Another important consideration is the fact that the number of sensory neurons in a mixed nerve is far higher than that of motor neurons. For the entire nerve supply of the upper extremity with all emerging spinal nerve roots the relation is 90–10%; in anatomical branches this relation can vary considerably.

In summary, we need to be aware of limitations in selectivity of reaching specific or even single neurons by electrical stimulation and must scrutinize interpretation of physiological responses. We need to respect that due to the size depending excitation threshold of nerve fibres fast, rapidly fatiguing MUs are primarily recruited at low stimulation intensities and fatigue-resistant MUs can only be co-recruited with growing stimulus strength ("inverse recruitment" in comparison to natural recruitment). On the other hand, this should not discourage us from taking advantage of the many positive opportunities FES is offering. With some background knowledge and smart handling of electrodes, parameters and intervention strategies, superb therapeutic and functional results can be accomplished.

▶ **Note** In neuromuscular electrical stimulation with growing intensity first only fast, rapidly fatiguing motor units are activated, at higher intensities fatigue-resistant MUs are co-recruited—inverse recruitment.

## 4.6 Role of the Parameter Frequency

A fundamentally different role than amplitude and pulse width, which control fibre recruitment, has the parameter frequency, or to be more precise, two quite different roles. On one hand, if afferent sensory nerve stimulation is addressed, frequency has a strong influence on spinal and supraspinal interneuron processing with its essential involvement in movement control as well as sensory perception. On the other hand, in neuromuscular electrical stimulation, frequency has strong influence in contraction dynamics and fatigue behaviour of the activated muscles.

As the recruitment order with increasing intensity starts with selectively activating the largest neurons at lowest threshold, initially only large sensory neurons are reached. This offers effective opportunities for reducing neuropathic pain, modifying spasticity and augment movement functions. For these applications, meticulous assessment of altered neural functions and individually optimized intensity and frequency values and appropriate electrode setups need to be configured.

If stimulation intensity is increased beyond the motor threshold, obvious responses are muscular contractions, though in the background sensory neurons are unavoidably co-activated at the same time. This can add positive, disturbing, or unobtrusive side effects, that may require some attention. For example, in patients with spinal cord injury in some cases neuromuscular FES training can be accompanied by undesirable increase of spasticity, whereas in other patients the same neuromuscular FES is accompanied by even a reduction of spasticity. But, with individual optimization of the application protocol it is possible to find satisfactory solutions in the majority of cases.

For neuromuscular FES the role of frequency is twofold:

1. The co-activation of afferent (sensory) neurons has a frequency-dependent influence on central interneuron processing.
2. The frequency of motor neuron activation strongly influences biomechanical and metabolic properties in the activated muscle.

For neuromuscular training or neuromuscular activation of paralyzed or weakened musculature so-called phasic stimulation patterns are applied, meaning that contraction is induced for limited time intervals followed by inactivation pauses. Consequently, additional parameters, as well as intensity and frequency, become relevant: activation and pause intervals (on/off time) and in general also ramp times for on-off-transitions, which make onset of muscle contractions and muscle deactivation smoother and more comfortable. Appropriate selection of the parameter sets for muscle building and maintenance has decisive influence on effectiveness of the training.

Specific parameter sets and application management are required for direct muscle stimulation that have lost their nerve supply. Differences to neuromuscular FES are addressed later in Sect. 4.7.

### 4.6.1  Application of Single Stimuli

Single stimuli or repetitive stimuli delivered with very slow repetition rate play an important role in neuromuscular testing procedures, e.g., recruitment threshold detection, but can also have relevance for fostering muscular perfusion or rebuilding of excitability of denervated muscle fibres.

A typically useful test frequency is 1 Hz, which is slow enough to rule out influence of most neurophysiological post-activation activities. It is useful for finding sensory and motor thresholds, as for example needed for proper adjustment of intensity for tonic afferent nerve stimulation. Motor threshold and saturation intensity define the control range for neuromuscular or muscle stimulation, both can be comfortably determined with slowly repeated single stimuli and intensity variation. Further, slowly repeated single stimuli are useful for tests on innervation respectively denervation status of muscles and excitability of denervated muscle fibres.

There is one aspect that needs some attention: single stimuli usually do not cause sensible discomfort even if delivered with very high intensity, but as soon as trains of stimuli with usual application frequencies are delivered discomfort is perceived at much lower intensity levels. Therefore, if sensory perception is intact it is not possible to determine a tolerable intensity maximum with single stimuli. It is strongly recommended to start with low intensity and determine the individual discomfort threshold with the intended application parameter set and slowly increased intensity.

### 4.6.2  Application of Low Frequencies

Pulse frequencies below 10 Hz are often applied for a warmup period ahead to neuromuscular FES training, in so-called "active relaxation" pauses between contractions or in a terminal active regeneration periods after exercise. Stimulation evokes no fused muscle contraction, but a shaking movement that can enhance muscle perfusion and support washout of metabolites.

### 4.6.3  Frequencies Eliciting Fused Contractions

Shortening the time between subsequent stimuli, which is equal to increasing frequency, conflates muscle responses from single twitches to unsteady compound "shaking contractions." With further increased frequency to a so-called "fusion frequency" a burst of stimuli induces a smooth tetanic contraction. Further growing frequency leads to gain in contraction force and onset speed, but at the same time rapid muscular fatigue phenomena, which cause problems in functional applications and can lead to metabolic overuse and even muscle damage (Fig. 4.4).

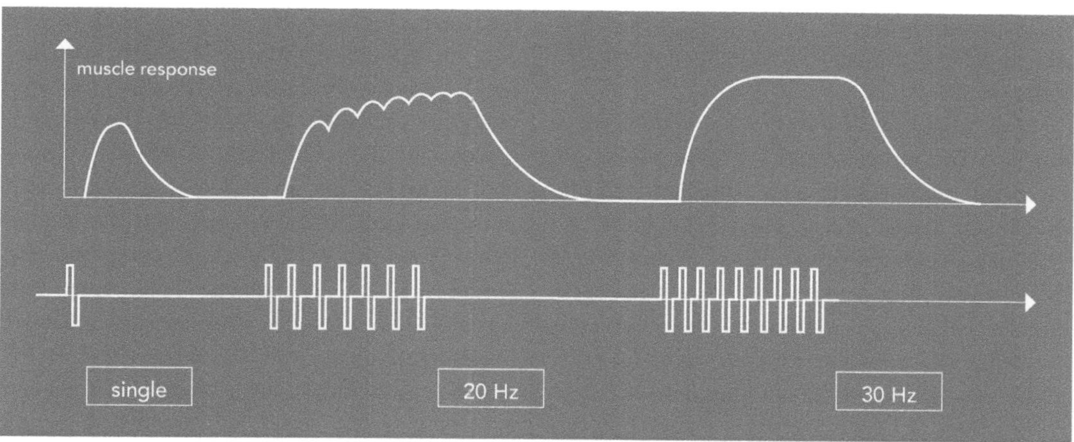


**Fig. 4.4** The muscle response to one stimulus is a compound twitch of all recruited muscle fibres. Growing repetition rate of stimuli results in merging twitches to unsteady ("shaking") and beyond "fusion frequency" tetanic contractions. The displayed curves stand for isometric contractions against a firm resistance

For most applications, a cautious start of training is recommended. Frequency should be selected for just starting to fuse in contraction, eventually with a residual minimal unsteadiness. Fusion frequency is not a sharp absolute value and influenced by metabolic factors in the muscle. Subjective perception of contraction smoothness usually starts in the range of 25–30 Hz and gets more pronounced with further increase. The recommendation of a cautious start of training also relates to strength and duration of contractions, relaxation pauses between contractions and strict avoidance of excessive fatigue. In the further course, length of training sessions, stimulation intensity, frequency and on-off timing can be adapted to a more intense training load in order to build muscles and gain in force and endurance.

## 4.7 Special Case FES of Denervated Muscles

Maintenance of denervated muscles is less for immediate functional restoration but rather for longer term improvements in quality of life and preserving health of utmost importance. Effective validated methods and instrumentation have not been available till the recent past, as outcome from the European R & D project RISE [1, 2]. The applicable parameters and intervention protocols differ substantially from those for neuromuscular muscle training, mainly due to differences in the electrically excitable membrane properties of nerve and muscle cells: action potentials travel along motor neurons with 50–100 m/s, whereas along healthy muscle fibres with only 2–5 m/s, in atrophied and degenerated muscle fibres far slower. This refers directly to suitable pulse parameters for eliciting action potentials on the respective membranes, for neurons pulses with a phase width of 100–1000 µs (0.1 to bis 1 ms) are most efficient. Longer pulses do not increase fibre recruitment in relation to intensity but lead to growing charge transfer across the electrode-tissue interface with unnecessary increase of safety risks. In direct comparison, even completely intact and well trained denervated muscles are not excitable with pulses below 15–20 ms per phase. With growing atrophy respectively, after longer denervation, degeneration of muscles the required pulse phase length increases towards 250 ms, in extreme case up to even 500 ms. It is strongly recommended to start stimulation of denervated muscles as early as possible after denervation on a regular basis, which is of vital importance for best possible maintenance of muscle in quantity and function. If excitability is high enough for shortest pulse length and inter-pulse pauses stimulation bursts with 25–30 Hz can elicit fused tetanic contractions [3] which is in turn essential for efficient training and functional use. Analogous principles like for neuromuscular FES training remain applicable (Fig. 4.5).

Main objective of training is maintenance of muscles for an anticipated re-innervation or, provided regular long-term application, comprehensive tissue preservation [4], mainly for effective decubitus prophylaxis. If atrophy, in the first year after denervation, or muscle degeneration, as usually beginning in the second year, are progressing longer, a longer minimal pulse width gets necessary for eliciting muscle twitch contractions, which make fused tetanic contractions impossible [4, 6]. There is a feasible option to recondition excitability of muscle fibres and reach a reduction of the necessary minimal pulse duration to an extend that re-enables stimulation-induced fused contractions and tetanizing rebuilding of muscle mass, force, and endurance, at least in part (Fig. 4.6). But there are limitations, which can be minimized with an early start and consequent compliance: the longer disuse is persisting the longer rebuilding will last and the severer limitations in achievable results get.

As a specific requirement for FES of denervated muscles, specific adaptations of stimulation parameters for test procedures and therapy protocols are of vital importance. Primarily, rectangular biphasic long-duration pulses above 15 ms per phase are necessary. For testing of the degree of denervation in incompletely denervated muscles and neuromuscular activation of residual motor units also short duration pulses with phase length below 1 ms can get relevant as complementary modality. There are important alternative pulse forms, biphasic long ramp shaped (exponential) pulses with phase length above 80–100 ms, which feature elevation of thresholds for nerve activation above those for denervated muscle fibres, based on an effect called "accommodation" (Fig. 4.7). Accommodation means that the fast-reacting electrical properties of neurons maintain an equilibrium of diffusion currents, when exposed to slowly raising electrical field strength, whereas the same field conditions induce electrical discharge in the less sensitive membrane of denervated muscle fibre.

▶ **Note** Long ramp shaped pulses with a phase length above 80–100 ms open the opportunity for activating denervated muscle fibres without co-activating near sensory or motor neurons.

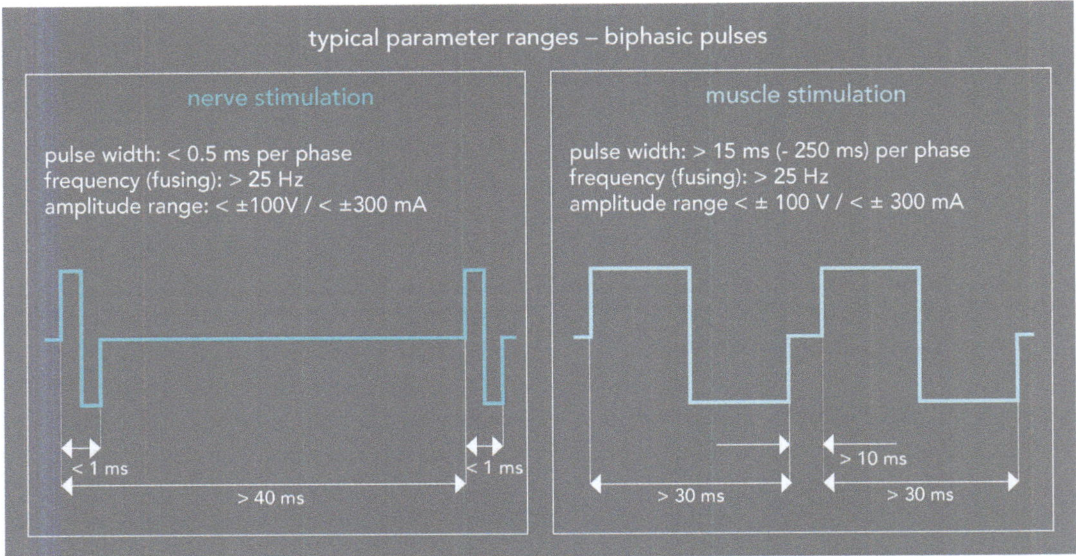



**Fig. 4.5** Parameter ranges for nerve and neuromuscular stimulation in comparison to those for direct stimulation of denervated muscles: the main difference is given in the necessary pulse width, with strong implication to training strategies and safety provisions

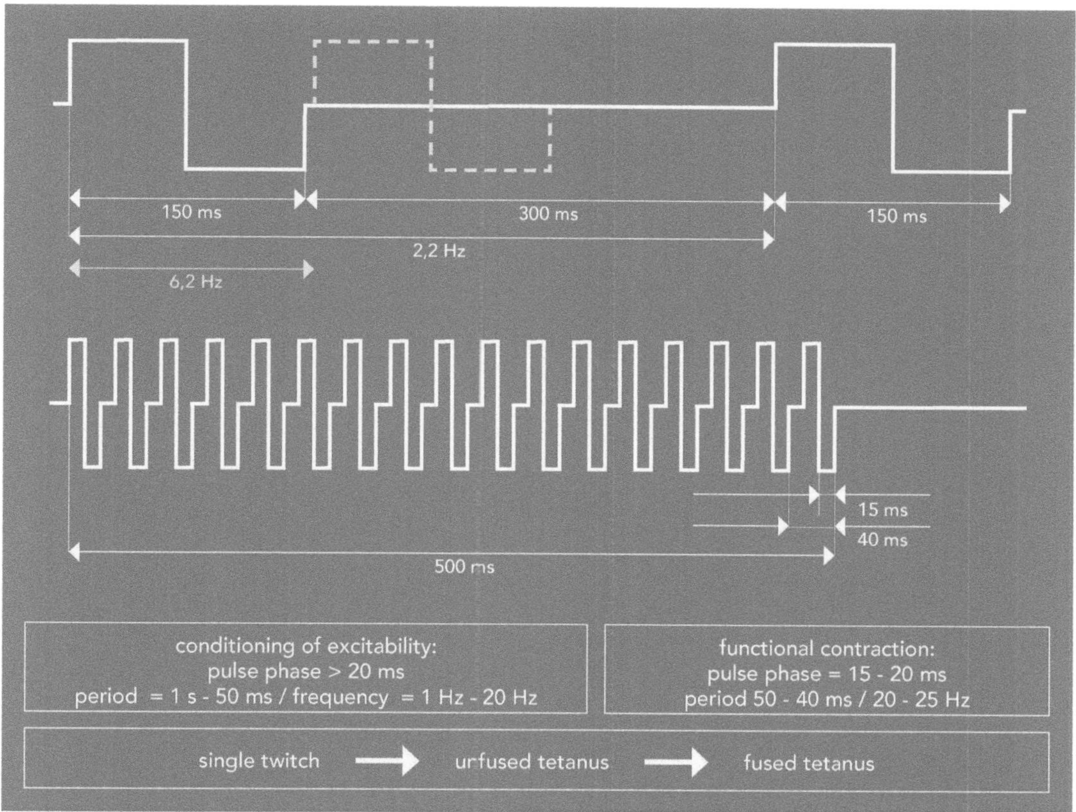


**Fig. 4.6** In electrical stimulation of denervated muscles it is challenging to accomplish fused tetanic muscle contractions, due to the required long stimulus duration. In dependence of inactivity time after denervation a prolonged period for rebuilding of muscle excitability, beginning with single twitch conditioning, is necessary

Ramp shaped pulses can also be applied with shorter phase duration, though accommodation effects can appear clearly reduced. Nevertheless, it is always worth trying if at least gradually reduced co-activation of sensory or motor neurons can be accomplished. Not to be underestimated: this pulse form can also reduce charge transfer per pulse, which is to some extend safety relevant (Fig. 4.8).

## 4.8 Electrode and Parameter Management for Testing and Treatment of Completely or in Part Denervated Muscles

The start of the first assessment should be as soon as possible after denervation, the earlier the better status of and the lower efforts for muscle maintenance will get. Electrode configuration should as far as possible cover the entire dermatome above the target muscle, as eliciting action potentials in each single muscle fibre are necessary for complete activation.

For the first test single pulses, or slow trains with 1 Hz, should be chosen for identifying intact MUs and estimating to what extend partly or complete denervation is given. If a considerable response appears, neuromuscular training of the still nerve supplied part can be considered with the goal of hypertrophy in innervated motor units and eventual promotion of reinnervation processes in other muscle parts.

In case the muscle is not reacting to short pulses, next tests with longer pulses should be undertaken, phase length chosen depending on the time since denervation, for acute cases in a range of 15–30 ms, for less recent cases gradually more, typically above 100 ms. Initially a maximal twitch contraction is to be searched by

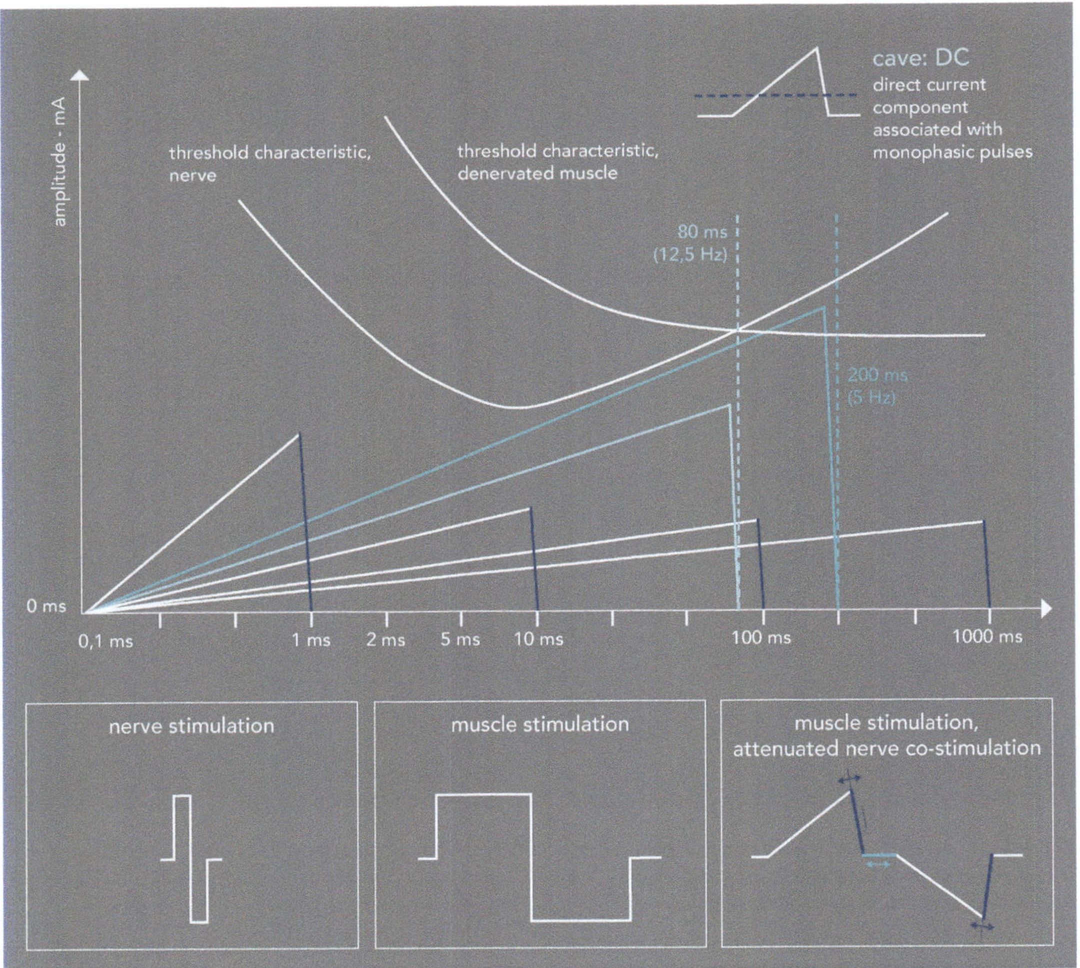


**Fig. 4.7** For testing and training of denervated muscles (completely or in part) short pulses for eventual residual MU activation, and long-duration rectangular and ramp shaped pulses for muscle fibre activation are needed. Ramp shaped pulse with phase lengths above 80–100 ms can provide an elevation of the threshold for neurons above threshold for denervated muscle fibres

increasing intensity and eventual lengthening of pulse width, next a stepwise reduction of pulse length is applied to find a threshold where a drop of reachable twitch strength occurs. For conditioning respectively training the shortest pulse width eliciting a substantial twitch is the best choice. For beginning therapy slow repetitive stimuli with contant intensity should be applied first for a period until visible weakening of responses is noticed. Later, based on regular follow-up tests, improvements in excitability and endurance should be noticeable, in time period dimensions of weeks.

As soon as excitability allows application of phase durations of 15–20 ms, a transition to tetanizing contractions and classical muscle building, but with special attendance to avoiding excessive fatigue and metabolic overload, can be considered [2, 5, 6].

If intact sensibility or disturbing co-activation of neighbouring innervated muscles limit the applicable stimulation intensity too much, ramp shaped long duration pulses can be considered as an alternative for the above outlined test and application procedures.

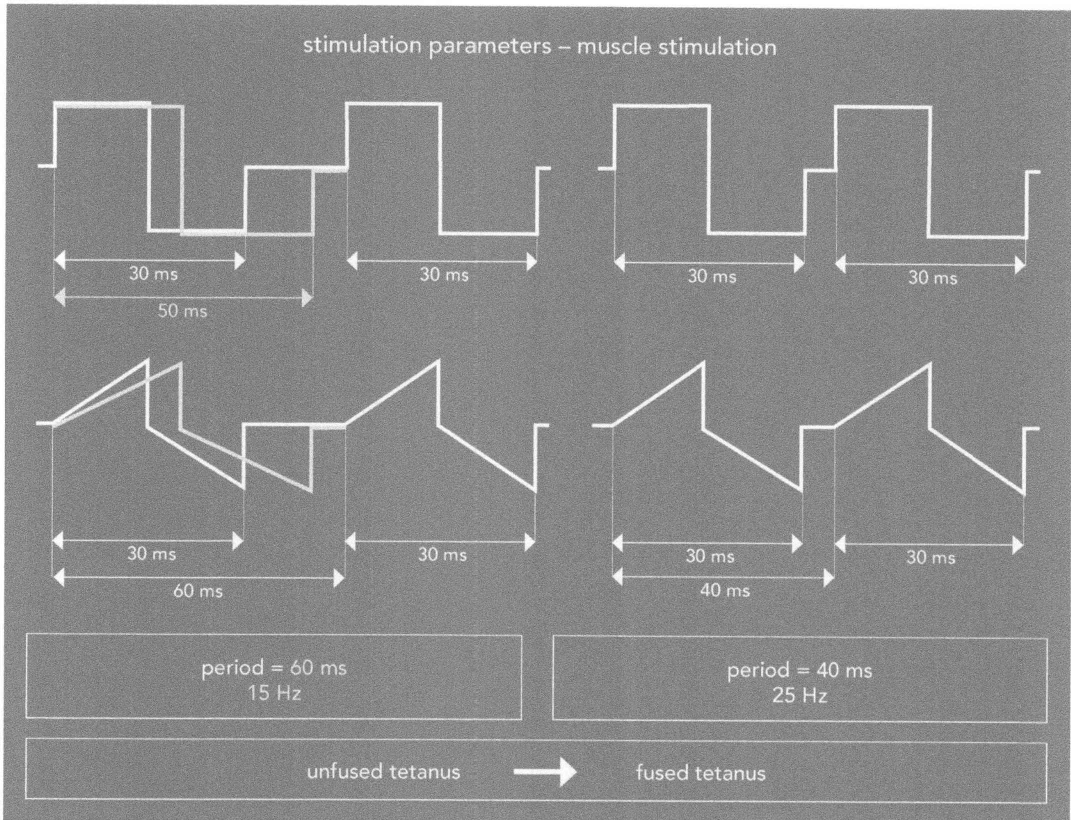


**Fig. 4.8** Ramp shaped pulses can provide advantages regarding reduction of coactivation of sensory and motor neurons in the same anatomical region. Charge transfer per pulse phase gets lower, associated with reduced risks of skin damage

# References


1. Kern H, Carraro U, Adami N, Biral D, Hofer C, Forstner C, Mödlin M, Vogelauer M, Pond A, Boncompagni S, Paolini C, Mayr W, Protasi F, Zampieri S. Home-based functional electrical stimulation rescues permanently denervated muscles in paraplegic patients with complete lower motor neuron lesion. Neurorehabil Neural Repair. 2010;24(8):709–21. [Epub ahead of print]
2. Gallasch E, Rafolt D, Kinz G, Fend M, Kern H, Mayr W. Evaluation of FES-induced knee joint moments in paraplegics with denervated muscles. Artif Organs. 2005;29(3):207–11.
3. Mayr W, Hofer C, Bijak M, Rafolt D, Unger E, Sauermann S, Lanmueller H, Kern H. Functional electrical stimulation (FES) of denervated muscles: exist-ing and prospective technological solutions. Basic Appl Myol. 2002;12:287.
4. Carraro U, Rossini K, Mayr W, Kern H. Muscle fiber regeneration in human permanent lower motoneuron denervation: relevance to safety and effectiveness of FES-training, which induces muscle recovery in SCI subjects. Artif Organs. 2005;29(3):187–91. PubMed PMID: 15725214
5. Kern H, Carraro U, Adami N, Hofer C, Loefler S, Vogelauer M, Mayr W, Rupp R, Zampieri S. One year of home-based daily FES in complete lower motor neuron paraplegia: recovery of tetanic contractility drives the structural improvements of denervated muscle. Neurol Res. 2010;32(1):5–12.
6. Kern H, Hofer C, Strohhofer M, Mayr W, Richter W, Stöhr H. Standing up with denervated muscles in humans using functional electrical stimulation. Artif Organs. 1999;23(5):447–52.

Klemens Fheodoroff

## 5.1 Goal Setting Theory—Essentials

Goals and goal setting have become standard interventions in neurorehabilitation [1]. Goals affect the rehabilitation process on several levels, both for service recipients (patients) and for service providers (therapists). In various reviews, it has been demonstrated that goal setting and goal agreements positively affect self-efficacy, health-related quality of life and the emotional state. Furthermore, goal agreements lead to a feeling of being actively involved in the rehabilitation process [2, 3].

Goals strengthen the work relationship between cooperating therapists and their patients, ensure that progresses achieved are measurable, help patients cope with anxiety and promote insight into and acceptance of limited restitution if necessary [4, 5]. Already in 2009, Wade postulated that goal setting should be a core competency of any member in a rehabilitation team [6].

### 5.1.1 Goal Sources and Comprehensibility of Goals

Goals can be set by the affected individuals themselves or by their significant others. They can be suggested by therapists and physicians or participatively set and agreed within a shared decision-making approach. All three of these methods seem to be equally effective [7]. Research has shown that, contrary to the self-determination theory, goals chosen by the patients themselves are not superior in enhancing the patients' performance than goals set by experts or set participatively [8]. If the reasoning behind expert goals is understandable and rational for the affected individuals, patients are ready to take necessary efforts to reach difficult goals as long as these goals do not interfere with the self-concept of the individual or the self-concept of the team [9, 10]. Consequently, *specificity of goals* positively correlates with the degree of goal commitment [11]. Understandable and straightforward goals are more likely to be followed than vague, unspecific goals. Mastery-type goals (*"to achieve something"*) stimulate self-efficacy and the search for solutions more than avoidance-type goals (*"to avoid something"*) both, for learning goals (*"develop strategies"*) and for performance goals (*"become better"*) [12].

▶ Goals that are incomprehensible to the affected persons cannot be pursued by them. Therefore, comprehensibility of goals to the individuals/significant others is a key factor for success.

To assess goal comprehensibility, the acronyms SMART and RUMBA have proven to be useful.

K. Fheodoroff (✉)
Gailtal Klinik Hermagor, Hermagor, Austria
e-mail: klemens.fheodoroff@kabeg.at


T. Schick (ed.), *Functional Electrical Stimulation in Neurorehabilitation*,
https://doi.org/10.1007/978-3-030-90123-3_5

**Table 5.1** Goal quality indicators: the RUMBA rule

| letter | main term | comment |
| --- | --- | --- |
| R | relevant | Relevant to the problem and meaningful for the affected person. |
| U | understandable | The goal is phrased in a comprehensible way. |
| M | measurable | The starting level and the final result can be measured easily with high reliability and validity. |
| B | behaviourable | The goal can be achieved through proactive behaviour. |
| A | achievable | The goal is achievable within existing barriers/resources. |

The term SMART has been derived from project management [13] but has since been used in many other areas, such as employee management and in rehabilitation [14]. The acronym stands for:

S: Specific
M: Measurable
A: Achievable
R: Relevant
T: Timed (typically refers to the current treatment cycle)

One example for a SMART goal is: "(To be able to) open/close/hold a bottle with the paretic hand—within 14 days." (For more examples see Table 5.2.)

*The* RUMBA rule additionally *emphasises* the comprehensibility of goals, also for lay persons [15] (Table 5.1).

Especially in the early stages of a disease, patients long to *"become the same person as before"* or to *"be able to walk normally again."* In goal setting theory, such goals are labelled as *"stretch goals."* Stretch goals are (on purpose or unintentionally) set at a very high level—practically out of reach with current resources. From the practitioner's point of view, it is useful to classify such stretch goals as *"very important to the patient, but very difficult/challenging from the experts view to be reached with current resources."* This allows introducing milestone goals that are more likely to be reached within given timeframes and resources. Stretch goals should always be accompanied by goals such as *"(being able to) realize internal barriers (i.e., body function impairments) for individual task performance."*

## 5.1.2 Self-Evaluation, Self-Efficacy, Self-Management and Goals

Goals that are deemed unimportant by the affected person will consequently not be pursued [16]. Therefore, goals should be meaningful and challenging. The following components were found to increase goal commitment in general and in patients in particular:

- **Significance** (= factors that make goal attainment important and desirable).
- **Achievability** (= factors that make a person confident that the goal can be attained with the available resources).
- **Complexity** of goals (= the difficulty to develop strategies for goal attainment).
- **Self-efficacy** (= one's confidence that one can do what is required to perform a given task / an activity and to reach a goal) [8, 17, 18].

The degree of self-efficacy particularly influences whether people stay committed to a course of action, especially when difficulties and setbacks occur. The optimum level of self-efficacy is slightly above the actual ability; if this is the case, people are most readily prepared to take on tasks and gain experience—in other words: to learn [18].

Furthermore, self-efficacy substantially influences self-regulation (= the ability to influence and control one's own feelings and moods through inner dialogue) as well as self-management [19, 20].

Self-management consists of four key processes [21]:

1. **Goal setting:** developing, prioritising, ranking, adopting, adapting or rejecting goals.
2. **Planning:** internal processes involved in preparing to pursue a goal.
3. **Striving/acting:** implementing measures to move toward or maintain a goal.
4. **Revision:** changing or disengaging from a goal.

### 5.1.3  Goals and Feedback

Feedback refers to the countless reactions (gestures, emotional vocal utterances, verbal or machine-supported feedback) that allow the person undergoing rehabilitation to draw conclusions about their current performance with regard to goal-directed behaviour. Feedback, hence, influences the learning process and/or the degree of goal attainment and also has affective consequences: People feel joy or disappointment depending on the feedback they receive on their performance—especially if said feedback is provided by accepted reference persons or experts. The mere fact that someone is observing the individual progress seems to reinforce performance [22].

Goals can be "achieved"—"partially achieved"—"not achieved" or "overachieved." Not all goals must be achieved. A "partially achieved" goal can justify the further need for treatment. Stretch goals (i.e., goals that can barely or not all be achieved within the given time frame or with the available resources) will frequently have to be evaluated as "not achieved."

However, evaluating a stretch goal as "not achieved" does not necessarily have to lead to disappointment and frustration but can contribute to accepting one's own limits and to letting go of unachievable goals [23–25].

## 5.2  International Classification of Functioning, Disability and Health (ICF)

In order to meet the complexity of neurological rehabilitation, a holistic perspective is needed that goes beyond purely medical (impairment-oriented) problem assessment. With the International Classification of Functioning, Disability and Health (ICF) [26], the World Health Organisation (WHO) has created a classification allowing to describe the influence of body function impairments (usually serving as internal barriers) as well as the influence of contextual factors (external barriers or facilitators) on capacity (what one can do under certain circumstances) and performance (what one does in his or her individual environment).

### 5.2.1  The Structure of ICF)

ICF) consists of two parts with two components each:

**Part 1:** Functioning and Disability with the two components: *Body Functions/Structures* and *Activities/Participation.*
**Part 2:** Contextual Factors with the two components: *Personal Factors* and *Environmental Factors.*

Alphanumeric codes are assigned to the individual elements to allow international comparison if used in different languages. The codes for body functions are indexed with the letter "b," the codes for body structures with the letter "s"; the codes for contextual factors with the letter "e" (for environmental factors); the codes for the component Activities/Participation with the letter "d" (for domains). If a construct is deemed to be an activity, the letter "d" is replaced by the letter

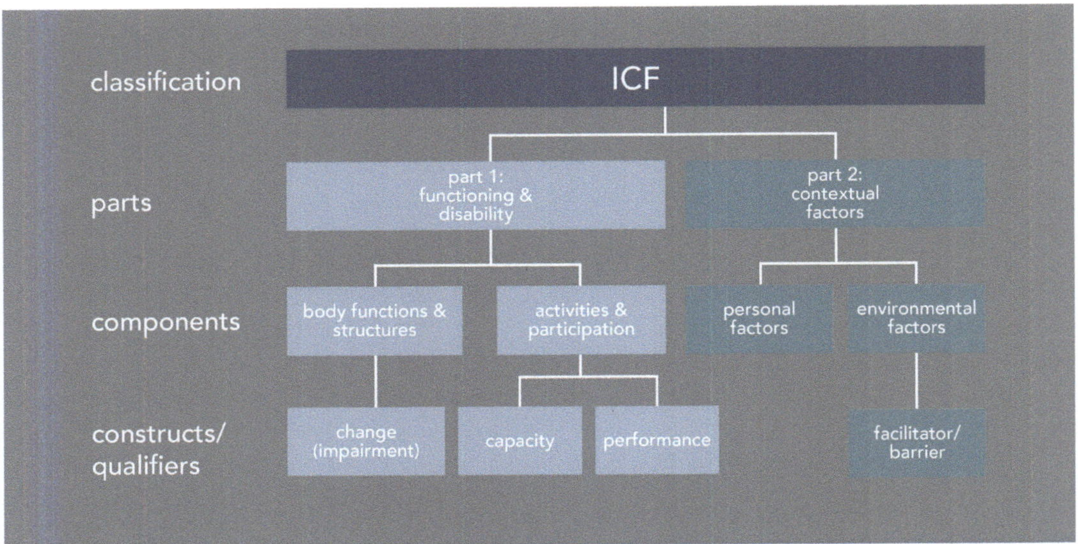



**Fig. 5.1** Structure of the ICF

"a" (activity); if a construct is classified as participation, the letter "d" is replaced by the letter "p" (participation) (Fig. 5.1).

In total, the classification consists of 1424 constructs structured hierarchically on up to four item levels. Depending on the clinical situation, an adequate level of detailing must be chosen. As a rule of thumb, the more severe the disability, the more general the construct can be chosen; the less severe, the more specific and detailed must the construct be to capture the level of disability. Thus, for a patient with severe paresis, the construct "d520 Caring for Body Parts" will sufficiently describe the situation and need for assistance/help, whereas for a Parkinson's patient with Parkinson's disease, the constructs: "d5203/d5204 Caring for Fingernails/Toenails" may still not be specific enough to describe tremor-related difficulties when cutting nails.

### 5.2.2 Capacity and Performance

To assess activity limitations (which is about "performing tasks/actions") and participation restrictions ("being involved in a life situation"), the constructs for *capacity* and *performance* are used.

*Capacity* refers to the (highest) level of ability of a person to execute a task or an action in a standard environment (e.g., a test environment). By varying the test environment, capacity can be assessed with or without support (qualifier 2 or 3, Fig. 5.2.). This approach corresponds to every standard examination and test situation in clinical routine. It allows to describe the outcomes of all kinds of interventions (with/without assistance/aids/adaptions) in a standardised way.

*Performance* refers to what a person does in his or her current environment. Because the current environment includes a societal context, performance can also be understood as *"involvement in a life situation"* or *"the lived experience"* [26]. Assessing performance requires observing a person's behaviour in different life situations as neutral/uninfluenced as possible—with all methodological difficulties associated with such an approach. However, the *"lived experience,"* the subjective experience of involvement (the *"sense of belonging"*), which is a central aspect in the definition of Participation, can only be measured by directly conferring with the affected person (using patient-reported outcome measures, PROMs or health-related quality-of-life instruments, HR-QoL). Information that reflects

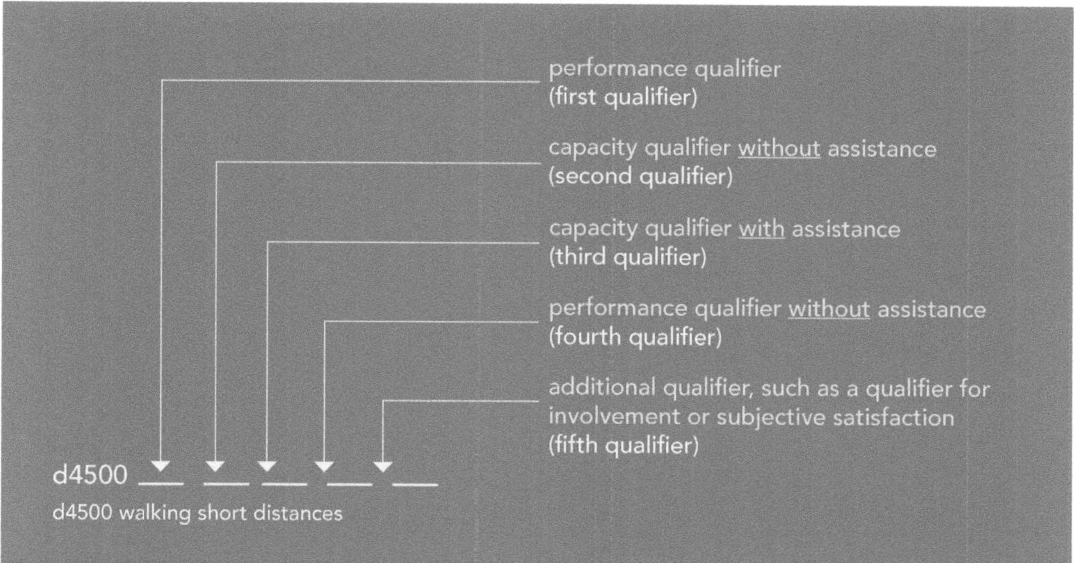


**Fig. 5.2** Coding activities (capacity) and participation (performance)

the feeling of individuals of involvement or satisfaction with their level of functioning is currently not coded in the ICF [26].

### 5.2.3 Contextual Factors

*Personal factors,* as one component of contextual factors, refer to the specific background and lifestyle of a person and include internal influences of the person that are not part of their health problem or condition. Examples for personal factors are age, gender, education, occupation, hobbies and (life) experience as well as individual attitudes and values (e.g., a high-performance expectation or a low readiness to learn). Some of these information are part of personal data; others should be recorded as part of individual history. Often, these narratives also include references to rehabilitation goals and promote cues for developing a new self-image.

*Personal factors* are not classified in the ICF because of the large social and cultural variance associated with them. One may use *"Temperament and Personality Functions"* (b126), *"Energy and Drive Functions"* (b130) and other mental functions if they impact on individual capacity and performance and if these factors affect the course of disease.

*Environmental factors* refer to the physical, social and attitudinal environment in which people live and conduct their lives. These factors can act as *facilitators* or *barriers*.

*Environmental factors* are of particular importance for scaling the severity of any disability. Whenever a person is able to get along with *general products and technologies*, he/she will be less impaired in his/her ability to act than if in need *special products and technologies*. For the description of clinical findings and goals, environmental factors (especially: facilitators) serve as modifiers (syntax: what is possible—under which circumstances?).

### 5.2.4 Top-Down or Bottom-Up?

In bottom-up approaches, the focus lies on detecting impaired body functions (muscle strength, muscle tone, movement control)—with the inherent assumption that disability develops linearly from these impairments (*"internal barriers"*). Here it is worth noticing that affected individuals themselves have only few possibilities to directly influence body function impairments. This is the domain of medical treatment (medication, brain and muscle stimulation or surgical interventions).

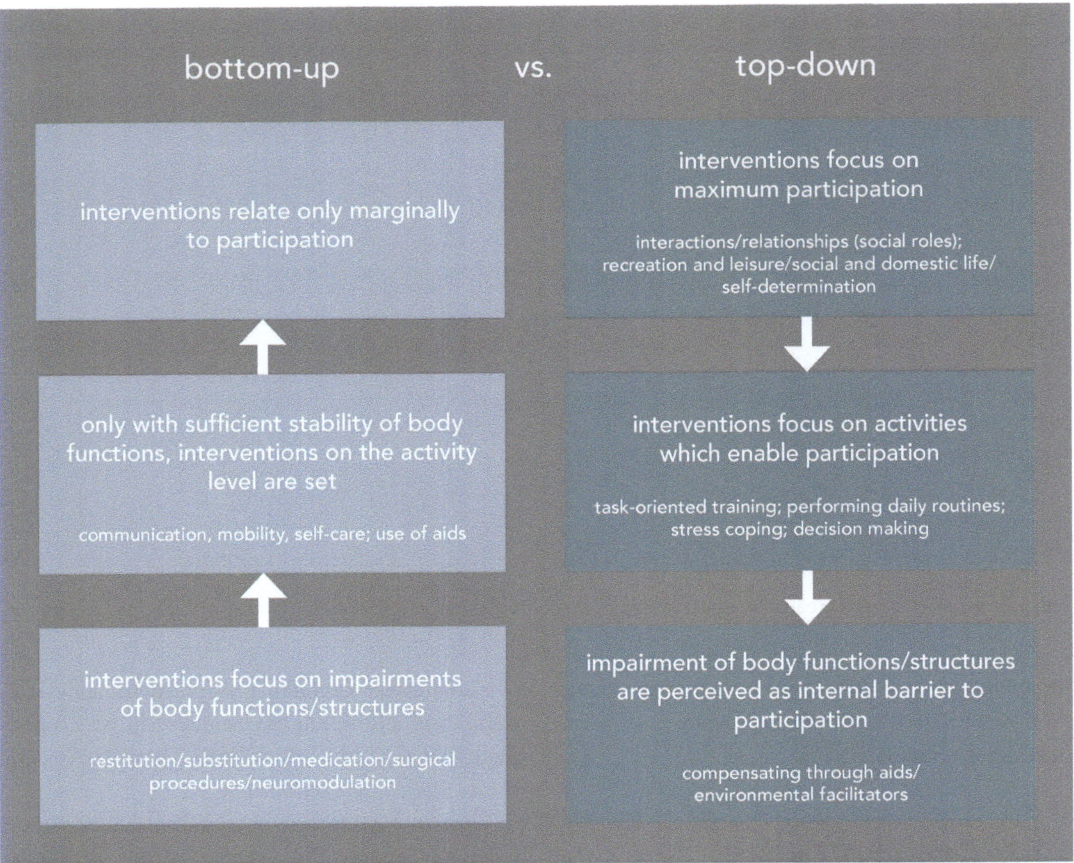



**Fig. 5.3** Bottom-up and top-down approaches in neurorehabilitation

In contrast, the top-down model promotes a participatory approach in medical history taking, evaluation of clinical findings and for treatment planning. The overarching goal is to achieve maximum self-determination and participation of the individuals affected. Starting with exploring the most important life areas an individual wants to actively participate in the near or distant future, current activity limitations and body function impairments are recorded as internal barriers. Based on this analysis, specific action goals focussing on individual behaviour and taking into account all inhibiting and facilitating factors can be set and agreed on with the team and the patients. Part of this process might be developing and practising strategies how to deal with body function impairments not likely to disappear in a given timeframe (Fig. 5.3).

### 5.2.5 ICF-Based Clinical Findings and Goals

For multi-/interdisciplinary evaluation and documentation of clinical findings and for goal setting/evaluation, the ICF is a natural choice for describing individual functioning in a given context at different timepoints. The classification enables the description of all consequences of disease. In a shared documentation, redundancy and fuzziness in scaling can be avoided easily. However, to be able to use the ICF to its full extent, the team needs an agreement on the number and measurability of relevant items to be recorded (and documented) in different clinical situations. Furthermore, constructs and items should be assigned to specific experts within a multidisciplinary team. Here, the choice of a discipline-specific mini core sets, i.e., the selection of mandatory items to be assessed by different team members, might be helpful in avoiding redundancies and overlaps. A brief core set can be found in Annex 9 [26].

Especially the Classification of Activities (capacity) is very useful for goal setting. [27, 28]. Considering the Guidelines for coding of environmental factors in Annex 2.3 [26], we recommend the following syntax for goal formulation:

- **What**: denominate action/task (using a verb phrase; including the relevant ICF codes if required).
- **How/under which circumstances**: denominate facilitators (aids, assistance).
- **By when**: Time frame up until the degree of goal achievement is evaluated, usually by the end of the current treatment cycle.

The examples in Table 5.2 exemplify this further.

### 5.2.6 Examples for ICF-Based Goals and Functional Electrical Stimulation (FES)

The following two patient examples illustrate how FES interventions can be incorporated in an ICF-based goal setting.

#### 5.2.6.1 Patient Example 1

A 72-year-old married retired teacher (*personal context factors*) suffering from the sequelae of an ischemic left middle cerebral brain artery stroke (*structure level*) shall return to her home and social environment after in-patient neurorehabilitation (*participation*). The stroke has caused a moderate hemiparesis of her right arm and leg (*body functions*) with limitations in grasping and releasing and in walking and climbing stairs (*tasks/actions*). Self-care and domestic life activities are limited with a need for assistance/support (*environmental contextual factor*) when dressing herself and when preparing meals/housekeeping.

To improve control of voluntary movements of the right arm (b760), an EMG-triggered multichannel electrical stimulation (EMG-MES)

under expert supervision has been established for a 2–4 weeks period (*see also Chap. 6*). After this treatment, the individual should be able to fix a bottle with the paretic hand while opening/closing the bottle cap with the left hand. To continue FES treatment at home—if necessary—the patient should be able to independently apply self-adhesive electrodes (d220) and arrange for assistance if needed (d730).

#### 5.2.6.2 Patient Example 2

A 61-year-old farmer suffering from a hypertensive right basal ganglia haemorrhage (*structure level*) developed a spastic plegia of the left arm and hand (*body functions*). He lives in a rural region and is well-integrated into social and family life (*environmental factors*). Due to the severe spasticity of left finger and hand flexors, washing and caring for the left hand is a difficult, nearly impossible task (*tasks/actions*). Moreover, the patient experiences moderate to severe pain in the affected hand. After inpatient rehabilitation, ongoing treatment is planned in the patient's home environment with support of his family. Currently, the patient's family members consider themselves unable to take care for the paretic arm due to severe pain when stretching the fingers and when cleaning the palm. To reduce forearm flexor spasticity, Botulinum toxin A (BoNT-A) injections in the forearm and finger flexors were delivered/applied. Immediately after the injections, cyclical electrical stimulation (ES) of the agonists (injected muscle group) was performed for 20–30 min. In the following days and weeks, FES of the antagonistic wrist and finger extensors was performed (for detailed information see Chap. 14, Sect. 14.3 of this book). Goals for these interventions were: to enable the patient to take care for the paretic arm (d570), to stretch the fingers against mild resistance (d210) and to fix objects in place with the paretic hand on a table (d440). The patient should also be able to independently wash and towel the left hand (d520). The patient and his family members agreed on these goals and interventions. The family members have been trained to continue *FES* therapy as part of daily routine at home (home therapy).

**Table 5.2** Examples for goal syntax

| d | task/action (what) | context (how) |
|---|---|---|
| d160 | focus attention | up to … minutes in a quiet/busy environment |
| d177 | make decisions (on … matter) | spontaneously/instructed/with assistance |
| d210 | perform stretching/movement/strengthening exercises | independently/prompted/instructed … |
| d220 | attach electrodes; activate the stimulator; … | independently/prompted/instructed/supervised/with assistance |
| d230 | plan/comply with breaks | spontaneously/prompted/instructed … in time before exhaustion/pain sets in … |
| d410 | stand up from a lying/sitting position | independently/holding onto sth./supervised/instructed/with guidance/with assistance … |
| d440 | grasp/let go of a bottle | spontaneously/with preparation/using a dynamic splint … |
| | secure in place a piece of paper | spontaneously/with preparation/instructed … |
| d450 | walk short distances (inside/outside the house) | self-supported with/without splint/cane with (continuous/intermittent) support/with (professional/lay) assistance |
| d455 | climb stairs | self-supported/using the handrail/alternating/step by step/with/without splint/stimulator/cane with (continuous/intermittent) support/with (professional/lay) assistance |
| d510 | hold the shower gel bottle when showering | spontaneously/with preparation/instructed … |
| d520 | apply lotion to your hands | spontaneously/with preparation/instructed … |
| d570 | take care for the paretic arm | spontaneously/prompted/controlled/instructed/with guidance … |
| d710 | make/keep eye contact | up to (duration)/in a quiet/busy environment/with preparation/initial touch etc. |
| | signal discomfort in care (or in any other situation if relevant) | spontaneously/prompted/skilled – familiar – unfamiliar persons |
| d720 | adhere to rules/agreements when changing position (or any other action if relevant) | spontaneously/prompted/skilled – familiar – unfamiliar persons |
| d730 | call for assistance to attach the electrodes (or any other action if relevant) | using call bell, beeper, mobile phone, … |

## 5.3  Summary

Using the ICF for evaluating clinical findings and for goal planning allows patients and practitioners to choose adequate intervention strategies and to evaluate the effectiveness of these interventions. In accordance with shared decision making, patients and their significant others are included in the goal decision. As functional electrical stimulation requires a high degree of self-initiative and/or initiative of family members, aspects of self-management are important for goal setting. Ideally, progress should always be evaluated using SMART goal statements. Finally, it is important to highlight that reaching a goal is not a clinical endpoint (except for a current treatment cycle), but rather a starting point for a higher level of independence and self-determination for the affected persons and their significant others.

## References


1. Siegert RJ, Levack WMM. In: Scherer MJ, Muller D, editors. Rehabilitation goal setting: theory, practice and evidence. 1st ed. Taylor & Francis Group: Boca Raton, FL; 2015.
2. Sugavanam T, Mead G, Bulley C, Donaghy M, van Wijck F. The effects and experiences of goal setting in stroke rehabilitation - a systematic review. Disabil Rehabil. 2013;35(3):177–90.
3. Levack WM, Weatherall M, Hay-Smith EJ, Dean SG, McPherson K, Siegert RJ. Goal setting and strategies to enhance goal pursuit for adults with acquired disability participating in rehabilitation. Cochrane Database Syst Rev. 2015;7:CD009727.
4. McGrath JR, Adams L. Patient-centered goal planning: A systemic psychological therapy? Top Stroke Rehabil. 1999;6(2):43–50.
5. Playford ED, Siegert R, Levack W, Freeman J. Areas of consensus and controversy about goal setting in rehabilitation: a conference report. Clin Rehabil. 2009;23(4):334–44.
6. Wade DT. Goal setting in rehabilitation: an overview of what, why and how. Clin Rehabil. 2009;23(4):291–5.
7. Gauggel S, Hoop M, Werner K. Assigned versus self-set goals and their impact on the performance of brain-damaged patients. J Clin Exp Neuropsychol. 2002;24(8):1070–80.
8. Locke EA, Latham GP. New developments in goal setting and task performance. New York/London: Routledge; 2013.
9. Locke EA, Latham GP. Goal setting theory: the current state. In: Locke EA, Latham GP, editors. New developments in goal setting and task performance. 1st ed. New York/London: Routledge; 2013. p. 623–30.
10. Day DV. Goals and self-regulation. In: Locke EA, Latham GP, editors. New developments in goal setting and task performance. 1st ed. New York/London: Routledge; 2013.
11. Seijts GH, Latham GP, Tasa K, Latham BW. Goal setting and goal orientation: an integration of two different yet related literatures. Acad Manag J. 2004;47(2):227–39.
12. Wood RE, Whelan J, Sojo V, Wong M. Goals, goal orientations, strategies, and performance. In: Locke EA, Latham GP, editors. New developments in goal setting and task performance. 1st ed. New York/London: Routledge; 2013.
13. Doran GT. There's a S.M.A.R.T. way to write managements's goals and objectives. Manag Rev. 1981;70(11):35–6.
14. Cott C, Finch E. Goal-setting in physical therapy practice. Physiother Can. 1991;43(1):19–22.
15. Braun JP, Mende H, Bause H, Bloos F, Geldner G, Kastrup M, et al. Quality indicators in intensive care medicine: why? Use or burden for the intensivist. Ger Med Sci. 2010;8:Doc22.
16. Locke EA, Latham GP. A theory of goal setting & task performance. Englewood Cliffs, N.J: Prentice Hall; 1990.
17. Bandura A. The nature and structure of self-efficacy. Self-efficacy: the exercise of control. New York: W.H. Freeman; 1997. p. 36–78.
18. Bandura A. The role of self-efficacy in goal-based motivation. In: Locke EA, Latham GP, editors. New developments in goal setting and task performance. first ed. New York/London: Routledge; 2013. p. 147–57.
19. Cicerone KD, Azulay J. Perceived self-efficacy and life satisfaction after traumatic brain injury. J Head Trauma Rehabil. 2007;22(5):257–66.
20. Erez A, Judge TA. Relationship of core self-evaluations to goal setting, motivation, and performance. J Appl Psychol. 2001;86(6):1270–9.
21. Austin JT, Vancouver JB. Goal constructs in psychology: structure, process, and content. Psychol Bull. 1996;120(3):338.
22. Ashford SJ, De Stobbeleir KEM. Feedback, goal setting, and task performance revisited. In: Locke EA, Latham GP, editors. New developments in goal setting and task performance. 1st ed. New York/London: Routledge; 2013.
23. Brands IM, Wade DT, Stapert SZ, van Heugten CM. The adaptation process following acute onset disability: an interactive two-dimensional approach applied to acquired brain injury. Clin Rehabil. 2012;26(9):840–52.
24. Brands I, Stapert S, Kohler S, Wade D, van Heugten C. Life goal attainment in the adaptation process after acquired brain injury: the influence of self-efficacy

and of flexibility and tenacity in goal pursuit. Clin Rehabil. 2014;29(6):611–22.

25. Scobbie L, McLean D, Dixon D, Duncan E, Wyke S. Implementing a framework for goal setting in community based stroke rehabilitation: a process evaluation. BMC Health Serv Res. 2013;13(1):190.

26. WHO. International classification of functioning, disability and health: ICF. Organization WH, editor. Geneva: World Health Organization; 2001.

27. Lohmann S, Decker J, Muller M, Strobl R, Grill E. The ICF forms a useful framework for classifying individual patient goals in post-acute rehabilitation. J Rehabil Med. 2011;43(2):151–5.

28. Constand MK, MacDermid JC. Applications of the international classification of functioning, disability and health in goal-setting practices in healthcare. Disabil Rehabil. 2014;36(15):1305–14.

# Functional Electrical Stimulation for Motor Function Disorders due to Damage to the Central Nervous System

**6**

Thomas Schick

Within central damages of the nervous system, stroke is one of the most common diseases of the brain and the second most common cause of death worldwide [1–3]. Out of 160,000 people affected every year in Germany, 100,000 survive the first year. These figures are comparable with other industrialized countries. About 80% are ischemic strokes. Twenty five percent of all patients are severely impaired and require assistance or care. In Germany, out of all patients who survive the acute phase in hospital, between one-third and one-half are admitted to a post-inpatient rehabilitation program [4]. Apart from ischemic strokes, people are diagnosed with hemorrhagic strokes, traumatic brain injuries, multiple sclerosis, spinal cord injuries, and neurodegenerative diseases such as Parkinson's disease and many others. The treatment of patients with damage of the first motor neuron, also known as upper motor neuron syndrome (UMNS), is a therapeutic focus in neurorehabilitation. Upper motor neuron (UMN) refers to the neuronal cell bodies together with the efferent nerve fibers that are responsible for innervation of skeletal muscles. The tasks of the UMN include the initiation of voluntary movement and body control. The nuclei of the UMN are located in the motor cortex of the brain. The axons travel predominantly as pyramidal tracts (tractus corticospinalis, TCS) to the spinal cord where they are switched into the anterior horn cell to the second motor neuron or "lower motor neuron" (LMN). The cell bodies of the LMN) are located in the gray matter of the spinal cord where the switching sites, the synapses, are located [5]. From there, the efferent tracts as spinal nerves are divided into A$\alpha$- and A$\gamma$-fibers to the extra- and intrafusal muscle fibers which are responsible for muscle contraction and receptor sensitivity.

The involuntary movements and the supporting and holding motor functions are mainly determined by the extrapyramidal system which is functionally different from the pyramidal system. The afferent and efferent nerve pathways run separately from those of the pyramidal pathways. It is not a coherent, closed system and is not uniformly defined in the literature. The following functions assigned to the extrapyramidal system are also referred to as the *striatal system* denoted: Striatum, globus pallidus, nucleus subthalamicus, nucleus ruber, and substantia nigra. In an extended sense, the cerebellum, the thalamic nuclei, the formatio reticularis, and the vestibular nuclei are assigned to the striatal system [6].

---

**Supplementary Information** The online version contains supplementary material available at [https://doi.org/10.1007/978-3-030-90123-3_6].

---

T. Schick (✉)
MED-EL, Department Neurorehabilitation
STIWELL, Innsbruck, Austria
e-mail: schick@neuro-reha.info

The consequences of damages to the UMN are very diverse and are described as UMNS with plus syndromes or minus syndromes, ipsilateral syndromes, and adaptive phenomena:

The *plus syndromes* are assigned to the afferent disorders, such as spasticity, relexifications, Babinski reflex, clonus, and spasms of the flexors/extensors, efferent disorders, such as tonic patterns, mass tendence, cocontraction, spastic patterns, and spastic dystonia.

*Minus syndromes* include force reduction. The patient is characterized by reduced speed of decontraction, reduced speed of force development, disturbance of dexterity, and high fatigability.

The *adaptive phenomena* are followed by effects to the musculature. These include atrophy, change in muscle fiber type, viscosity change, sarcomere loss, and shortening of the muscle-tendon unit. Impairment of dexterity is also common on the less affected side and is referred to as ipsilateral syndrome.

Table 6.1 summarizes the UMNS and shows the complexity of the possible effects in motor-disordered neurological patients [7].

The adaptive phenomena with dysfunctional muscle physiology, symptoms of spasticity, paresis/plegia, and ataxia are discussed in the following sections (Sects. 6.1.1, 6.1.2, 6.1.3, and 6.1.4) in particular.

The possible deficits can affect in an activity-oriented classification in particular:

- Postural control.
- Locomotion.
- Grasping and manipulation.
- Gestures and facial expressions.
- Speaking and swallowing.

The therapeutic treatment approach is thus multi-layered and can include a structure- and function-oriented as well as activity- and action-oriented approach. In addition, it is particularly important to improve the patient's motivation [7]. Stroke patients with accompanying neurological symptoms in addition to the motor disorder such as anosognosia, apraxia, neglect, or somatosensory deficits have a less favorable prognosis. The

therapy approaches with FES for neglect or somatosensory deficits are presented in Chap. 9.

## 6.1 Introduction to Symptom-Related Functional Electrical Stimulation

In the previous section, the potential consequences of UMNS were presented. The use of FES can effectively treat many of these deficits when used in a targeted therapeutic manner. A prerequisite, however, is background knowledge on its effective problem-centered use. In addition to a differentiation of the existing damage patterns, it requires the resulting objective of the therapy in rehabilitation.

The therapeutic use of FES can extend from the structural and functional level to the execution of actions at the activity level. Structural aspects of treatment, such as improved blood circulation, improved trophism, or pain reduction of affected body regions, etc., represent a desirable side effect of the repeated electrical stimulation, but are rarely seen as the primary therapeutic focus of neurorehabilitation in UMNS. Rather, under the aspects of neuromodulation and motor learning with the resulting possible changes in cortical plasticity, active, goal- and task-oriented training contents with a high degree of problem-solving strategies are necessary.

**Summary**
FES combined with task-oriented training promotes problem-solving strategies and thus supports motor learning in patients with upper motor neuron damage.

Recent reviews and meta-analyses indicate strong evidence that FES combined with task-oriented training improves upper extremity voluntary activity in acute and subacute stroke patients [8] and shows a greater therapeutic effect on upper extremity activity than training without FES [9]. A recent guideline from the *American Stroke Association (ASA)* recommends FES in

**Table 6.1** Summary of upper motor neuron syndrome (UMNS) and illustration of the complexity of its potential implications in motor-disordered neurological patients

| plus symptoms | minus symptoms | adaptive symptoms | ipsilateral symptoms |
|---|---|---|---|
| **1 AFFERENT DISORDERS**<br>disinhibited spinal reflexes | | change in the muscle | |
| **HYPERREFLEXIA**<br>increased sensitivity of phasic muscle stretch reflexes | power reduction | atrophies | decreased dexterity of the ipsilateral hand |
| **CLONUS**<br>increased sensitivity of phasic muscle stretch reflexes | decreased power development speed | change muscle fiber type | |
| **SPASTICITY**<br>increased sensitivity of tonic muscle stretch reflexes | decreased decontraction speed | change of viscosity | |
| **FLEXORS-EXTENSORS SPASMS**<br>increased sensitivity of cutaneous and nociceptive reflexes | decreased dexterity | loss of sarcoma | |
| **BABINSKI**<br>increased sensitivity of cutaneous and nociceptive reflexes | high fatigability | muscle tendon unit shortening | |
| **2 EFFERENTE DISORDERS**<br>modified supraspinal output due to damaged pyramidal tracts | | change of elasticity of the muscle fascia | |
| **TONIC PATTERNS**<br>disinhibition of vestibular spinal activity | | | |
| **MASS TENDENCY**<br>lack of power is compensated by mass activation | | | |
| **COCONTRACTION**<br>lack of movement control is compensated by cocontraction | | | |
| **SYNKINESIA**<br>compensatory activation of ipsilateral tract systems | | | |
| **SPASTIC DYSTONIA**<br>tonic muscle contraction at rest | | | |

combination with task-oriented training in stroke rehabilitation [10].

Functional improvements after stroke have been shown to depend on both the number of daily therapy hours and the number of weekly therapy days [11, 12]. The therapy density of several hours with daily repetition appropriate for motor learning can be effectively supported and implemented with FES. In suitable cases and with good compliance of the patient or, if applicable, his relatives, the method can be continued by the patient at home or therapeutically accompanied in the context of outpatient therapy beyond the course of rehabilitation. A comprehensive description of home therapy can be found in Chap. 17.

The appropriate choice of FES procedure from the patient's point of view depends on the desired and necessary level of treatment and, in particular, on the severity of the disorder. The Fugl-Meyer Assessment (FMA; 0–66 points) is regularly used in studies, but less so in routine clinical practice, to assess the degree of impairment to the upper extremity after a stroke., In addition to its function to measure the impairment after a stroke, this assessment allows to classify the severity degree of the upper extremity impairment. The latter is divided into four categories: "severe", "severe to moderate", "moderate to mild", and "mild" [13]. Table 6.2 describes the classification of a patient's severity based on the FMA and the associated impairments.

In order to ensure the desired effective use of FES for the patient, the various forms of FES treatment should be adapted to the severity of the patient's impairment. Table 6.3 compares the main areas of application of the different FES methods on the basis of the severity classification and the therapeutic objective. Of course, there is a smooth transition between categories.

The goal of all interventions is to achieve the most constant neuronal networking possible through intensive practice. This results in skilled motor actions under changing contextual conditions [14]. Independent, active, repetitive movements are of central importance in these modern therapy concepts under aspects of motor learning and the neuroplastic changes to be aimed at [7] and are thus to be preferred to purely passive, mostly cyclical forms of stimulation.

Thus, the stimulation forms of transcutaneous electrical nerve stimulation (TENS), neuromuscular electrical stimulation (NMES) [15], and cyclic functional electrical stimulation (cFES) [16] are frequently used as primarily repetitive, but passive stimulation methods for the motorically more severely affected patients in the subacute and chronic phase after a stroke. In the latter described therapy methods, the focus is not on the respective voluntary

**Table 6.2** describes the classification of a patient's severity based on the FMA and the associated impairments

| points 0-66 | severity | impairment |
| --- | --- | --- |
| 0-15 | severe | Severe impairment with no hand, wrist, or multi-joint movement. Minimal movement limited to single joint extensor and flexor muscle synergies. |
| 16-34 | severe to moderate | Severe impairment without movement due to synergies and movement restrictions of individual joint extensor and flexor synergies, hand, wrist or multi-joint movements. |
| 35-53 | moderate to mild | Moderate impairment with limited movements due to synergies and partial impairment due to synergies of single joint extensors and flexors and hand, wrist and multi-joint movements. |
| 54-66 | mild | Minimal impairment with the ability to perform movements from synergy with full movement of the arm. |

**Table 6.3** Compares the main uses of the different FES methods based on severity classification (FMA) and treatment goal

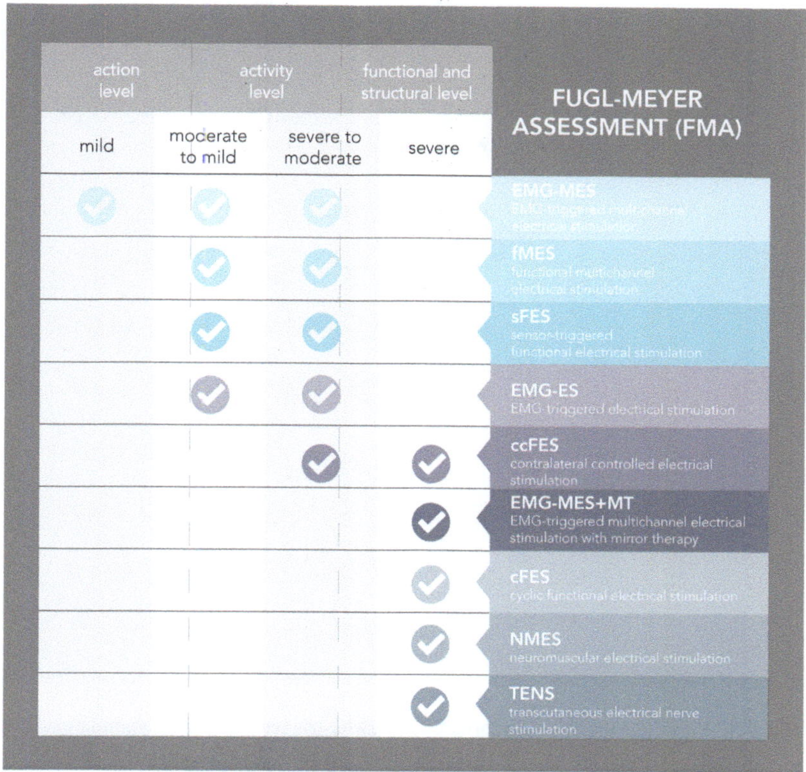

| action level | activity level | functional and structural level | | FUGL-MEYER ASSESSMENT (FMA) |
| mild | moderate to mild | severe to moderate | severe | |
| --- | --- | --- | --- | --- |
| ✓ | ✓ | ✓ | | **EMG-MES** EMG-triggered multichannel electrical stimulation |
| | ✓ | ✓ | | **fMES** functional multichannel electrical stimulation |
| | ✓ | ✓ | | **sFES** sensor-triggered functional electrical stimulation |
| | ✓ | ✓ | | **EMG-ES** EMG-triggered electrical stimulation |
| | | ✓ | ✓ | **ccFES** contralateral controlled electrical stimulation |
| | | | ✓ | **EMG-MES+MT** EMG-triggered multichannel electrical stimulation with mirror therapy |
| | | | ✓ | **cFES** cyclic functional electrical stimulation |
| | | | ✓ | **NMES** neuromuscular electrical stimulation |
| | | | ✓ | **TENS** transcutaneous electrical nerve stimulation |

movement initiation and execution, but increasingly on structural and only partly functional deficits. Peripheral or afferent electrical stimulation (PES/AES) has been studied in the past and shows at least short-term changes in handgrip strength after intervention [17]. Authors describe the benefit as preparatory or adjuvant to other active rehabilitation procedures [18]. This topic and the influence on neuropsychological symptoms such as neglect are discussed in Chap. 9.

In recent years, there has been an increasing demand for the combination of functional stimulation and task-oriented therapy methods to improve motor outcome [15]. In moderately to severely affected hemiparetic patients, therapeutic methods such as contralateral controlled functional electrical stimulation (ccFES) use the less affected side via motion sensors integrated into cuffs to trigger simultaneous movement on the affected side of the body [19].

To optimize the necessary active cooperation of the patient in modern FES, EMG signals are used to pulse an initial movement triggered by the patient (Fig. 6.1).

> ▶ **Motor learning requires the active participation of the patient. EMG-triggered stimulation promotes patient-triggered impulse and movement initiation and thus decisively supports the motor learning process.**

Here, the movement effects can be strengthened if they are performed in combination with a patient-adapted, clear, functional, and problem-solving task with electrical support of individual muscle groups required for this action.

The combination of EMG-triggered multichannel electrical stimulation (EMG-MES) with optimized visual motion feedback using mirror therapy (ST) (EMG-MES+ST) achieved significant, clinically relevant motor improvements in subacute stroke patients [20]. This therapy-relevant treatment approach for mostly severely affected stroke patients is discussed in Sect. 14.2 and elaborated in detail in Sect. 6.3.3.

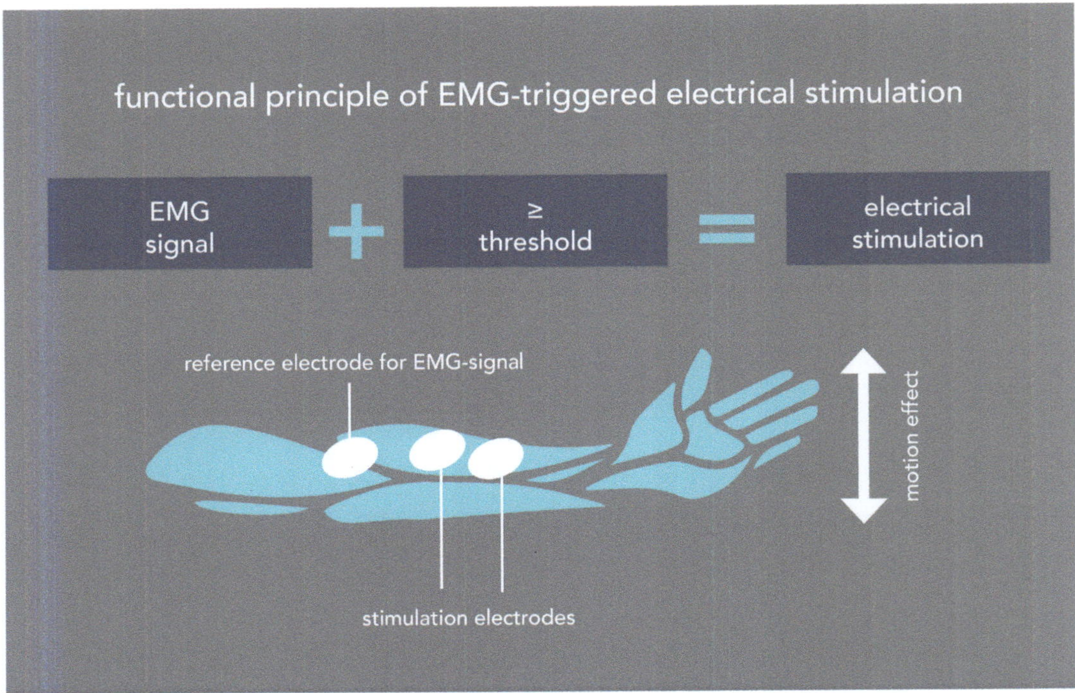



**Fig. 6.1** Illustrates the operating principle of EMG-triggered electrical stimulation (EMG-ES)

Stimulation forms triggered with switches or motion sensors (sFES) are often used therapeutically to support mobility during walking, also in the sense of a myoelectric orthosis. Depending on the number of stimulation channels, functions to improve the stance or free leg phase during walking are possible. Severely affected patients, on the other hand, usually benefit from multichannel electrical stimulation (MES) or contralateral EMG or sensory triggering via the less affected leg, Sensory triggering over the less affected limb or unilaterally over less severely affected limb segments. Thus, multichannel electrical stimulation can also be usefully applied in these patients. If the rehabilitative objective is specifically to improve activities of daily living such as the grasping, manipulation and transport of objects, or the mobility of the patient, the EMG-triggered electrical stimulation (EMG-ES), the contralateral controlled functional electrical stimulation (ccFES), and the EMG-MES procedures are used clinically. This is also true for ipsilateral symptoms like disturbance of dexterity, reduction of plus symptoms like spasticity, cocontraction or mass tendency on the affected side or minus symptoms like paresis, strength reduc-

tion, strength endurance, and coordination deficits. A review of EMG-triggered stimulation after stroke [21], which included 26 studies with 782 patients, described robust significant effects in follow-up after EMG-ES intervention, both at the level of damage and function, especially in the chronic phase. This was defined here as more than 3 months after stroke occurrence. According to the authors, it is a good option for the treatment of severely to moderately affected stroke patients.

The enormous biomechanical complexity of the hand is reflected in its distinct cortical representation in the motor cortex and requires an intact corticospinal tract for fine motor control [22]. If this tract is massively destroyed by a stroke, contralesional motor-cortical recreation becomes more important. Depending on the severity, from moderately to severely affected patients, the contralesional cortex takes over the main motor compensation [23]. Stroke affects hand motor function more than elbow or shoulder motor function, and only less than half of patients achieve adequate hand function after 6 months [24].

Positive effects on activities of daily living (ATL) that persisted 2 months after the intervention were described in a review [25]. Evidence is found that EMG-ES in combination with rehabilitative interventions is superior in terms of upper extremity limitations. This is true for the post-acute rehabilitation phase after stroke and for the chronic phase [26].

EMG-MES is regularly used in rehabilitation of severely to moderately [27] to mildly affected patients to improve functions with task-oriented training of the upper extremity after stroke. It is also well suited for use in the home setting as a post-inpatient rehabilitation measure [28]. The restoration of lost functions with the goal of an improved activity level is focused. Of course, EMG-MES is not limited to the upper extremities but offers a variety of useful therapeutic interventions including the trunk and the lower extremities to improve postural stability, control, and mobility.

In summary, the FES procedures with patient-intended triggering, the following can be achieved, e.g., by EMG or sensor triggering with several stimulation channels, mostly severely to moderately affected, but also mildly affected patients benefit greatly.

**Summary**
Patients who are severely to mildly motor-impaired benefit from EMG-MES.

Due to the complexity of movement-synchronous multichannel stimulation during walking with the aid of functional multichannel electrical stimulation (FMES), this therapy method is regularly used primarily in the clinical setting [29]. The 1- to 2-channel mobile electrical stimulation devices with different sensor technology for movement triggering or control have proven to be suitable as myoelectric orthoses for the care of neurological patients with UMNS and foot lift and knee joint control deficits. Electrical stimulation is also used for stroke patients. The sole of the foot of the affected leg is used successfully in the early gait rehabilitation to trigger the withdrawal reflex, in conjunction with an increase of stance stability on the non-affected leg, in walking speed and distance and to initiate movement [30].

The therapeutic interventions of FES are not exclusively dependent on the severity, but also on the symptom expression. Therapeutic treatment options with FES for the plus and minus symptoms described

in Sect. 6.1, the adaptive and ipsilateral symptoms, but also rehabilitation-relevant symptoms such as pain or swelling can be found in Table 6.4. This shows an overview of the different electrical stimulation approaches and their symptom-dependent areas of application. The therapeutic focus of the individual stimulation methods differs considerably.

## 6.1.1 Adaptive Phenomena with Dysfunctional Muscle Physiology

There is literature on muscle physiology that describes adaptive phenomena and the structural consequences after a central brain damage, e.g., stroke. The changes range from decreased oxidative capacity [31], an increased prevalence for sarcopenia [32] to increased fatigable muscle fibers [33] weakness, such as muscle-fiber length, decrease of pennation angle, muscle atrophy, and tendon compliance [34].

Other authors describe the greatly reduced muscle mass compared to the unaffected side and the resulting muscle weakness with an increase of intramuscular fat [35]. For structural deficits such as swelling or functional deficits due to adaptive symptoms, in particular, NMES including TENS or cFES can also be used sensibly.

A meta-analysis investigated different therapy methods to improve strength in chronic stroke patients [36]. Here, other therapy methods such as forced resistance training for strengthening the knee joint extensors were shown to be more effective than electrical stimulation. This is not surprising, since the focus by means of FES in neurorehabilitation should not be primarily on the structural but rather on the functional and, even better, on the activity-related level. The principles of motor learning and thus the influence on neuronal plasticity should clearly be focused and not the purely structural approach with a pure improvement of strength.

Therapeutically relevant motor target sets, EMG-MES in particular, serve this purpose. This is because under the aspects of motor learning, in addition to, e.g., repetition, above all task- and problem-solving-oriented approaches are therapeutically very well implemented and can be combined well. The importance and the advantage of a task-oriented treatment with EMG-ES compared

**Table 6.4** Functional electrical stimulation procedures for upper motor neuron syndrome

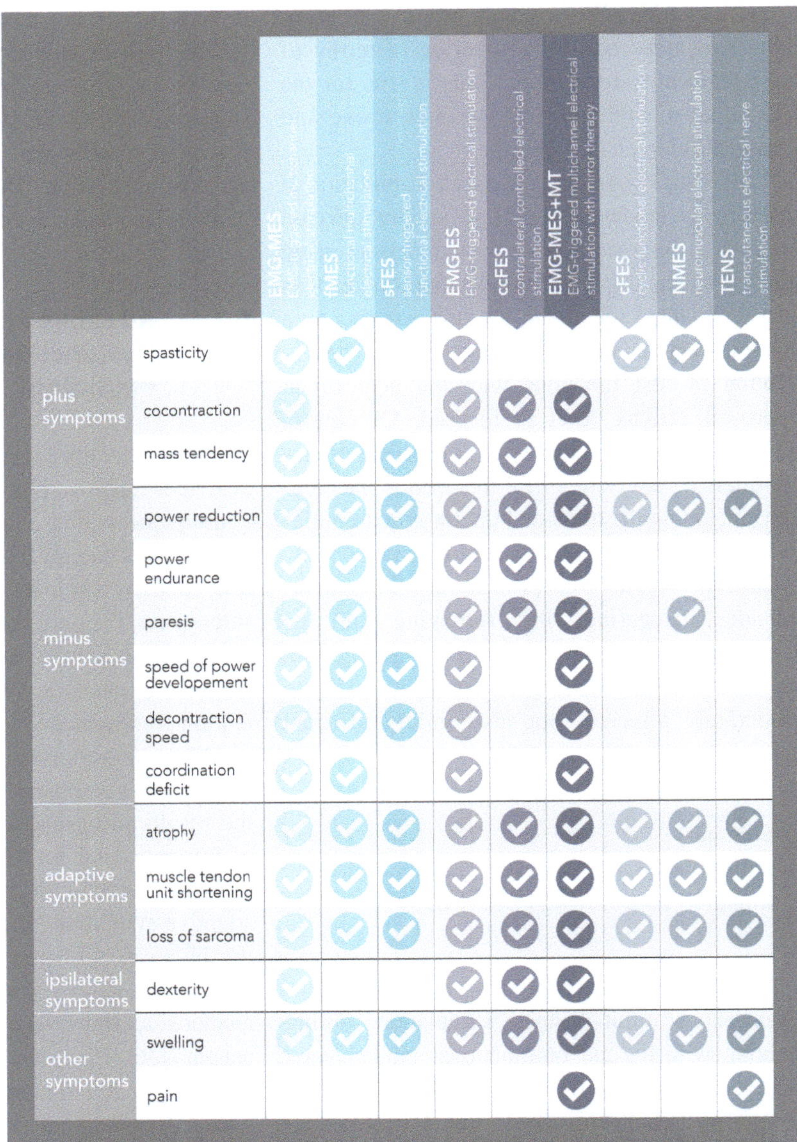

| Group | Symptom | EMG-MES (EMG-triggered multichannel electrical stimulation) | fMES (functional multichannel electrical stimulation) | sFES (sensor-triggered functional electrical stimulation) | EMG-ES (EMG-triggered electrical stimulation) | ccFES (contralateral controlled electrical stimulation) | EMG-MES+MT (EMG-triggered multichannel electrical stimulation with mirror therapy) | cFES (cyclic functional electrical stimulation) | NMES (neuromuscular electrical stimulation) | TENS (transcutaneous electrical nerve stimulation) |
|---|---|---|---|---|---|---|---|---|---|---|
| plus symptoms | spasticity | ✓ | ✓ |  | ✓ |  |  | ✓ | ✓ | ✓ |
|  | cocontraction | ✓ |  |  | ✓ | ✓ | ✓ |  |  |  |
|  | mass tendency | ✓ | ✓ | ✓ | ✓ | ✓ | ✓ |  |  |  |
| minus symptoms | power reduction | ✓ | ✓ | ✓ | ✓ | ✓ | ✓ | ✓ | ✓ | ✓ |
|  | power endurance | ✓ | ✓ | ✓ | ✓ | ✓ | ✓ |  |  |  |
|  | paresis | ✓ | ✓ |  | ✓ | ✓ | ✓ |  | ✓ |  |
|  | speed of power developement | ✓ | ✓ | ✓ | ✓ |  | ✓ |  |  |  |
|  | decontraction speed | ✓ | ✓ | ✓ | ✓ |  | ✓ |  |  |  |
|  | coordination deficit | ✓ | ✓ |  | ✓ |  | ✓ |  |  |  |
| adaptive symptoms | atrophy | ✓ | ✓ | ✓ | ✓ | ✓ | ✓ | ✓ | ✓ | ✓ |
|  | muscle tendon unit shortening | ✓ | ✓ | ✓ | ✓ | ✓ | ✓ | ✓ | ✓ | ✓ |
|  | loss of sarcoma | ✓ | ✓ | ✓ | ✓ | ✓ | ✓ | ✓ | ✓ | ✓ |
| ipsilateral symptoms | dexterity | ✓ |  |  | ✓ | ✓ | ✓ |  |  |  |
| other symptoms | swelling | ✓ | ✓ | ✓ | ✓ | ✓ | ✓ | ✓ | ✓ | ✓ |
|  | pain |  |  |  |  |  | ✓ |  |  | ✓ |

to cFES for the improvement of shoulder function was shown in a randomized controlled trial [37].

### 6.1.2 Paresis and Plegia

Paralysis of the musculature, also referred to as paresis if incomplete and as plegia if complete, usually means a considerable restriction for neurological patients with UMNS. The effects on functionality and activity allow only very limited freedom of action and activity.

Participatory competence. Paresis is much more common in UMNS than complete plegia, which is more common in LMNS, i.e., peripheral nerve damage. Muscular weakness causes patients to fail at everyday movements. Depending on the degree of severity, they then compensate for the loss of function more on the less affected side. In addition to achieving the best possible functional competence on the paretic side of the body, the therapy goal can also be to improve dexterity on the less affected ipsilesional side of the body.

Patients with residual functions are particularly suitable for EMG-ES and EMG-MES in rehabilitation and outpatient therapy, as they can still initiate a movement independently and the electrical stimulation provides an additional positive incentive for the possible execution of the movement. A successfully performed action on the activity level and thus a successful problem-solving approach increases the patient's motivation level considerably.

**Summary**
Successful handling of patients with paresis in UMNS by means of individual and targeted EMG-MES can have a marked motivational effect and support them in developing further task-specific problem-solving approaches.

If several stimulation channels can be used therapeutically, not only simple joint movements but also complex, relevant movement sequences are electrically stimulated and thus supported. Sections 6.3 and 6.4 contain a variety of practical therapy suggestions for EMG-MES and explain the special features and the usefulness of the precise and individual use of modern electrical stimulation devices.

### 6.1.3 Spastic Movement Disorder

A spastic movement disorder is defined as an increase in muscle tension due to rapid stretching of the muscle. The symptom, which occurs in the context of UMNS, usually shows up with a time lag a few weeks after the event. Spasticity develops in 38% of stroke patients. A spastic movement disorder occurs when the activation of the descending extrapyramidal pathways predominates over the inhibitory control functions. In addition, the following phenomena often occur [7]:

- **Reflex irradiation:** spreading of the excitation on adjacent muscle groups,
- **Reduced reciprocal inhibition:** reduced decontraction of antagonistic muscle groups,
- **Clonus:** muscular activation and deactivation caused by a stretch stimulus.

The treatment of spastic movement disorders in UMNS with the aid of FES pursues different therapeutic approaches. On the one hand, stimulation of the antagonist or antagonistic functional chains, on the other hand, stimulation of the spastic muscle itself. In many cases, it is more effective in the medium term to select equipment and forms of stimulation in such a way that a patient is supported, for example, in performing movements from a flexion synergy through either active or electrical stimulation in an assistive and repetitive way.

In preparation for such a treatment approach, selected stimulation frequencies can also be applied to the tonic agonist (i.e., the affected) muscles to detonate them, which in certain cases makes the antagonistic movement possible in the first place. Proven frequencies for muscular fatigue are "low-frequency fatigue" (LFF < 10 Hz) [38, 39] or "high-frequency fatigue" (HFF > 50 Hz) [40] In the treatment of spastic movement disorders of extremities, the functional aspect is not always the primary goal. Rather, in selected cases, a structural approach is initiated, which can then progressively transition to a treatment emphasizing function and improvement of activity. A review and meta-analysis of NMES in stroke patients with 27 randomized trials and nearly 940 cases showed an improvement in spasticity and an increase in range of motion [41]. The authors concluded that targeted electrical stimulation, also in combination with other interventions, is a good rehabilitative therapy option. Pronounced forms can additionally be treated with botulinum neurotoxin (BoNT) (Sect. 14.3).

**Summary**
The treatment of spastic movement disorders focuses on the functional aspect. In the longer term, functional changes can be achieved by targeted activation of antagonistic movement patterns using FES. Due to the rather short-term therapy effects, the direct stimulation of spastic muscles with suitable frequencies should ideally be used as a precursor to therapy.

### 6.1.4 Ataxia

Ataxia is an impairment of movement coordination (fine tuning of movements; Greek: "a-taxis"—disorder) [42]. The cause can be hereditary, acquired, or idiopathic.

The prerequisite for coordinated movements is the complex interaction of the cerebrum and cerebellum, the brain stem, the spinal cord, the afferent and efferent nerve structures and the musculature.

If there is a malfunction in one of these functional areas, this may lead to uncontrolled, overshooting, or erratic movements. Structures such as the cerebellum, the pons, or the capsula interna can lead to overshooting and uncontrolled movements when damaged. Patients with multiple sclerosis or after craniocerebral trauma are frequently affected by ataxia. Cerebral infarctions may also lead to ataxic hemiparesis [43]. These can affect arms or legs with limb ataxia or manifest within the trunk. If the ataxia manifests primarily in stance or gait function, it is referred to as stance or gait ataxia. Depending on the site of damage, a distinction is made between *cerebellar* ataxia with cause in the cerebellum that can also lead to ipsilateral dysmetria and intention tremor [43], and *spinal* ataxia, where the cause originates from the spinal cord. In addition, damage to sensitive nerve structures, such as polyneuropathy, may also occur. The consequence is sensory ataxia.

Not only the intermuscular coordination between different muscle groups, but also the intramuscular coordination in the muscles themselves may be impaired. Ataxia in cerebellar damage can have a negative effect on vocal articulation like ataxic dysarthria or on eye-gaze coordination [43].

As a treatment, the focus is on regular professional counseling. Rehabilitation interventions such as physiotherapy, occupational therapy, or speech therapy focus on active measures to promote coordination.

A study including patients with spinocerebellar ataxia (SCA, a neurodegenerative disease) in direct comparison with healthy subjects documented an increase in cortical excitability after 30 min of electrical stimulation of the median nerve. The authors conclude that their findings are relevant to the use of electrical stimulation to increase cortical motor excitability in motor rehabilitation of cerebellar dysfunction [44]. Thus, it is plausible to assume that targeted FES can also promote coordinative control functions. EMG-MES supports coordinative movements relevant in everyday life. In this case, EMG triggering for movement initiation by the patient should also be used if possible, in order to improve voluntary and thus patient-directed movement control.

By using multichannel electrical stimulation, the muscular coordination of agonists and antagonists in functional chains can be improved in a way that controlled movement can be performed and the relearning of coordinative functions is supported.

> **Summary**
> EMG-MES supports movements relevant in everyday life and the muscular coordination of agonists and antagonists in their functional chains. Thus, movement control in ataxia can be improved.

## 6.2 Symptom-Related Functional Parameter Setting

In the following practice section (Sects. 6.3 and 6.4), examples of EMG-MES are presented and the possible parameter settings are discussed in detail. The importance of parameter adaptations for the performance of activities and movements will be explained (Fig. 6.1). The following parameter settings will be discussed in particular (Fig. 6.2):

- Intensity.
- Frequency.
- Pulse width.
- Plateau-pause Times.
- Rise time of the pulses.
- Fall time of the pulses.
- Second contractions.
- EMG trigger threshold.
- Intensity.

**Intensity:** The intensity or amplitude of the current pulse determines the desired motor response. In order to achieve an adequate motor response for functional movement execution, it is essential in most cases to choose an intensity that is not only sensory, but also motor-sensitive. If a patient reacts very sensitively to the electrical stimuli, it is possible to start with lower intensities and then adjust them step by step to the therapeutic needs. Reducing the pulse width can also reduce the sensitive load and consequently increase the required intensity. It should be noted that once the motor threshold has been reached, the sensitive load due to the current stimulus no longer increases to the same extent.

**Frequency:** The frequency describes the number of individual current pulses per second and is expressed in the unit Hertz (Hz). In addition to the intensity, it is the decisive factor in determining whether a complete contraction of the muscles is achieved. A complete or tetanic contraction is achieved at more than 20 Hz. Frequencies around 30–35 Hz are commonly used in FES and EMG-MES. However, higher frequencies of up to 50 Hz are also useful without causing excessive fatigue. Higher frequencies can lead to more intensive contraction due to increased recruitment of muscle fibers and thus to a stronger training effect directly on the muscle.

**Pulse width:** FES including the EMG-MES in UMNS regularly uses short pulse widths in the microsecond range (<1000 µs = 1 ms) to stimulate the motor unit. The muscular responses occur through electrical stimulation of the efferent nerve structures and not the muscle itself. The pulse widths most commonly used in therapy and in studies with FES and EMG-MES are usually between 250 and 400 µs.

**Plateau and pause times:** An important role is given to the individual setting of the stimulation times, referred to as plateau times and pause times represent the most important aspect of the therapy. In order to simulate a function or activity with the support of electrical stimulation in a way that is suitable for everyday life, the therapist should set the required stimulation times. The sequence of the muscle groups or functional chains involved in this movement can be mapped accordingly in the suitable electrical stimulation device. Thus, during a planned movement, different muscle groups can be stimulated in a staggered or overlapping sequence.

**Rise/fall times:** Modern and suitable electrical stimulation devices not only allow individual adjustment of the plateau-pause times among the different stimulation channels, but also different rise and fall times for each individual channel. The rise and fall times to be set for the stimulations differ according to the required movements. In many cases, a longer rise time leads to a more coordinated and less chopped execution of movements. This option can also be useful in the treatment of spasticity to avoid unwanted reflex responses. The individual parameter adaption offers immense possibilities for experienced therapists and their patients. If one plans to perform a movement against or with the force of gravity (e.g., when lifting an object above shoulder level), a significant extension of the drop time prevents a sudden, uncontrolled drop of the arm.

**Second contractions:** For some activities, it may be necessary or advantageous to perform a stimulation a second time within a stimulation cycle in mostly reciprocal movement sequences. For this purpose, a second contraction can be set on up to four channels in modern electrical stimulation devices.

**EMG trigger threshold:** Patient-specified pulse triggering with automatic determination of the trigger threshold should be the standard for electrical stimulation devices in neurorehabilitation. This means that during movement initiation, the patient has to exert a certain amount of self-activity in order to start the movement and to receive electrical stimulation to support task performance. Since the activity level of patients varies greatly, this requires an individual and adapted determination of the trigger threshold. The activity level of a patient changes regularly during ongoing electrical stimulation therapy. In some cases, this can manifest itself in an increase in activity during therapy. Here an adaption and thus an increase in the trigger threshold value are reasonable. Fatigue effects can also make it necessary to lower the trigger threshold. Depending on the type of device, this readjustment can be performed automatically or manually by the therapist or patient. The movement triggering can also be carried out on the less affected limb or in a less affected proximal or distal limb section, if this makes sense from a therapeutic point of view.

▶ **It may be crucial for the therapy success to select and adjust suitable stimulation parameters on an individual basis, such as:**
▶ **Intensity.**

- ▶ **Frequency.**
- ▶ **Pulse width.**
- ▶ **Plateau and pause times.**
- ▶ **Trigger threshold.**
- ▶ **Rise and fall times.**
- ▶ **Second contraction.**

In the modern and contemporary form of EMG-MES, the focus is not on current-induced muscular contractions to improve muscle strength, but on the successful execution of an individual task or problem. The positive feedback of a successfully performed action on the activity level can have a strong emotional and motivational aspect in addition to the motor aspect. Therefore, EMG-MES is an important component in the neurorehabilitative care of patients with various neurological disorders.

The fear occasionally expressed by critics that parameter adjustment takes up too much therapy time can be contradicted both by practical experience and by scientific work. In a controlled study, therapeutically relevant effects were documented on the basis of the documented net treatment time or stimulation time of the patients on an average of almost 20 min in a 30 minutes session with a bilateral four-channel system of the upper extremities [20]. The remaining treatment time comprised set-up times, including preparation and post-processing and patient positioning, and was only partly used for parameter adaption. Another RCT on EMG-MES compared to cNMES, published in 2022, showed even longer net treatment times of almost 24 min on average out of a total treatment time of 30 minutes [45].

The practical examples of the listed parameter adaptations are prepared in detail in the following two sections. It is explicitly emphasized that the listed stimulation patterns are only therapy examples and can be adapted variably, individually, and flexibly to the patient. Electrical stimulation devices, which allow an individualizable and very versatile parameter adaptation to the patient's needs and have a simple operator guidance, have become established in therapy. It is advisable to use only high-quality self-adhesive electrodes for functional programs involving movements and sequences of movements. These are characterized by a very thin and flexible surface and good adhesion even after several therapy sessions. With appropriate care and cool storage, they can usually be used many times on the same patient. Depending on the region to be stimulated, the appropriate electrode size needs to be selected. In many cases, unsuitable electrodes have a direct negative effect on the patient and an influence on the treatment process and the result. It should also be noted that the skin surface is free of moisture and grease and hair in the stimulation area should be removed at an early stage in advance if necessary.

Table 6.5 provides an overview of the options for symptom-dependent therapy.

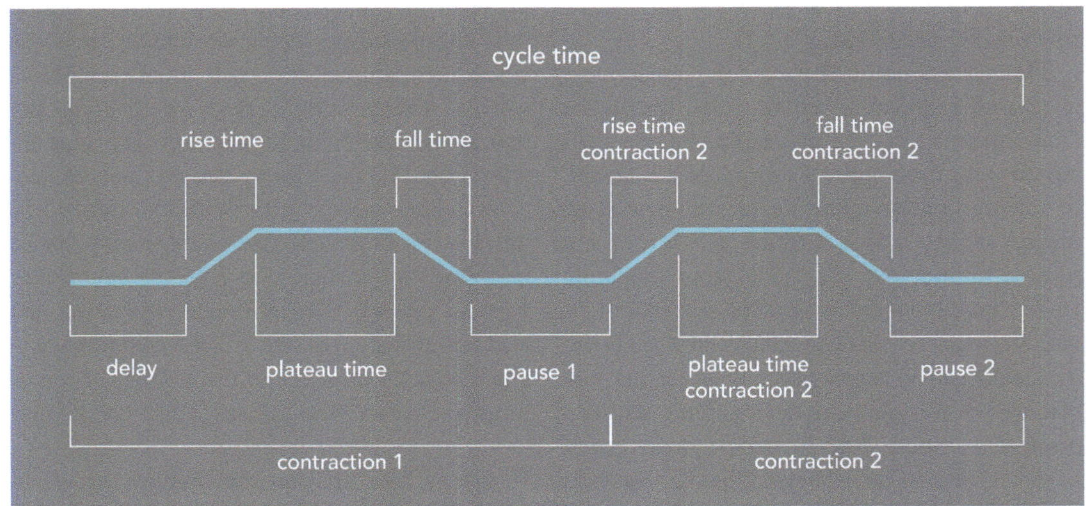


**Fig. 6.2** Describes the different stimulation phases within a stimulation cycle, as illustrated by practical examples in the following practical sections

**Table 6.5** provides an overview of the options for symptom-dependent therapy

| | paresis & plegia | spastic syndrome | ataxia |
| --- | --- | --- | --- |
| move object to mouth | ✓ | ✓ | ✓ |
| grasp and release object | ✓ | ✓ | ✓ |
| grasp bilateral with mirror | ✓ | | |
| wipe unilateral | ✓ | | ✓ |
| arm support unilateral | ✓ | ✓ | ✓ |
| grasp and move an object | ✓ | ✓ | ✓ |
| shoulder stabilization with subluxation | ✓ | | |
| grasp and lift the arm more than 90° | ✓ | ✓ | ✓ |
| forearm supination/pronation | ✓ | | ✓ |
| key grip | ✓ | | ✓ |
| tripod grip | ✓ | | ✓ |
| spherical grip | ✓ | | ✓ |
| opposition grip | ✓ | | ✓ |
| bridging | ✓ | | ✓ |
| ankle joint coordination | ✓ | ✓ | ✓ |
| stand up unilateral | ✓ | | ✓ |
| stand up and step | ✓ | | ✓ |
| stand up bilateral | ✓ | | ✓ |
| single leg stance | ✓ | | ✓ |
| lunge from standing position | ✓ | | ✓ |
| walk with rollator | ✓ | ✓ | ✓ |

## 6.3  EMG-MES to Improve Arm/Hand Function

To increase comprehensibility, practical examples of EMG-MES for the upper extremities to improve arm/hand functions (in this section) are separated from those for the lower extremities for therapy and improvement of postural control and mobility (Sect. 6.4). FES appears to be a promising tool for improving UL function in post-stroke patients, according to a recent narrative review [46]. The activities presented represent selected examples of therapy, are highly variable depending on the needs of the patient, and in many cases require individualization. Furthermore, countless of the therapy options are conceivable and applicable in everyday therapy.

EMG-MES is excellent for improving motor function of the upper extremities and trunk muscles and the activity levels in the clinical setting, which leads to an innovative approach in numerous neurorehabilitation facilities.

The stimulation parameters adapted to the respective activities are explained in detail.

### 6.3.1 Move Object to Mouth

The aim of this activity is to enable the patient to grasp objects such as a glass, a cup or food such as an apple and move them to the mouth so that they can be put down again in a controlled manner. The wrist extensor (extensor carpi radialis longus muscle) is chosen to initiate the movement to ensure hand function control. The finger flexors (flexor digitorum superficialis muscle) follow with a delay of 1 s and the elbow flexors (biceps brachii muscle) and the flexors of the shoulder joint (deltoideus muscle, pars clavicularis) with a further delay of 1 s. The prolonged drop time allows the eccentric and controlled release of the elbow and shoulder joint flexors with the force of gravity for safer object placement. The selected frequency and pulse width is suitable for muscular activation and prevents premature fatigue of the paretic muscles (Table 6.6, Fig. 6.3 and Video 6.1).

### 6.3.2 Grasp and Release Object

The therapeutic focus of this activity is on the activated stretching of the fingers I–V (extensor digitorum muscle; extensor pollicis longus muscle) to open the hand. Subsequently, the object is grasped by the flexor muscles (flexor digitorum superficialis muscle; flexor pollicis longus muscle), and a second contraction again activates the extension of the thumb and fingers II–V for release. The length of the pause time depends on the task. If the focus is on the repetitive approach and the patient is able to grasp a big number of objects while function is already present or beginning, the pause time can be reduced accordingly. Several affected patients usually require longer pause times. A longer rise

time for the finger extensors is useful in cases of severe spasticity or reflex tendency of the flexors. The selected frequency and pulse width are suitable for muscular activation and prevent premature fatigue of the paretic muscles (Table 6.7, Fig. 6.4 and Video 6.2).

### 6.3.3 Grasp Bilateral with Mirror

This activity has been shown to improve arm/hand function in stroke patients with high motor impairment [20]. A bilateral grasping movement is performed. Using the wrist extensors (extensor carpi radialis longus muscle) and the finger flexors (flexor digitorum superficialis muscle), which follow with a 1-s delay, the desired movement is performed. EMG triggering takes place via the less affected side. The mirror is directed toward the less affected side and thus mirrors the grasping movement of this hand. Both the use of the mirror illusion and a low EMG trigger threshold that allows synchronous movement of the affected hand to match the visual feedback are crucial. The therapist positions the affected hand in an appropriate starting position and does not provide tactile support during the movement. The intensity of the current should be selected to make the tactile-kinesthetic information as comparable as possible on both sides. In severely impaired patients, the frequency and pulse width are selected in a way that premature fatigue of the paretic musculature is mostly avoided (Table 6.8, Fig. 6.5 and Video 6.3).

### 6.3.4 Wipe Unilateral

Wiping is a very practical everyday activity with a synergistic and antagonistic sequence of movements. The patient sits at the table with the affected arm resting on it. He/She grasps, e.g., a cloth or towel, and performs a wiping movement during stimulation. The cloth or towel prevents additional friction effects and thus allows the wiping movement in a simplified manner. The prolonged rise and fall times overlap and thus lead to a coordinated movement. In this example, the infraspina-

**Table 6.6** Stimulation parameters for the activity "Move object to mouth"

### MOVE OBJECT TO MOUTH
objective: grasp and hold an object, then move it to the mouth and put it down again

| frequency: 35 Hz<br>pulse width: 300 µs | contraction 1 | | | | |
| --- | --- | --- | --- | --- | --- |
| | delay | rise time | plateau time | fall time | pause 1 |
| **channel 1**<br>M. extensor carpi radialis longus | 0 | 1 | 8 | 2,5 | 4,5 |
| **channel 2**<br>M. flexor digitorum superficialis | 1 | 1 | 7 | 2,5 | 4,5 |
| **channel 3**<br>M. biceps brachii | 2 | 1,5 | 5 | 2,5 | 5 |
| **channel 4**<br>M. deltoideus, Pars clavicularis | 2 | 1,5 | 5 | 2,5 | 5 |

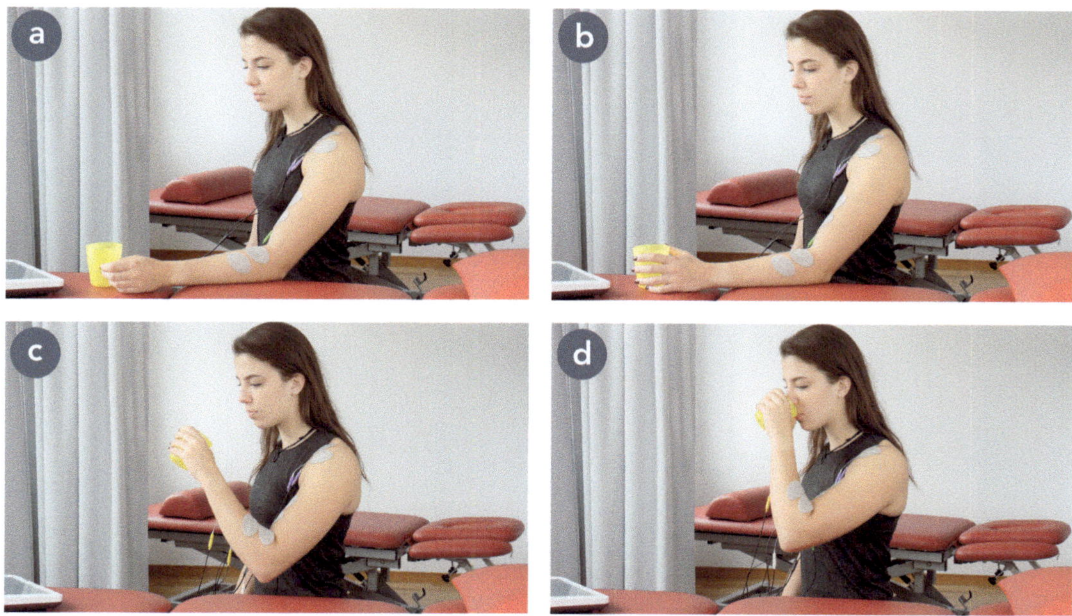

**Fig. 6.3** Movement sequence of the activity "Move object to mouth"

**Table 6.7** Stimulation parameters for the activity "Grasp and release object"

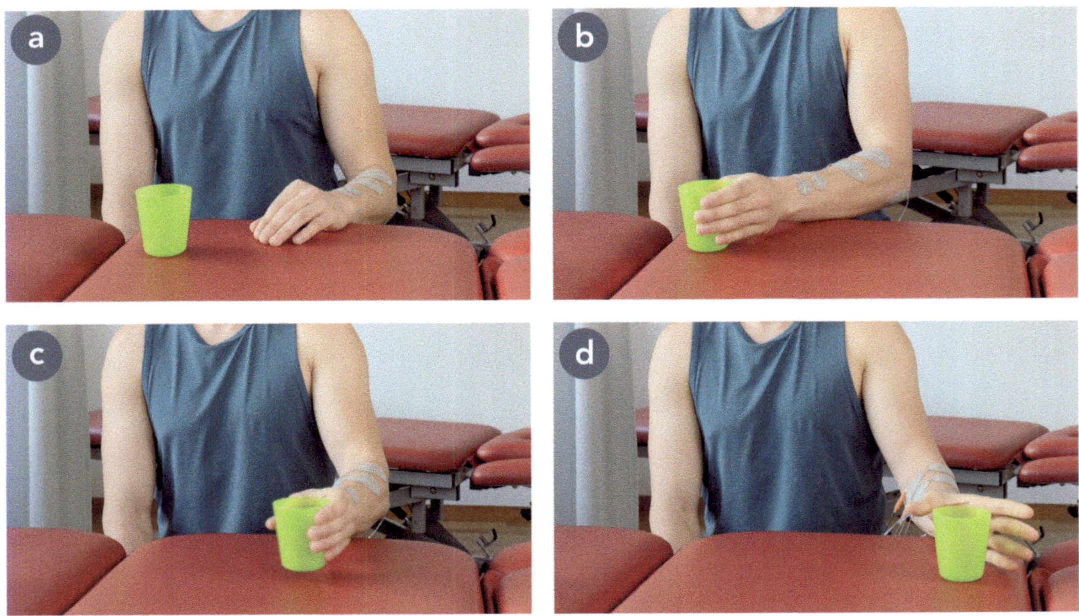



| frequency: 35 Hz<br>pulse width: 300 µs | contraction 1 | | | | | contraction 2 | | | |
|---|---|---|---|---|---|---|---|---|---|
| | delay | rise time | plateau time | fall time | pause 1 | rise time c2 | plateau time c2 | fall time c2 | pause 2 |
| channel 1<br>M. extensor digitorum | 0 | 1 | 2 | 1 | 2 | 1 | 2 | 1 | 4 |
| channel 2<br>M. extensor pollicis longus | 0 | 1 | 2 | 1 | 2 | 1 | 2 | 1 | 4 |
| channel 3<br>M. flexor digitorum superficialis | 2 | 1 | 3 | 1 | 7 | 0 | 0 | 0 | 0 |
| channel 4<br>M. flexor pollicis longus | 2 | 1 | 3 | 1 | 7 | 0 | 0 | 0 | 0 |

**Fig. 6.4** Movement sequence of the activity "Grasp and release object"

**Table 6.8** Stimulation parameters for the activity "Grasp bilateral with mirror"

### GRASP BILATERAL (with mirror)
objective: movement initiation of the affected hand using a bilateral grasping movement, additional use of the mirror illusion of the less affected hand

| frequency: 35 Hz<br>pulse width: 300 µs | contraction 1 | | | | |
| --- | --- | --- | --- | --- | --- |
| | delay | rise time | plateau time | fall time | pause 1 |
| **channel 1** M. extensor carpi radialis longus | 0 | 1,5 | 3 | 1,5 | 6 |
| **channel 2** M. flexor digitorum superficialis | 1 | 1,5 | 2 | 1,5 | 6 |
| **channel 3** M. extensor carpi radialis longus | 0 | 1,5 | 3 | 1,5 | 6 |
| **channel 4** M. flexor digitorum superficialis | 1 | 1,5 | 2 | 1,5 | 6 |

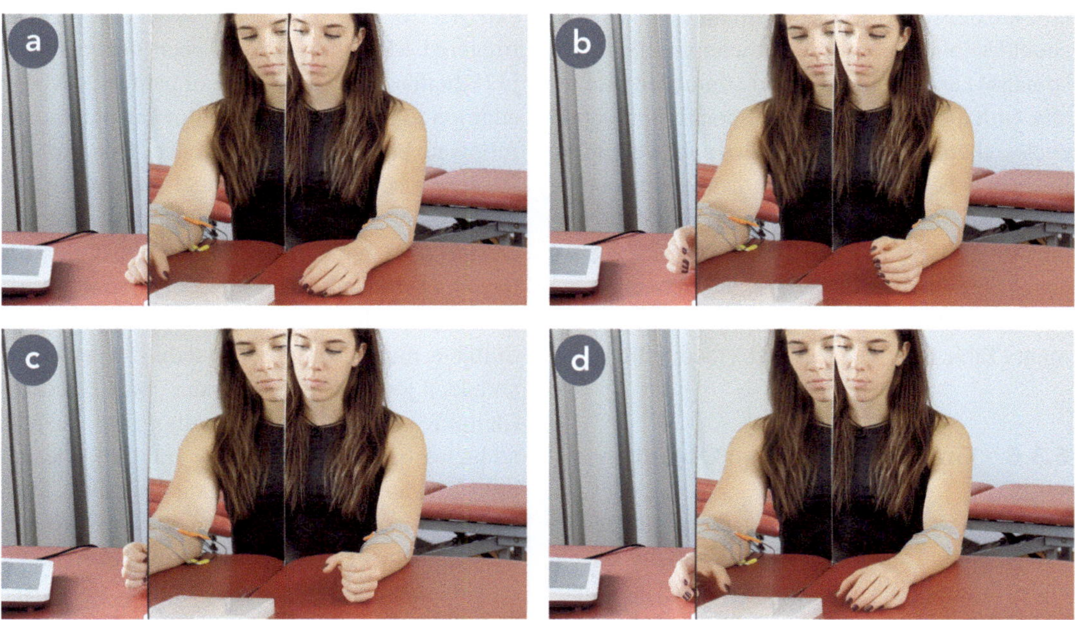

**Fig. 6.5** Movement sequence of the activity "Grasp bilateral with mirror"

tus muscle functions as the shoulder joint external rotator. Alternatively, the teres minor muscle can also be used here. This is followed by an extension, internal rotation in the shoulder joint (latissimus dorsi muscle) or, alternatively, the teres major muscle followed by an adduction movement through the chest muscles (pectoralis major muscle). The movement is completed by an extension in the elbow joint (triceps brachii muscle). If the pause times are reduced to a minimum and the EMG trigger threshold is selected low, almost continuous alternating and superimposed stimulations and thus the wiping movement can be produced (Table 6.9, Fig. 6.6 and Video 6.4).

### 6.3.5  Support Arm Unilateral

This activity has a high everyday relevance for a large number of patients with a wide range of complaints. When standing up from a seated position, for example, extension of the wrist (extensor digitorum muscle) with simultaneous optimal finger extension ensures the necessary ventral weight shift. Alternatively, in the absence of finger joint extension, the wrist extensor (extensor carpi radialis longus muscle) can be selected. If the symptoms are bilateral, the finger or wrist extensors can be dispensed with the elbow extensors (triceps brachii muscles) and the shoulder joint extensors (deltoidei muscles, pars spinalis) can also be used and stimulated bilaterally with a short delay of 1 s. Shorter stimulation cycles should rather be selected when standing up than when supporting on a treatment table. Short rise times can be helpful to facilitate support to standing in a timely manner. If the arms are to bear more body weight, the frequency can be increased to 50 Hz to increase muscle recruitment (Table 6.10, Fig. 6.7 and Video 6.5).

### 6.3.6  Grasp and Move an Object

In addition to the grasping activity, the seated patient should move the object spatially on the table surface before releasing it again. This stimulation pattern is suitable for guiding a patient out of his flexion synergy into an antagonistic movement. The movement is initiated with the wrist extensor (extensor carpi radialis longus muscle). With a delay of 1 s, the finger flexors (flexor digitorum superficialis muscle) come into action. After that, the elbow extensor (biceps brachii muscle) and the shoulder joint flexor (deltoideus muscle, pars clavicularis) are activated for a further second. In this movement, the focus could also be placed on finger extension for active grasping and late release, which would be emphasized by a second contraction. The selected frequency and pulse width is well suited for muscular activation and prevents early fatigue of the paretic muscles (Table 6.11, Fig. 6.8 and Video 6.6).

### 6.3.7  Shoulder Stabilization (with Shoulder Subluxation)

Patients with hemiplegia or hemiparesis sometimes suffer from complications such as shoulder subluxation, which in many cases is accompanied by a significant pain syndrome. Since movement is often painful in the early phase, activity can be performed in a sitting position with weight bearing of the arm by resting the forearm. From this position, smaller movements in the shoulder joint can be trained, especially in the direction of external rotation. The success of this EMG-triggered MES has already been demonstrated [37]. In this study, the degree of pain improved in addition to function, so the following parameters follow up based on this experience. This explains the long rise and fall times and the plateau and pause times. The delay for the external rotator can be used for a stroke-free external rotatory movement like pushing away a balloon. It should still be possible to select a low trigger threshold. Suitable muscle groups for stabilization in the shoulder joint are the shoulder joint extensors (deltoid muscle, pars spinalis), the scapula adductor (rhomboideus major muscle), the initial shoulder joint abductor (supraspinatus muscle), and the shoulder joint external rotator (infraspinatus muscle). To avoid movement-induced pain, a prolonged rise time can be used with the arm in an adapted position. A reduction

**Table 6.9** Stimulation parameters for the activity "Wipe unilateral"

### WIPE UNILATERAL
objective: wiping movement with the affected arm while sitting at the table

| frequency: 35 Hz<br>pulse width: 300 µs | contraction 1 | | | | |
|---|---|---|---|---|---|
| | delay | rise time | plateau time | fall time | pause 1 |
| **channel 1**<br>M. infraspinatus | 0 | 1,5 | 2 | 1,5 | 6 |
| **channel 2**<br>M. latissimus dorsi | 2 | 1,5 | 2 | 1,5 | 4 |
| **channel 3**<br>M. pectoralis major | 4 | 1,5 | 2 | 1,5 | 2 |
| **channel 4**<br>M triceps brachii | 6 | 1,5 | 2 | 1,5 | 0 |

alternative channel 1: M. teres minor, channel 2: M. teres major

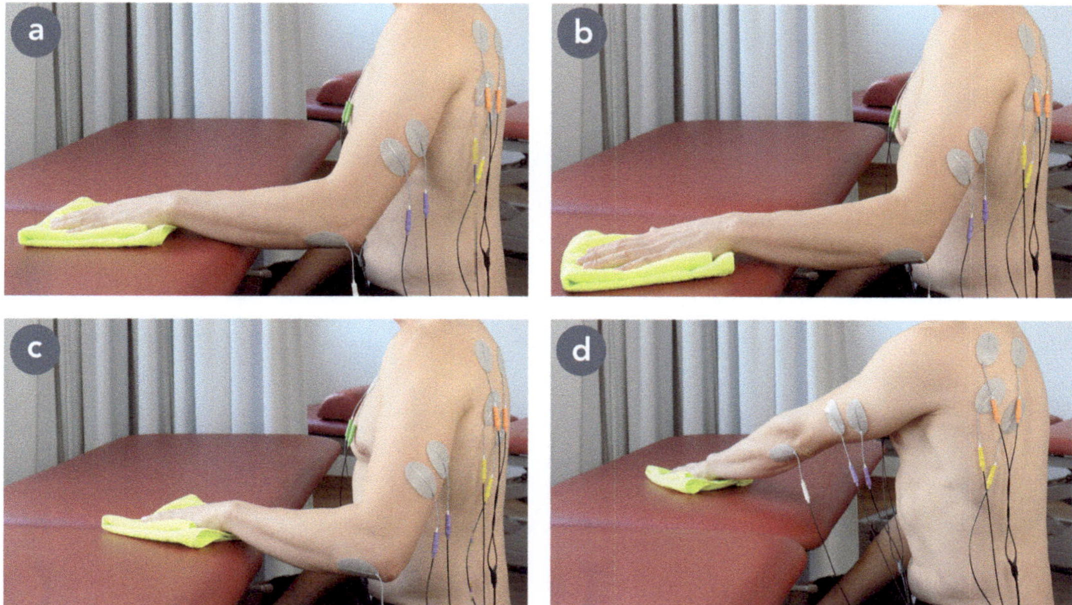

**Fig. 6.6** Movement sequence of the activity "Wipe unilateral"

**Table 6.10** Stimulation parameters for the activity "Support arm unilateral"

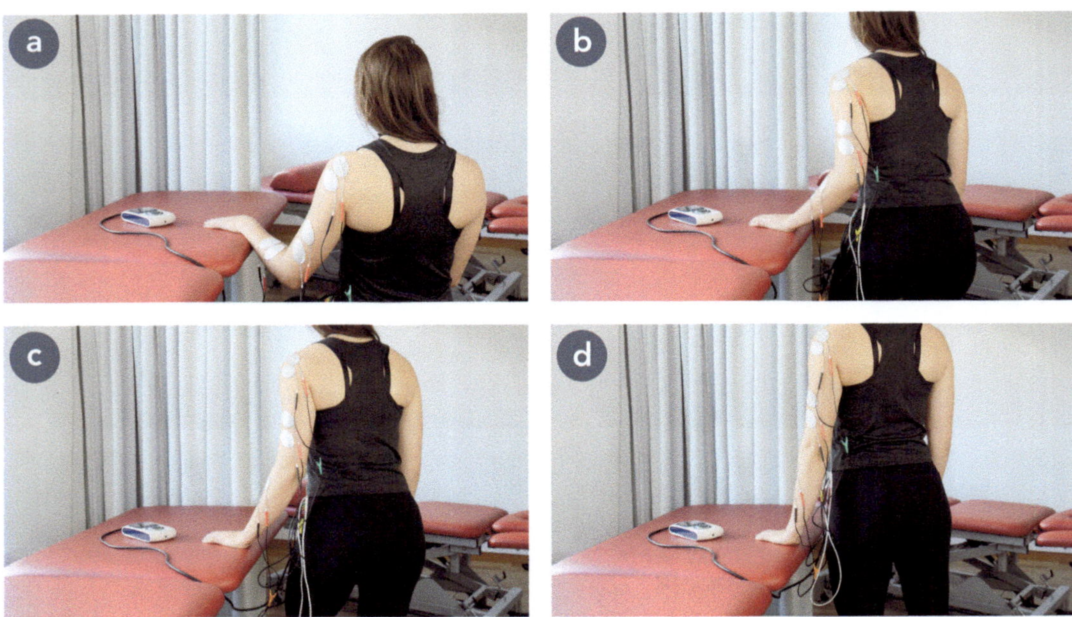



**Fig. 6.7** Movement sequence of the activity "Support arm unilateral"

**Table 6.11** Stimulation parameters for the activity "Grasp and move an object"

| GRASP AND MOVE AN OBJECT | | | | | |
| objective: grasping an object and moving it on a tabletop | | | | | |
| **frequency: 35 Hz**<br>**pulse width: 300 μs** | contraction 1 | | | | |
| | delay | rise time | plateau time | fall time | pause 1 |
| **channel 1**<br>M. extensor carpi radialis longus | 0 | 1 | 4 | 1 | 4 |
| **channel 2**<br>M. flexor digitorum superficialis | 1 | 1,5 | 3 | 1 | 4 |
| **channel 3**<br>M triceps brachii | 2 | 1,5 | 2 | 1 | 3,5 |
| **channel 4**<br>M. deltoideus , Pars clavicularis | 2 | 1,5 | 2 | 1 | 3,5 |

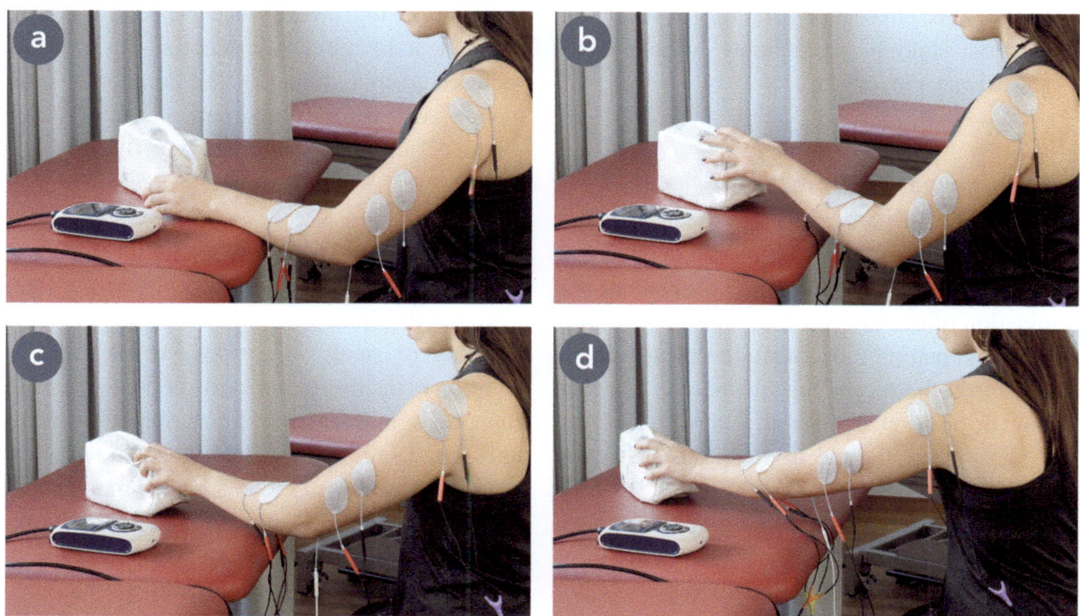

**Fig. 6.8** Movement sequence of the activity "Grasp and move an object"

of the pulse width can reduce the sensory load caused by the stimulation in an existing pain situation and, if necessary, allows a higher intensity for a better motor response (Table 6.12, Fig. 6.9, and Video 6.7).

### 6.3.8 Grasp and Lift Arm More Than 90°

For patients with moderate to mild shoulder function deficits, this activity can be used to train reaching a level with the arm or hand above shoulder girdle level. Task-oriented objects should be used to clarify the task and the degree of goal achievement. The anterior shoulder joint flexor (deltoideus muscle, pars clavicularis) starts the movement by flexing the arm in the shoulder joint. The scapula muscle (rhomboideus major muscle) stabilizes the scapula, while the external rotator (infraspinatus muscle) supports the external rotation necessary for elevation. Alternatively, to the rhomboideus major muscle, the serratus anterior muscle has also proven to be effective and additionally emphasizes scapular rotation. With a further delay, the elbow extension (triceps brachii muscle) takes place to enable the targeting of the hand. Since this movement involves long levers against the force of gravity, the fall time should be chosen long enough to prevent the arm from falling prematurely (Table 6.13, Fig. 6.10 and Video 6.8).

### 6.3.9 Forearm Supination/ Pronation

The activity allows alternating pronation and supination of the forearm like for screw turning. For the supinating movement, the most suitable supinator is the biceps brachii muscle. The arm should be positioned in elbow joint with less than 90° flexion and the electrodes positioned more distally on the biceps brachii muscle. This emphasizes less the flexion and more the supinator component. Alternatively, the supinator muscle can be selected. However, since it is located deeper, it is usually more difficult to localize and

more challenging to reach for successful electrode position. As a result, unwanted movements of other muscle groups, such as the elbow flexors, can often be stimulated as well. Slightly prolonged and partially overlapping rise and fall times for a short time reduce the possibility of increasing muscle tension of the reflex-enhanced musculature. The pronator (pronator teres muscle) is located in the proximal quarter of the ventral forearm and, although low-lying, can be stimulated well and specifically. If the EMG threshold is low, continuous sequences of movements are chosen, and a stimulation close to the action can be achieved (Table 6.14, Fig. 6.11 and Video 6.9).

### 6.3.10 Key Grip

This gripping function can be used in everyday life to pick up and hold an object such as a key. The thumb adductor (adductor pollicis muscle) fixes the object with only a short delay (1 s) by exerting pressure on the loosely fisted hand. The wrist extensor (extensor carpi radialis longus muscle) stabilizes the wrist, and the long finger flexor (flexor digitorum superficialis muscle) ensures the slightly fisted hand position and thus enables simultaneously bringing the thumb and index finger together. Extended rise times allow the patient to arbitrarily adapt his grip to the required grasping function. The duration of stimulation and pause times depend on the task (Table 6.15, Fig. 6.12 and Video 6.10).

### 6.3.11 Tripod Grip

The tripod grip is well suited to the purposeful grasping of small objects in everyday life. In addition to the fine motor skills of the fingers 1–3 (opponens pollicis muscle; lumbricalis manus muscles, Digiti II-III), the stabilization in the wrist (extensor carpi radialis longus muscle) is a prerequisite. A short delay of 1 s is sufficient for the flexor muscles in the metacarpophalangeal joints in many cases. The electrode position can be chosen exclusively on the dorsal side distally

**Table 6.12** Stimulation parameters for the activity "Shoulder stabilization (with shoulder subluxation)"

**SHOULDER STABILIZATION (with subluxation)**
objective: stabilization of the plegic shoulder joint in subluxation with or without pain

| frequency: 35 Hz<br>pulse width: 200 μs | contraction 1 | | | | |
|---|---|---|---|---|---|
| | delay | rise time | plateau time | fall time | pause 1 |
| **channel 1** M. deltoideus, Pars spinalis | 0 | 1,5 | 11,5 | 2 | 5 |
| **channel 2** M. rhomboideus major | 1 | 2 | 9 | 2 | 6 |
| **channel 3** M. supraspinatus | 1 | 2 | 9 | 2 | 6 |
| **channel 4** M. infraspinatus | 2 | 2 | 8 | 2 | 6 |

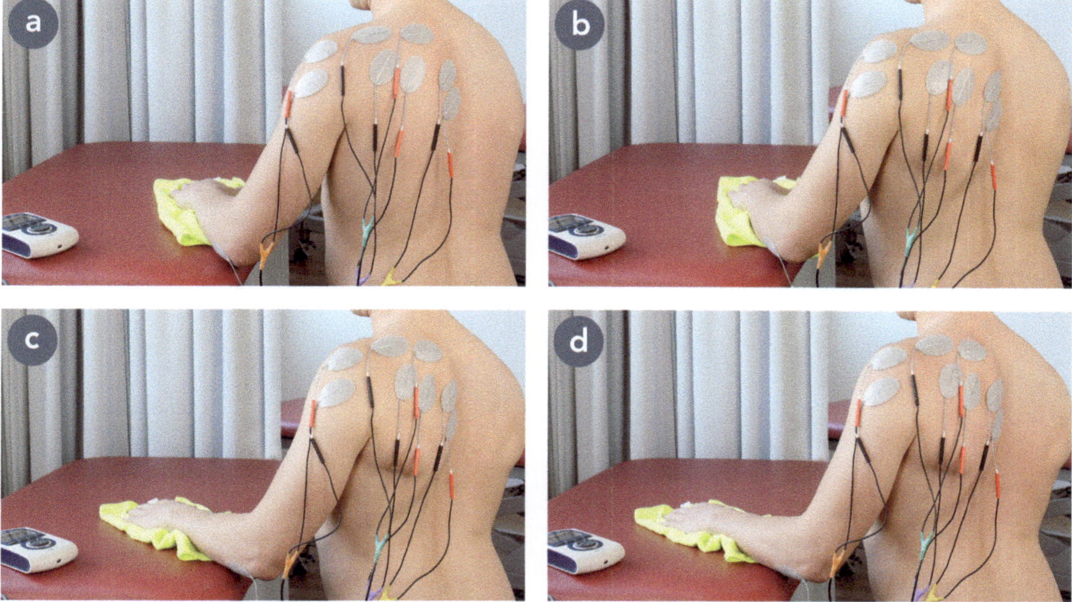

**Fig. 6.9** Movement sequence of the activity "Shoulder Stabilization with shoulder subluxation"

**Table 6.13** Stimulation parameters for the activity "Grasp and lift arm more than 90°"

| GRASP AND LIFT THE ARM MORE THAN 90°<br>objective: lift the object and move it to a higher level | | | | | |
| --- | --- | --- | --- | --- | --- |
| frequency: 35 Hz<br>pulse width: 300 µs | contraction 1 | | | | |
| | delay | rise time | plateau time | fall time | pause 1 |
| **channel 1**<br>M. deltoideus, Pars clavicularis | 0 | 1 | 5 | 2,5 | 6 |
| **channel 2**<br>M. rhomboideus major | 1 | 1 | 3 | 2,5 | 7 |
| **channel 3**<br>M. infraspinatus | 1 | 1 | 3 | 2,5 | 7 |
| **channel 4**<br>M. triceps brachii | 2 | 1 | 2 | 2,5 | 7 |

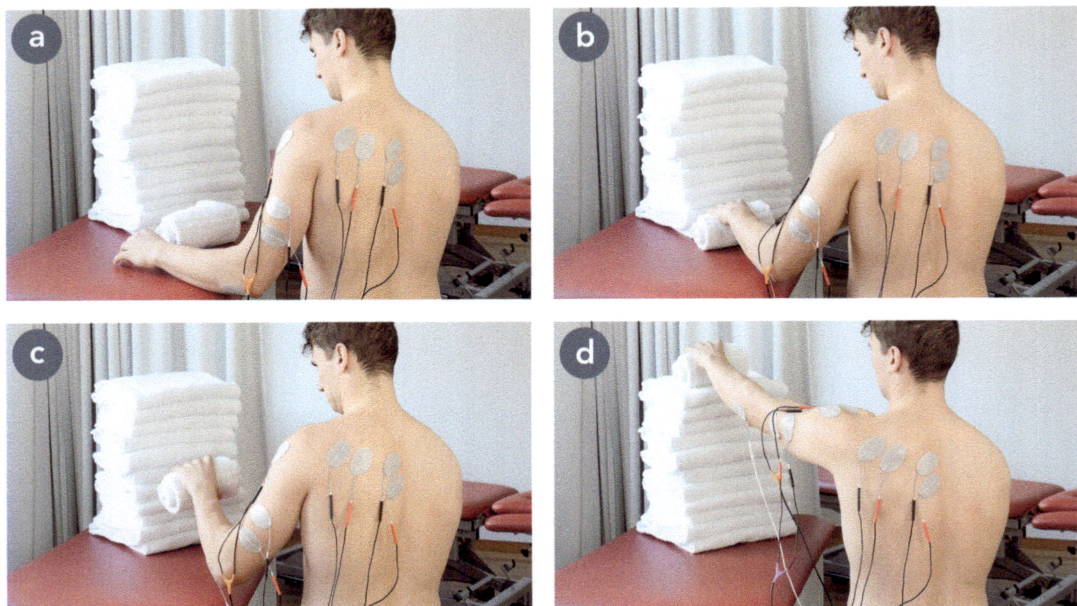

**Fig. 6.10** Movement sequence of the activity "Grasp and lift arm more than 90°"

**Table 6.14** Stimulation parameters for the activity "Forearm supination/pronation"

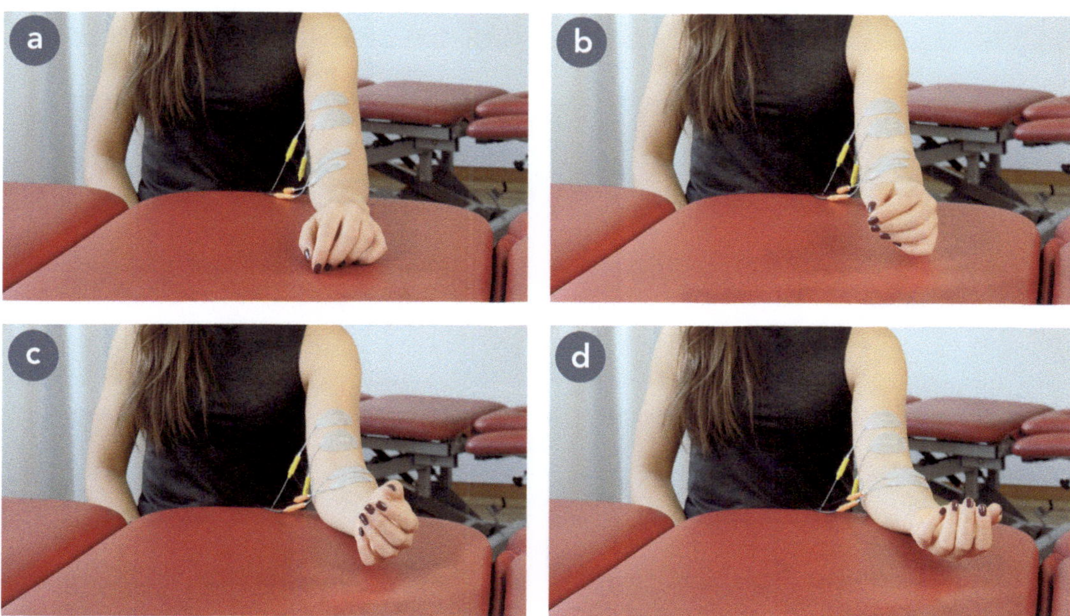



| frequency: 35 Hz<br>pulse width: 300 µs | contraction 1 | | | | |
|---|---|---|---|---|---|
| | delay | rise time | plateau time | fall time | pause 1 |
| channel 1<br>M. biceps brachii | 0 | 1 | 2 | 1 | 3 |
| channel 2<br>M. pronator teres | 3 | 1 | 2 | 1 | 0 |



**Fig. 6.11** Movement sequence of the activity "Forearm supination/pronation"

on the hand or alternatively dorsally on the back of the hand and at the same time palmar of the hand. The rise time is 1 s in order not to provoke an excessive tonus of the flexors in case of reflex-increased finger and wrist flexors. The activity can be very well integrated into task-oriented training if the patient is able to grasp and transport objects. In this case, a shorter pause time can be selected accordingly (Table 6.16, Fig. 6.13, and Video 6.11).

**Table 6.15** Stimulation parameters for the activity "Key grip"

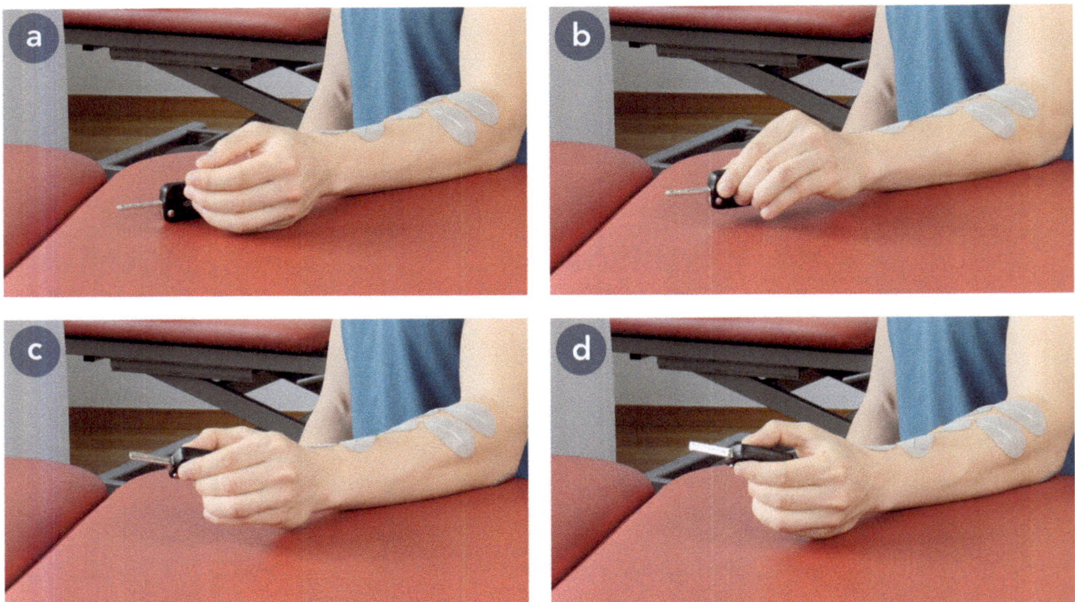

KEY GRIP
objective: holding objects between thumb and hand

| frequency: 35 Hz<br>pulse width: 300 µs | contraction 1 | | | | |
| --- | --- | --- | --- | --- | --- |
| | delay | rise time | plateau time | fall time | pause 1 |
| channel 1<br>M. extensor carpi radialis longus | 0 | 1 | 4 | 1,5 | 3 |
| channel 2<br>M. adductor pollicis | 1 | 2 | 3 | 1,5 | 2 |
| channel 3<br>M. flexor digitorum superficialis | 1 | 2 | 3 | 1,5 | 2 |

**Fig. 6.12** Movement sequence of the activity "Key grip"

**Table 6.16** Stimulation parameters for the activity "Tripod grip"

| TRIPOD GRIP | | | | |
|---|---|---|---|---|
| objective: merging the thumb with the index and middle finger to grasp small objects | | | | |

| frequency: 35 Hz<br>pulse width: 300 µs | contraction 1 | | | | |
|---|---|---|---|---|---|
| | delay | rise time | plateau time | fall time | pause 1 |
| **channel 1**<br>M. extensor carpi radialis longus | 0 | 1 | 3 | 1,5 | 3 |
| **channel 2**<br>Mm. lumbricales manus (Digiti II–III) | 1 | 1 | 2 | 1,5 | 3 |
| **channel 3**<br>M. opponens pollicis | 1 | 1 | 2 | 1,5 | 3 |

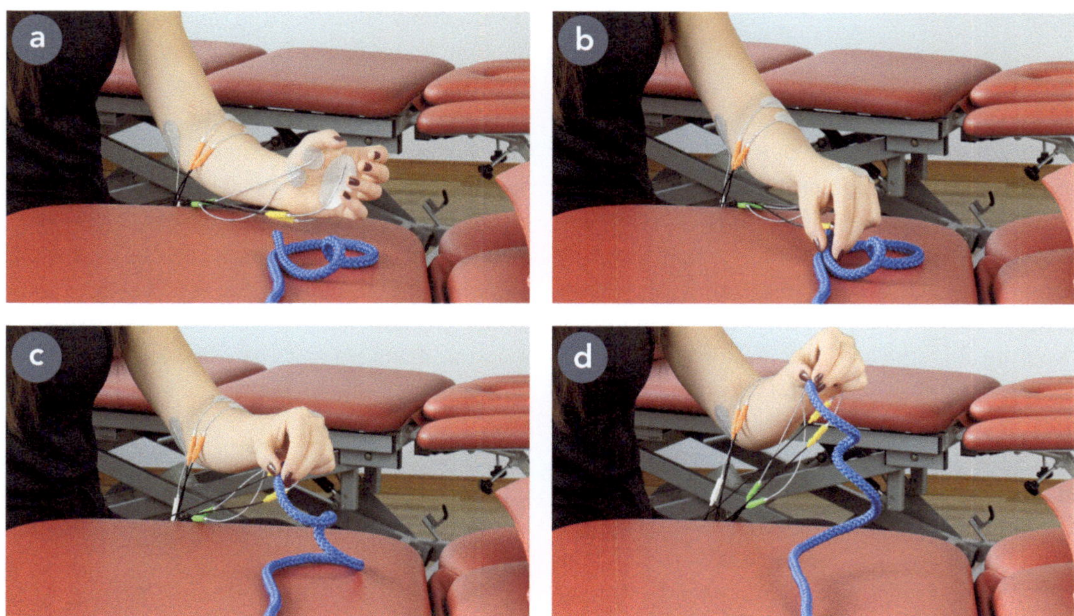

**Fig. 6.13** Movement sequence of the activity "Tripod grip"

### 6.3.12 Spherical Grip

The spherical grip is used, for example, to grasp and lift an object from above. It differs from the tripod grip because all fingers are used when grasping a larger object, such as a ball. The current intensity of the wrist extensor (extensor carpi radialis longus muscle) should be selected only high enough to stabilize the wrist, but not to achieve a dorsiflexion above 0 degrees. Typically, the wrist is slightly flexed. The lumbrical muscles adduct and flex in the base joint with simultaneous extension in the middle and end joints of the fingers. The electrode position can be chosen exclusively on the dorsal side distally on the hand or alternatively dorsally on the dorsum of the hand and simultaneously palmar of the hand. An application of the electrodes exclusively on the palmar side of the hand is usually inferior to the dorsal application technique in practice. Stimulation of the lumbrical muscles on the dorsal side of the hand has proven to be successful in many cases (Table 6.17, Fig. 6.14 and Video 6.12).

### 6.3.13 Opposition Grip

Depending on the shape and form of the object to be grasped, the anatomy of the human hand allows the thumb to be positioned in relation to the fingers II-V. In the form of finger insertion shown here, the tips of the thumb should be brought together at the same time as the tip of the little finger. The opposition grip is used as an alternative grip movement for picking up very small objects. Depending on the length of the pause following the stimulation phase, the activity can be used for repetitive picking up of small objects in therapy. After triggering and subsequent stabilization of the wrist by the wrist extensor (extensor carpi radialis longus muscle), the two digiti I (opponens pollicis muscle) and V (opponens digiti minimi muscle) are opposed with a delay of 1 s (Table 6.18, Fig. 6.15 and Video 6.13).

## 6.4 EMG-MES to Improve Postural Control and Mobility

Postural control and mobility are key motor goals in neurorehabilitation at the functional and activity level. The EMG-MES-supported activities described in the following are clinically relevant and have already proven themselves in practice many times.

In some of the exercise examples described here, a higher frequency was deliberately chosen to achieve a higher degree of recruitment of the muscle fibers. This is necessitated by the fact that activities such as standing up require greater force development against the force of gravity. The application of EMG-MES to the lower extremities and trunk allows the use of larger stimulation electrodes. This leads to an increase in the stimulation area and thus to an increased recruitment of muscle fibers to overcome gravity.

### 6.4.1 Bridging

This activity is designed to improve the range of motion from the supine position in preparation for a transfer in bed or from bed to a seat. The legs are ankled during this activity. The movement is initiated via a posterior tilt of the pelvis by EMG-triggered electrical bilateral stimulation of the gluteus maximus muscle. With a very short delay of 0.5 s, bilateral stimulation of the quadriceps femoris muscles occurs for additional overcoming of gravity. When lowering the pelvis, a fall time extended to 2 s can be selected for better eccentric control. In this example, a higher frequency (50 Hz) was chosen to recruit more muscle fiber portions during electrical stimulation (Table 6.19, Fig. 6.16 and Video 6.14).

### 6.4.2 Ankle Joint Coordination

Training of active ankle dorsiflexion (tibialis anterior muscle) and plantar flexion (gastrocnemius muscle) by patient-initiated impulse trig-

**Table 6.17** Stimulation parameters for the activity "Spherical grip"

SPHERICAL GRIP<br>objective: grasping an object from above with all fingers with slightly bent,<br>but stabilized wristk

| frequency: 35 Hz<br>pulse width: 300 µs | contraction 1 | | | | |
| --- | --- | --- | --- | --- | --- |
| | delay | rise time | plateau time | fall time | pause 1 |
| channel 1<br>M. extensor carpi radialis longus | 0 | 1,5 | 5 | 1 | 5 |
| channel 2<br>Mm. lumbricales manus (digiti II–V) | 1 | 1,5 | 4 | 1 | 5 |
| channel 3<br>M. opponens pollicis | 1 | 1,5 | 4 | 1 | 5 |

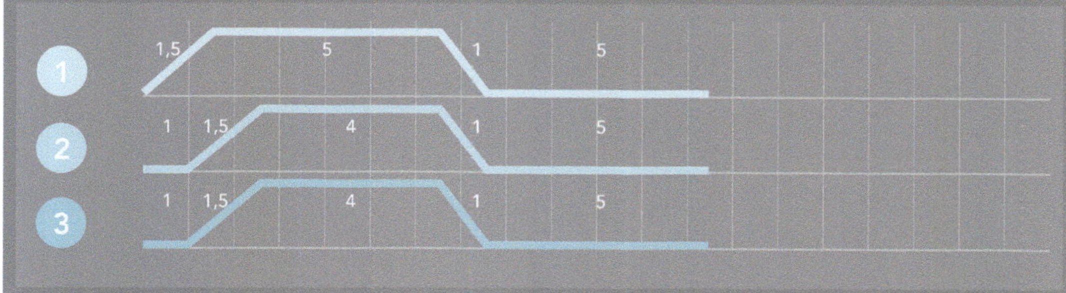

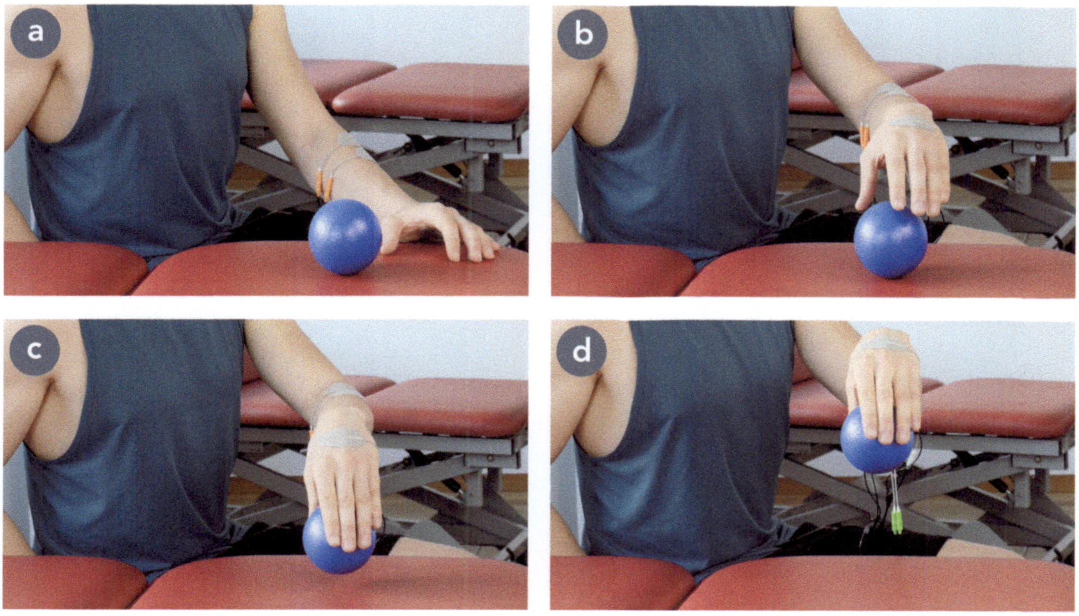

**Fig. 6.14** Movement sequence of the activity "Spherical grip"

**Table 6.18** Stimulation parameters for the activity "Opposition grip"

| OPPOSITION GRIP objective: merging the thumb with the little finger to optionally pick up small objects | | | | | |
| --- | --- | --- | --- | --- | --- |
| frequency: 35 Hz pulse width: 300 µs | contraction 1 | | | | |
| | delay | rise time | plateau time | fall time | pause 1 |
| channel 1 M. extensor carpi radialis longus | 0 | 1 | 4 | 1 | 4 |
| channel 2 M. opponens pollicis | 1 | 1 | 3 | 1 | 4 |
| channel 3 M. opponens digiti minimi | 1 | 1 | 3 | 1 | 4 |

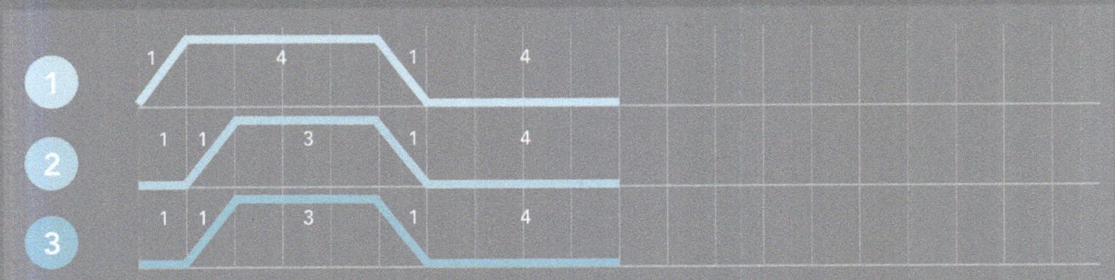

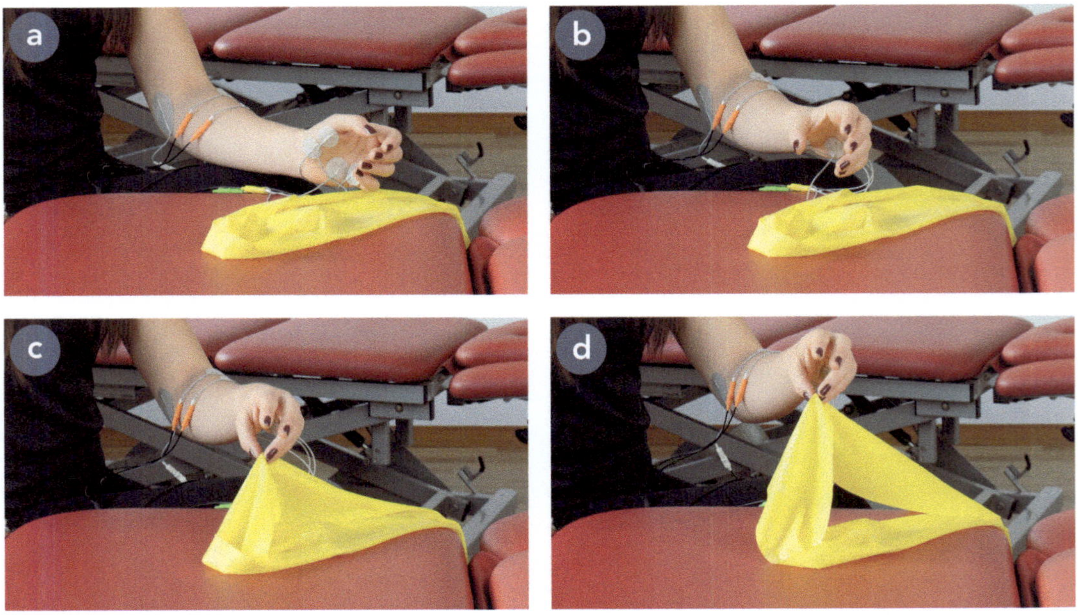

**Fig. 6.15** Movement sequence of the activity "Opposition grip"

gering in a sitting position or optionally in a standing position with a standing leg phase on the affected side and the side that should be trained.

Long rise and fall times allow dynamic movement through superimposition and avoid an unwanted increase in tone in hypertonic or reflex

**Table 6.19** Stimulation parameters for the activity "Bridging"

| BRIDGING<br>objective: lifting the pelvis in supine position with the legs in an upright position and changing the position | | | | | |
|---|---|---|---|---|---|
| frequency: 50 Hz<br>pulse width: 300 µs | | | contraction 1 | | |
| | delay | rise time | plateau time | fall time | pause 1 |
| **channel 1** M. gluteus maximus | 0 | 1 | 4 | 2 | 5 |
| **channel 2** M. gluteus maximus | 0 | 1 | 4 | 2 | 5 |
| **channel 3** M. quadriceps femoris | 0,5 | 1 | 3,5 | 2 | 5 |
| **channel 4** M. quadriceps femoris | 0,5 | 1 | 3,5 | 2 | 5 |

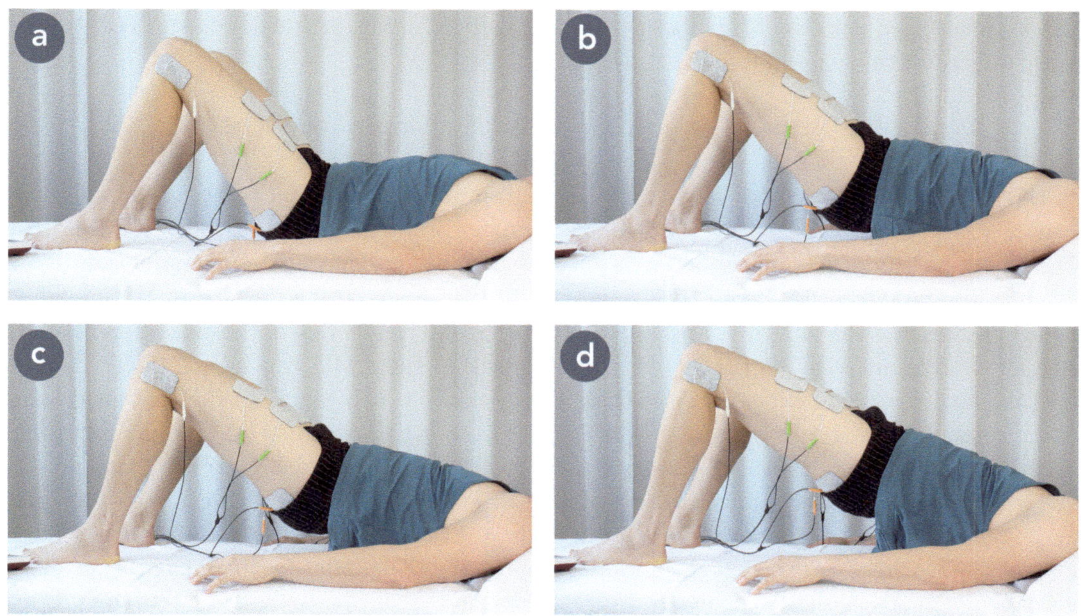

**Fig. 6.16** Movement sequence of the activity "Bridging"

enhanced muscle groups. Multichannel stimulation allows not only the dorsal extensor and plantar flexor components, but also inversion and eversion (extensor digitorum longus muscle; peronaeus longus muscle) to be specifically included in the movement sequence and trained alternately (Table 6.20, Fig. 6.17 and Video 6.15).

### 6.4.3 Stand Up Unilateral

The patient sits on a chair or stool with the feet in a walking position and the affected leg placed backward. This leads to weight transfer to this side when standing up. After active triggering of the dorsal extensor (tibialis anterior muscle), the body's center of gravity is moved over the ankle joint as an axis of rotation while the punctum fixum of the affected foot is present. This is followed by the antigravitational working muscle groups (quadriceps muscle; gastrocnemius muscle). To prevent unwanted knee joint recurvature on the affected side, the biceps femoris muscle from the ischiocrural muscle group is additionally activated with a time delay of 1 s to stabilize the knee joint. In order not to trigger the activity immediately after reaching the stance, a longer pause time can be selected as shown. Furthermore, a higher frequency (50 Hz) has been selected here for improved muscle recruitment (Table 6.21, Fig. 6.18 and Video 6.16).

### 6.4.4 Stand Up and Step

The patient starts from a sitting position via a stepping position in which the affected leg is positioned backward. The activity of the tibialis anterior muscle starts by triggering the EMG threshold and supports the forward displacement of the center of gravity over the ankle joint. The quadriceps femoris muscle works antigravitatorily and is supported by the biceps femoris muscle at the end of the movement to prevent possible knee joint recurvature. The second contractions for the quadriceps femoris muscle and tibialis anterior muscles on the affected side support the equilat-

eral play leg phase with active knee joint extension, active ankle joint dorsiflexion, and subsequent holding and eccentric release of the foot lifts in the "Initial Contact" to "Loading Response" phases. In this example, a higher frequency (50 Hz) is also selected for improved muscle recruitment (Table 6.22, Fig. 6.19 and Video 6.17).

### 6.4.5 Stand Up Bilateral

Patients with a significant strength restriction of the muscle groups in the thigh and trunk required for standing up receive significant muscular support, but also sensory guidance during the movement sequence. In this activity, the selection of the largest possible electrode pairs for the thigh muscles (quadriceps femoris muscles) on both sides should be considered. In this way, the largest possible proportion of contractile muscle fibers can be recruited by the stimulation. It is recommended to place the electrodes in the middle to lower third of the thoracic spine. Depending on the position of the electrodes, stimulation of the deep back extensors (erector spinae muscle) also reaches superficial muscle groups of the trapezius muscle, pars transversa or pars ascendence, which are responsible for retraction of the shoulder girdle and adduction of the two scapulae (Table 6.23, Fig. 6.20 and Video 6.18).

### 6.4.6 Single Leg Stance

To initiate the stance leg, the patient shifts his center of gravity toward the affected side. The patient "experiences" the increased stability in the stance leg during the electrical stimulation after EMG triggering of the quadriceps femoris muscle. The EMG trigger threshold must be selected in a way that tensing the quadriceps muscle while standing allows the threshold value to be exceeded. To reach as many muscle parts as possible, the largest possible electrodes should be used on the gluteal and thigh muscles. The plateau time can be selected depending on the activity of the playing leg phase. In this example, a time-delayed stimula-

**Table 6.20** Stimulation parameters for the activity "Ankle joint coordination"

**ANKLE JOINT COORDINATION (for foot lift weakness)**
objective: alternating dorsiflexion and plantarflexion of the ankle joint with simultaneous inversion and eversion.

| frequency: 35 Hz<br>pulse width: 300 μs | contraction 1 | | | | |
| --- | --- | --- | --- | --- | --- |
| | delay | rise time | plateau time | fall time | pause 1 |
| **channel 1**<br>M. tibialis anterior | 0 | 1,5 | 3 | 2 | 4,5 |
| **channel 2**<br>M. extensor digitorum longus | 0 | 1,5 | 3 | 2 | 4,5 |
| **channel 3**<br>M. gastrocnemius | 4,5 | 1,5 | 3 | 2 | 0 |
| **channel 4**<br>M. peroneus longus | 4,5 | 1,5 | 3 | 2 | 0 |

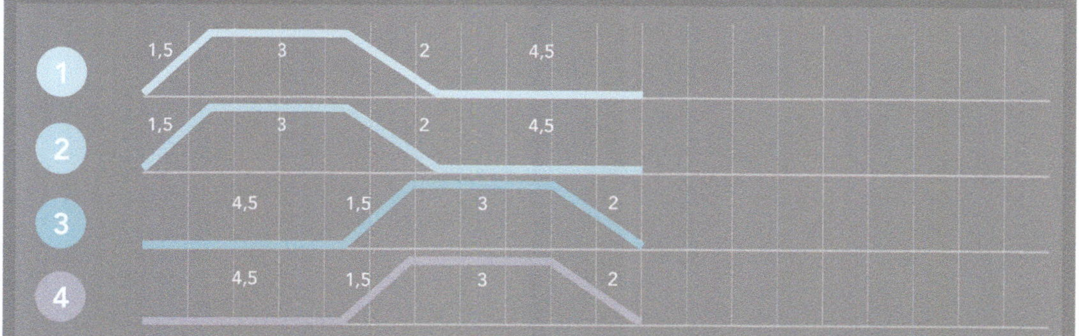

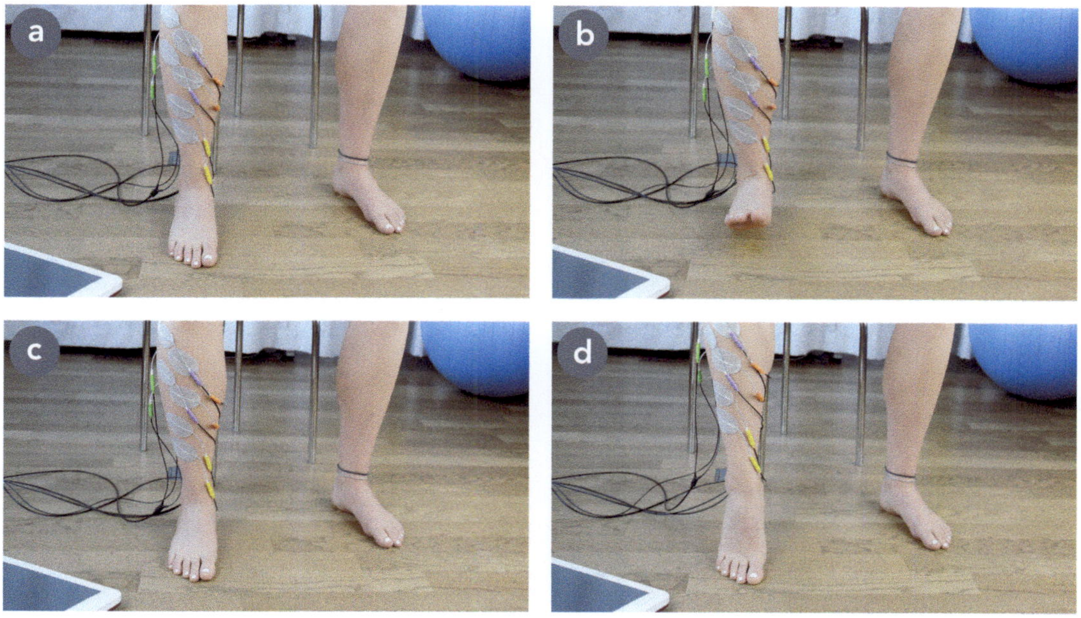

**Fig. 6.17** Movement sequence of the activity "Ankle joint coordination"

**Table 6.21** Stimulation parameters for the activity "Stand up unilateral"

## STAND UP UNILATERAL (stimulation of the affected side)

objective: to stand up from the seat using the affected leg - the activity of the tibialis muscle supports the shifting of the center of gravity over the axis of rotation of the ankle joint

| frequency: 50 Hz<br>pulse width: 300 µs | contraction 1 | | | | |
| --- | --- | --- | --- | --- | --- |
| | delay | rise time | plateau time | fall time | pause 1 |
| **channel 1**<br>M. tibialis anterior | 0 | 0,5 | 1 | 0,5 | 14 |
| **channel 2**<br>M. quadriceps femoris | 0,5 | 0,5 | 2 | 2 | 11 |
| **channel 3**<br>M. gastrocnemius | 0,5 | 0,5 | 2 | 2 | 11 |
| **channel 4**<br>M. biceps femoris | 1 | 0,5 | 1,5 | 2 | 11 |

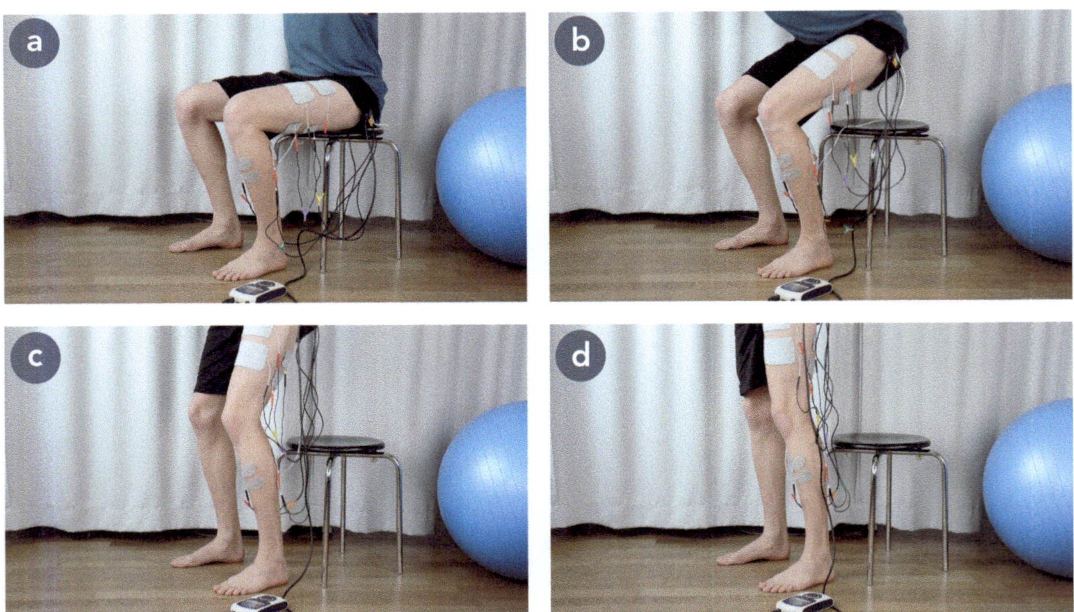

**Fig. 6.18** Movement sequence of the activity "Stand up unilateral"

**Table 6.22** Stimulation parameters for the activity "Stand up and step" on affected side with a second contraction

## STAND UP AND STEP ON AFFECTED SIDE (with 2nd contraction)

objective: stand up from step position, affected leg is placed in a backward position, step triggering with affected leg, second contractionen for M. tibialis und M. quadriceps femoris

| frequency: 50 Hz<br>pulse width: 300 µs | contraction 1 | | | | | contraction 2 | | | |
|---|---|---|---|---|---|---|---|---|---|
| | delay | rise time | plateau time | fall time | pause 1 | rise time c2 | plateau time c2 | fall time c2 | pause 2 |
| **channel 1** M. tibialis anterior | 0 | 0 | 1,5 | 0 | 2 | 0,5 | 1,5 | 1 | 6 |
| **channel 2** M. quadriceps femoris | 0 | 1 | 1,5 | 0,5 | 1 | 0,5 | 1 | 1 | 6 |
| **channel 3** M. biceps femoris | 1,5 | 1 | 2 | 0,5 | 8 | 0 | 0 | 0 | 0 |

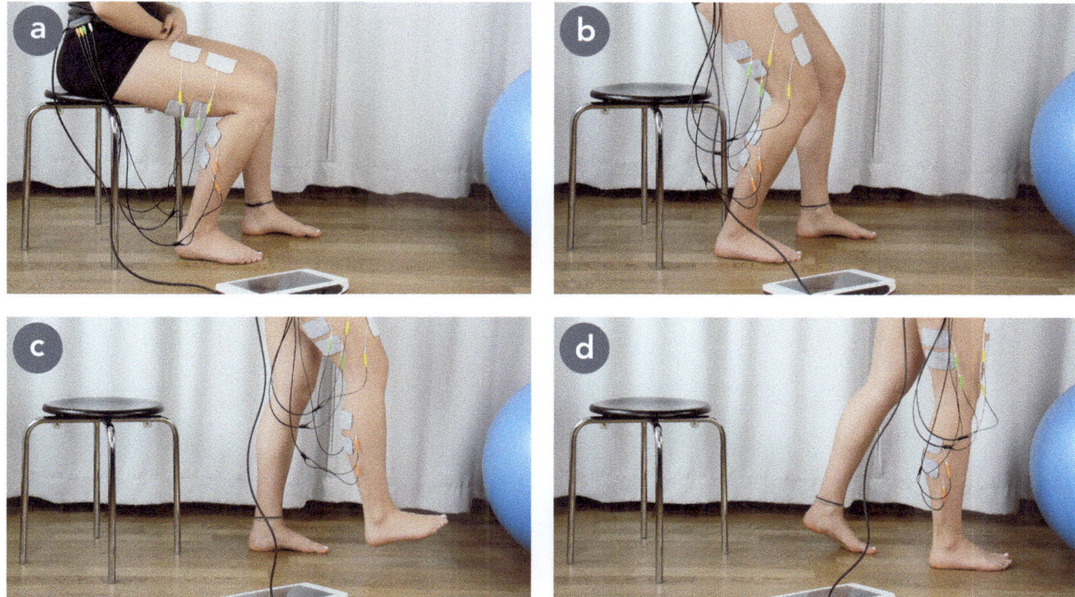



**Fig. 6.19** Movement sequence of the activity "Stand up and step" with a second contraction

**Table 6.23** Stimulation parameters for the activity "Stand up bilateral"

**STAND UP BILATERAL (torso/leg)**
objective: standing up bilaterally from sitting position with extensor involvement of the torso

| frequency: 50 Hz<br>pulse width: 300 µs | contraction 1 | | | | |
|---|---|---|---|---|---|
| | delay | rise time | plateau time | fall time | pause 1 |
| **channel 1**<br>M. quadriceps femoris | 0 | 1 | 3 | 2 | 10 |
| **channel 2**<br>M. quadriceps femoris | 0 | 1 | 3 | 2 | 10 |
| **channel 3**<br>M. erector spinae | 1 | 1 | 2 | 2 | 10 |
| **channel 4**<br>M. erector spinae | 1 | 1 | 2 | 2 | 10 |

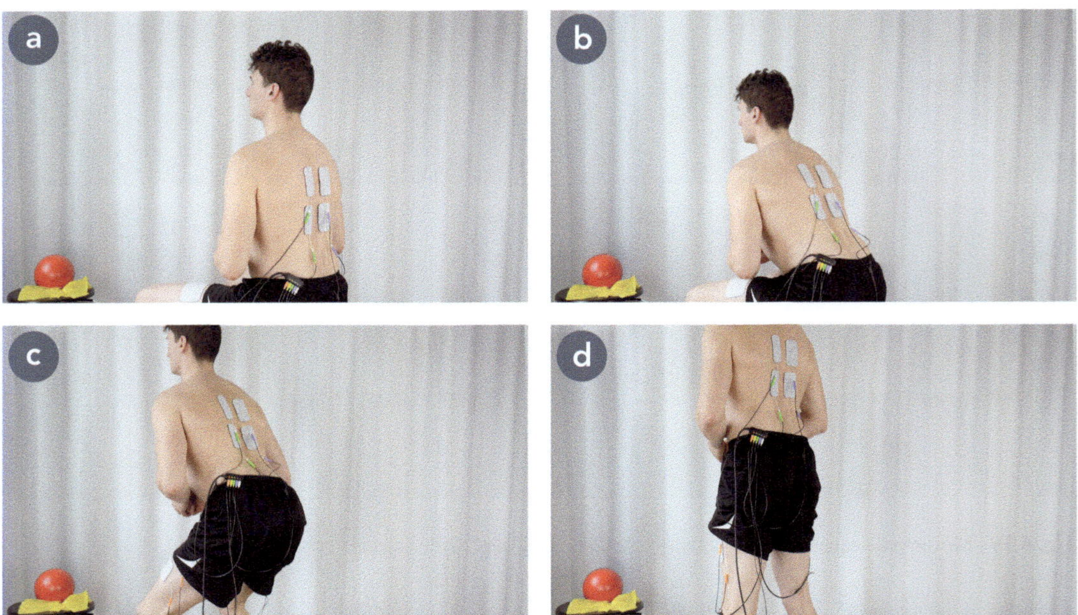

**Fig. 6.20** Movement sequence of the activity "Stand up bilateral"

tion is deliberately omitted in favor of an immediate stimulation of all muscle groups involved for the purpose of improved stability. In this initial position, an additional activity with the less affected upper extremity or lower extremity is appropriate. The use of an external focus of attention, for example, through the use of a ball or balloon, can reinforce motor learning (Table 6.24, Fig. 6.21 and Video 6.19).

### 6.4.7  Lunge from Standing Position

The activity is initiated from a standing position. The patient takes a step forward with the affected leg, puts more weight on the anterior leg in a stepping position (quadriceps femoris muscle) in order to then slow down the forward shift of the center of gravity over the area of support with this leg (gastrocnemius muscle; biceps femoris muscle). The rise time is chosen to be short enough (0.5 s) to allow a timely muscular response for movement control. EMG triggering is provided by the muscular responses of the quadriceps femoris muscle. The appropriate height of the trigger threshold must be observed. Attention must be paid to an adapted size when selecting the electrodes (Table 6.25, Fig. 6.22, and Video 6.20).

### 6.4.8  Walk with a Rollator

In this therapy sequence, involving the affected arm and hand, a supporting and pushing activity is performed as part of the activity "Walking with a rollator". In this way, the arm and hand are meaningfully integrated into a support activity, whereby the focus is primarily on the continuation of the gait movement. The wrist extensor (extensor carpi radialis muscle) and the finger flexors (flexor digitorum superficialis muscle) can be used to grasp the rollator handle. Support is provided in the elbow joint by the extensor (triceps brachii muscle) and in the shoulder joint by the shoulder flexor (deltoideus muscle, pars clavicularis). In many cases of hemiparetic gait, this function leads to a visible increase in gait symmetry with a simultaneous decrease in circumduction of the leg and a resulting increase in walking speed. Short rise time (0.5 s) and fall time (0 s) allow almost continuous stimulation of the arm during walking. The low frequency (35 Hz) prevents the muscles from fatiguing too quickly. Furthermore, it should be noted that the EMG trigger threshold is selected low in this case so that the patient can be continuously mobile on the rollator without a big effect on his hand function (Table 6.26, Fig. 6.23 and Video 6.21).

**Table 6.24** Stimulation parameters for the activity "Single leg stance"

| SINGLE LEG STANCE | | | | | |
| --- | --- | --- | --- | --- | --- |
| objective: securing the supporting leg on the affected side | | | | | |
| frequency: 50 Hz<br>pulse width: 300 μs | contraction 1 | | | | |
| | delay | rise time | plateau time | fall time | pause 1 |
| channel 1<br>M. quadriceps femoris | 0 | 1 | 10 | 1,5 | 7,5 |
| channel 2<br>M. gluteus medius | 0 | 1 | 10 | 1,5 | 7,5 |
| channel 3<br>M. biceps femoris | 0 | 1 | 10 | 1,5 | 7,5 |
| channel 4<br>M. gastrocnemius | 0 | 1 | 10 | 1,5 | 7,5 |

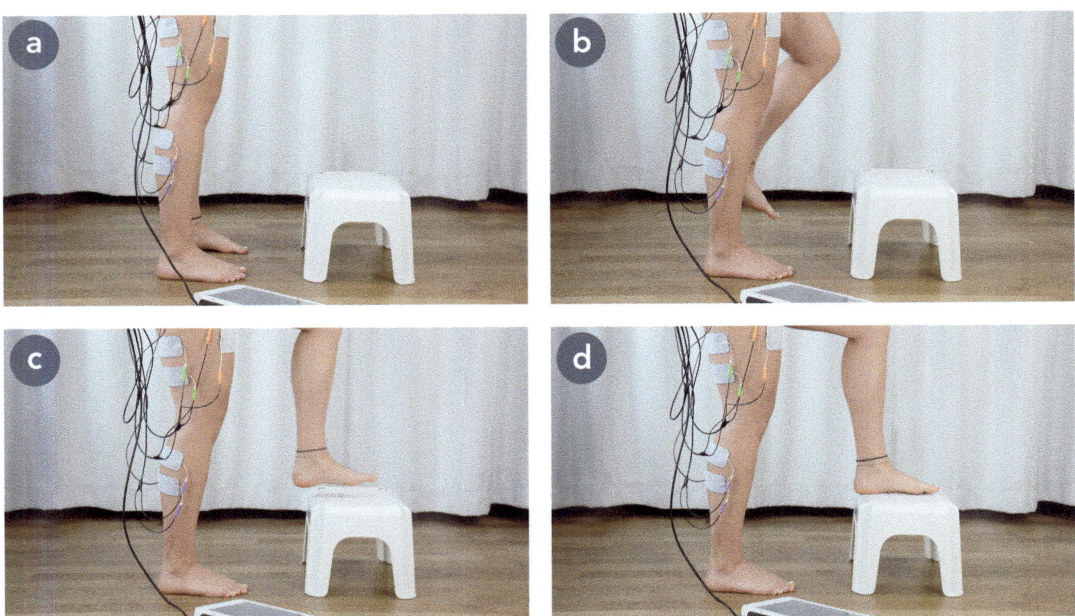

**Fig. 6.21** Movement sequence of the activity "Single leg stance"

**Table 6.25** Stimulation parameters for the activity "Lunge from standing position"

### LUNGE FROM STANDING POSITION
objective: performing a lunge from a standing position

| frequency: 50 Hz<br>pulse width: 300 µs | contraction 1 | | | | |
| --- | --- | --- | --- | --- | --- |
| | delay | rise time | plateau time | fall time | pause 1 |
| channel 1<br>M. quadriceps femoris | 0 | 0,5 | 3 | 0,5 | 5 |
| channel 2<br>M. gastrocnemius | 0,5 | 0,5 | 2,5 | 0,5 | 5 |
| channel 3<br>M. biceps femoris | 0,5 | 0,5 | 2,5 | 0,5 | 5 |

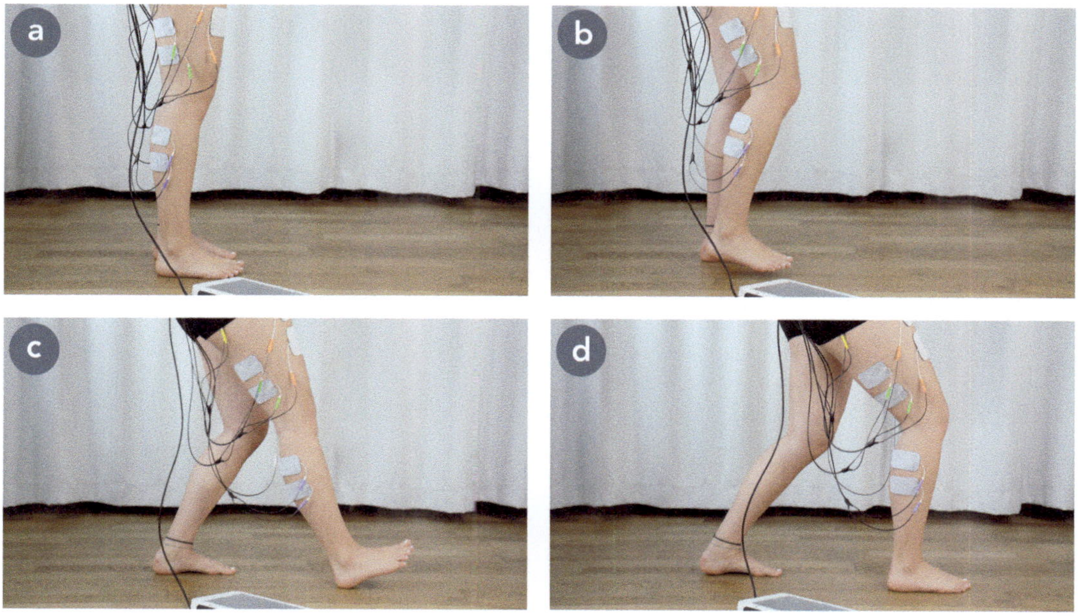

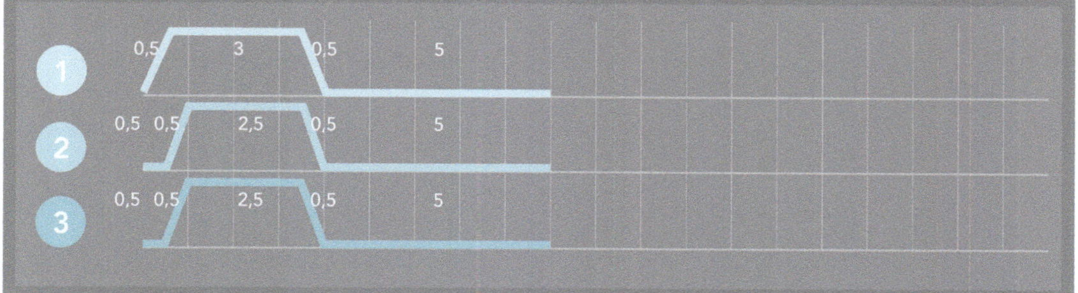

**Fig. 6.22** Movement sequence of the activity "Lunge from standing position"

**Table 6.26** Stimulation parameters for the activity "Walk with rollator"

**WALK WITH ROLLATOR**
objective: to walk safely with the rollator, using the affected arm and hand

| frequency: 35 Hz<br>pulse width: 300 µs | contraction 1 | | | | |
|---|---|---|---|---|---|
| | delay | rise time | plateau time | fall time | pause 1 |
| **channel 1**<br>M. extensor carpi radialis longus | 0 | 0,5 | 19,5 | 0 | 0 |
| **channel 2**<br>M. flexor digitorum superficialis | 0 | 0,5 | 19,5 | 0 | 0 |
| **channel 3**<br>M. triceps brachii | 0,5 | 0,5 | 19 | 0 | 0 |
| **channel 4**<br>M. deltoideus, Pars clavicularis | 0,5 | 0,5 | 19 | 0 | 0 |

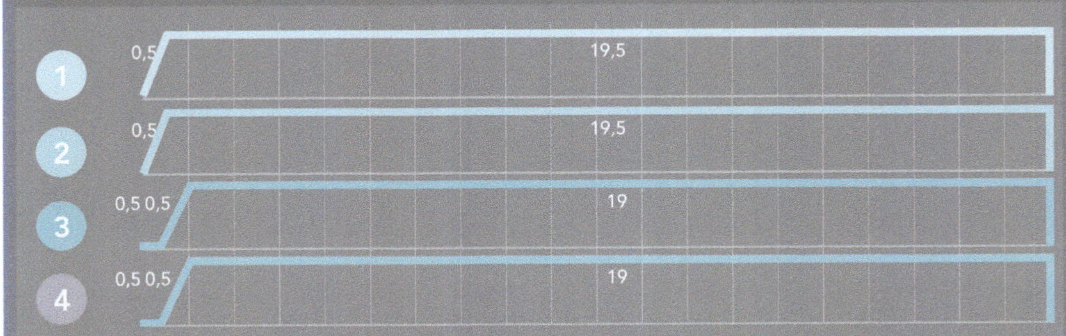

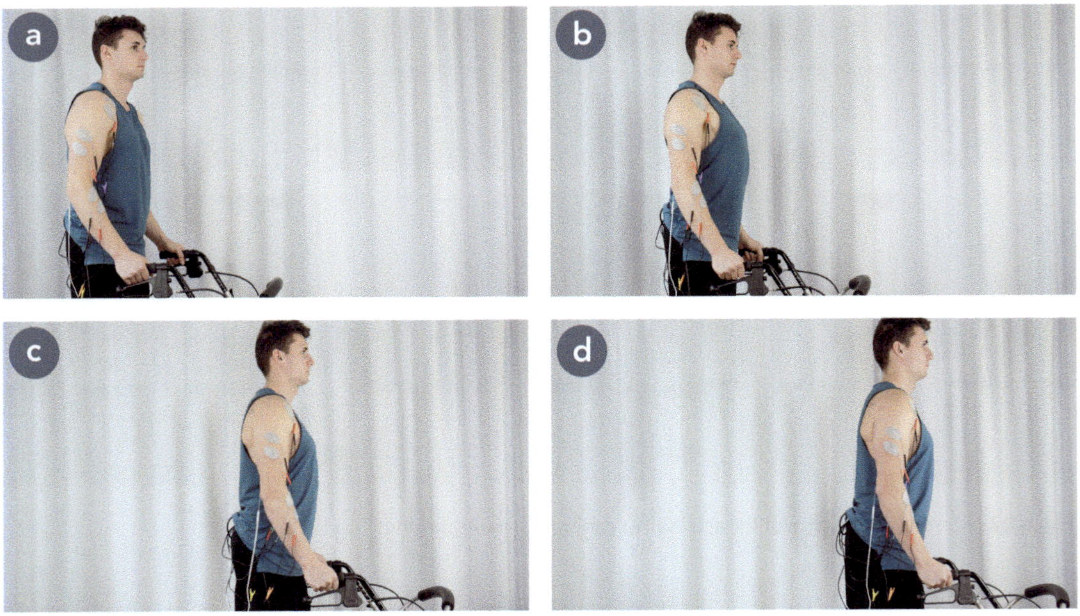

**Fig. 6.23** Movement sequence of the activity "Walking with a rollator"

## References


1. Nelles G. Neurologische rehabilitation. In: Neuronale Plastizität. Stuttgart: Georg Thieme Verlag; 2004. p. 356.
2. van Cranenburg B. Wiederherstellung nach Hirnschädigung. Theorie und Praxis der interdisziplinären Neurorehabilitation, vol. 2. Auflage. München: Kiener Verlag; 2014. p. 441.
3. World Health Organization. Global Health Estimates 2016: Deaths by Cause, Age, Sex, by Country and by Region, 200–2016. http://www.who.int/healthinfo/global_burden_disease/en/cited. 2016, Geneva: s.n., 2018.
4. Robert Koch Institut (Hrsg.). Gesundheit in Deutschland. Gesundheitsberichterstattung des Bundes. Gemeinsam getragen von RKI und Destatis. RKI. Berlin : s.n., 2015. S. 1–516. DOI: https://doi.org/10.17886/rkipubl-2015-003.
5. Trepel, M. Neuroanatomie. Struktur und Funktion. vol. 7 Ausgabe. München Jena : Urban & Fischer/Elsevier GmbH, 2017. S. 408. Bde. ISBN 3–437–41297-3, ISBN 3-437-41297-3.
6. Bähr M, Frotscher M. Neurologisch-topische Diagnostik, vol. 9. Auflage. Stuttgart: Georg Thieme Verlag KG; 2009. p. 59.
7. Fries W, Freivogel S. Motorische rehabilitation Kapitel 16. In: Frommelt P, Lösslein H (Hrsg.), Neurorehabilitation. Berlin, Heidelberg: Springer Verlag GmbH, 2010.
8. Foley N, Mehta S, Jutai, J. Upper extremity interventions. In: Teasell R (Hrsg.) Evidence based review of stroke rehabilitation. 16. Ausgabe. Heart & Stroke Foundation Canadien Partnership for stroke recovery. 2014, pp. 1–208.
9. Howlett OA, et al. Functional electrical stimulation improves activity after stroke: a systematic review with meta-analysis. Arch Phys Med Rehabil. 2015;96(5):934–43.
10. Winstein CJ, et al. Guidelines for adult stroke rehabilitation and recovery: a guideline for healthcare professionals from the American Heart Association/American Stroke Association. Stroke. 2016;47(6):e98–169.
11. Wang H, et al. Daily treatment time and functional gains of stroke patients during inpatient rehabilitation. PM&R. 2013;5(2):122–8.
12. Kapadia N, Moineau B, Popovic M. Functional electrical stimulation therapy for retraining reaching and grasping after spinal cord injury and stroke. Front Neurosci. 2020;14:718.
13. Woytowicz J, et al. Determining levels of upper extremity movement impairment by applying a cluster analysis to the Fugl-Meyer assessment of the upper extremity in chonic stroke. Arch Phys Med Rehabil. 2017;98(3):456–62.
14. Shumway-Cook A, Woollacott MH. Motor control: theory and practical applications. Philadelphia, PA: Lippincott Williams & Wilkins; 2001. p. 614.
15. Chae J, Sheffler L, Knutson J. Neuromuscular electrical stimulation for motor restoration in hemiplegia. Top Stroke Rehabil. 2008;15(5):412–26.
16. Coscia M, et al. Neurotechnology-aided interventions for upper limb motor rehabilitation in servere chronic stroke. Brain. 2019;142:2182–97.
17. Schabrun SM, Hiller S. Evidence for the retraining of sensation after stroke: a systematic review. Clin Rehab. 2009;23(1):27–39.
18. Golaszewski S, Frey V. Neuromodulationin der neurorehabilitation nach Schlaganfall. Jatros Neurol Psychiartrie. 2019;3:12–8.
19. Knutson JS, et al. Contralaterally controlled functional electrical stimulation for recovery of elbow extension and hand opening after stroke: a pilot case series study. Am J Phys Med Rehab. 2014;93(6):528–39.
20. Schick T, et al. Synergy effects of combined multichannel EMG-triggered electrical stimulation and mirror therapy in subacute stroke patients with severe or very severe arm/hand paresis. Restor Neurol Neurosci. 2017;35(3):319–32.
21. Monte-Silva K, et al. Electromyogram-Related neuromuscular electrical stimulation for restoring wrist and hand movement in poststroke hemiplegia: a systematic review and meta-analysis. Neurorehabil Neural Repair. 2019;33(2):96–111.
22. Hlustik P, et al. Somatotopy in human primary motor and somatosensory hand representations revisited. Cereb Cortex. 2001;11(4):312–21.
23. Hamzei F, et al. The effect of cortico-spinal tract damage on primary sensorimotor cortex activation after rehabilitation therapy. Exp Brain Res. 2008;190:329–33.
24. Kwakkel G, et al. Probability of regaining dexterity in the flaccid upper limb: impact of severity of paresis and time since onset in acute stroke. Stroke. 2003;34(9):2181–6.
25. Eraifej J, et al. Effectiveness of upper limb functional electrical stimulation after stroke for the improvement of activities of daily living and motor function: a systematic review and meta-analysis. Syst Rev. 2017;6(1):40.
26. Hatem SM, et al. Rehabilitation of motor function after stroke: a multiple systematic review focused on techniques to stimulate upper extremity recovery. Front Hum Neurosci. 2016;10:442.
27. von Lewinski F, et al. Efficacy of EMG-triggered electrical arm stimulation in chronic hemiparetic stroke patients. Restor Neurol Neurosci. 2009;27(3):189–97. https://doi.org/10.3233/RNN-2009-0469.
28. Gabr U, Levine P, Page SJ. Home-based electromyography-triggered stimulation in chronic stroke. RCT Clin Rahabil. 2005;19(7):737–45.
29. Hesse S, Werner C. Funktionelle Elektrosstimulation. In: Frommelt Lösslein (Hrsg.) Neurorehabilitation. vol. 2. Auflage. Berlin Heidelberg: Springer Verlag GmbH, 2010.
30. Spaich EG, et al. Rehabilitation of the hemiparetic gait by nociceptive withdrawal reflex-based func-

tional electrical therapy: a randomized, single-blinded study. J NeuroEng Rehabil. 2014;11:81.

31. Compagnat M, et al. Predicting the oxygen cost of walking in hemiparetic stroke patients. Ann Phys Rehabil Med. 2018;61(5):309–14.

32. Ryan AS, et al. Sarcopenia and physical function in middle-aged and older stroke survivors. Arch Phys Med Rehabil. 2017;98(3):495–9.

33. Severinsen K, et al. Skeletal muscle fiber characteristics and oxidative capacity in hemiparetic stroke survivors. Muscle Nerve. 2016;53(5):748–54.

34. Gray V, Rice CL, Garland SJ. Factors that influence muscle weakness following stroke and their clinical implications: a critical review. Physiother Can. 2012;64(4):415–26.

35. Akazawa N, et al. Muscle mass and intramuscular fat of the quadriceps are related to muscle strength in non-ambulatory chronic stroke survivors: a cross-sectional study. PLoS One. 2018;13(8):e0201789.

36. Wist S, Sattelmayer J, Sattelmayer M. Muscle strengthening for hemiparesis after stroke: a meta-analysis. Ann Phys Rehabil Med. 2016;59(2):114–24.

37. Jeon S, Kim Y, Jung K, Chung Y. The effects of electromyography-triggered electrical stimulation on shoulder subluxation, muscle activation, and function in persons with stroke: a pilot study. NeuroRehabil. 2017;40:9–75.

38. Keeton RB, Binder-Macleod SA. Low frequency fatigue. Phys Ther. 2006;86:1146–50.

39. Garcia, MA, et al. Is the frequency in somatosensory electrical stimulation the key parameter in modulating the corticospinal excitability of healthy volunteers and stroke patients with spasticity? Neural Plast 2016; Article ID 3034963, p. 11.

40. Jones DA, Bigland-Ritchie B, Edwards RHT. Excitation frequency and muscle fatigue:mechanical responses during voluntary and stimulated contractions. Exp Neurol. 1979;64:414–27.

41. Stein C, et al. Effects of electrical stimulation in spastic muscles after stroke: systematic review and meta-analysis of randomized controlled trials. Stroke. 2015;46(8):2197–205.

42. Patten J. Neurological differential diagnosis, vol. 2. London: Springer; 1996.

43. Ackermann H. Ataxien: assessment und management. In: Frommelt P, Lösslein H, editors. Neurorehabilitation, vol. 2. Berlin, Heidelberg: Springer Verlag; 2010.

44. Chen CC, et al. Neuromuscular electrical stimulation of the median nerve facilitates low motor cortex excitability in patients with spinocerebellar ataxia. J Electromyogr Kinesiol. 2015;25(1):143–50.

45. Schick T, Kolm D, Leitner A, Schober S, Steinmetz M, Fheodoroff K. Efficacy of four-channel functional electrical stimulation on moderate arm paresis in subacute stroke patients—results from a randomized controlled trial. Healthcare. 2022;10(4):704.

46. Sousa A, et al. Usability of functional electrical stimulation in upper limb rehabilitation in post-stroke patients: a narrative review. Sensors (Basel, Switzerland). 2022;22(4):1409.

Michaela M. Pinter

## 7.1 Introduction

Stroke is the most common cause of permanent disability in adulthood. Every year, 15 million people worldwide suffer a stroke, and about one-third have consecutive residual motor deficits [1]. Regaining the ability to walk after a stroke is a primary goal for many of those affected and thus an essential aspect in stroke rehabilitation [2, 3]. A large proportion of stroke patients, about 50%, have no walking function in the acute phase and about 12% require assistance to walk in the acute phase [4]. About 60% of initially non-ambulatory stroke patients are able to walk independently after 3 months of training in a rehabilitation facility, compared with only 39% of stroke patients treated in an acute facility. This evidence emphasizes the need for specific rehabilitation after stroke [5].

Gait deficits after stroke include a range of spatial, temporal, and kinematic deviations from normal gait, such as reduced speed, prolonged stance phase on the unaffected leg, reduced hip, knee, and ankle flexion during swing phase, and reduced knee extension and ankle stability during early stance on the affected leg [6]. Gait-oriented training is often used after stroke and it has been shown that, above all, walking speed and walking distance can be increased or enhanced by specific training [7]. Training of lower limb paresis after stroke typically consists of physiotherapy with the aim of strengthening the muscles of the lower limb, walking on different surfaces, walking on a treadmill as well as balance and coordination training [8–13].

About 10–20% of stroke patients who are able to walk again suffer from insufficient forefoot elevation in the swing phase on the affected leg – a so-called drop-foot when walking – and are consequently limited in their walking speed and distance and thus in danger to fall. Affected by a so-called "drop-foot"and the associated difficulties in walking are not only stroke patients, but also patients after brain injury, after spinal cord injuries and with multiple sclerosis [14].

Supporting the gait-oriented training described above, functional electrical stimulation (FES) of the peroneal nerve has been increasingly frequently used since its introduction by Liberson et al. (1961) [15]. Several studies support the motor remission of lower limb paresis after stroke by daily use of FES of the peroneal nerve [16–18]. FES is applied for weakness of forefoot elevation after stroke, in multiple sclerosis, after traumatic brain injury, and in traumatic paraplegic syndromes, among other conditions [19].

In the following chapter, in addition to the application of the FES, the effect on functional mobility induced by functional electrical stimula-

M. M. Pinter (✉)
Danube-University Krems, Department for Clinical Neuroscience and Prevention, Krems, Austria
e-mail: michaela.pinter@donau-uni.ac.at

tion of the peroneal nerve will be reflected on the basis of both semiquantitative and quantitative gait parameters. In the description of the effect of the FES, the differentiation between the "orthotic" effect and the "therapeutic" effect induced by long-term use of functional electrical stimulation of the peroneal nerve should be taken into account.

## 7.2 Functional Electrical Stimulation of the Peroneal Nerve-Method

Compared to the beginning of FES of the peroneal nerve in the sixties, the indication is unchanged. The clinical indications for which FES is frequently used are listed in Table 7.1.

The FES of the peroneal nerve is used to actively support the locomotor sequence in the swing phase during walking. Single-channel stimulators or dual-channel stimulators are used depending on whether there is isolated or predominantly a weakness in dorsal extension of the foot or additionally a weakness in hip flexion during the swing phase.

The FES is triggered either by a foot switch (placed on the heel) or by an accelerometer (integrated into the cuff).

Lifting the heel off the ground activates electrical stimulation of the peroneal nerve and tibialis anterior muscle via the pressure-sensitive foot switch (wired or wireless), and stops electrical stimulation at the end of the swing phase when the heel is placed on the ground via the pressure-sensitive foot switch (Fig. 7.1).

The accelerometer acts in a similar way; electrical stimulation is triggered by bending the knee at the beginning of the swing phase and stopped at the beginning of the stance phase when the knee is extended (Fig. 7.2).

In order to achieve an optimal synchronization of the gait pattern, the adaptation of the stimulation parameters such as rising ramp, follow-up time and falling ramp according to the walking speed is important additionally to the pulse width (Fig. 7.3). The following principles should be applied: The higher the walking speed the lower the rise ramp and extension time should be. However, if there is spasticity at the initiation of the swing phase, the rising ramp should be lengthened. If there is instability in the affected ankle joint, both the extension time and the falling ramp should be lengthened to support the affected ankle joint in the stance phase.

The stimulation parameters commonly used for FES of the peroneal nerve are listed in their range in Table 7.2.

In all currently available stimulation devices, the frequently applied stimulation parameters are already preset – this simplifies the handling of the stimulators during the testing phase. An essential condition for long-term FES therapy is a positive response in the testing of the FES of the peroneal nerve.

**Table 7.1** Indications for functional electrical stimulation

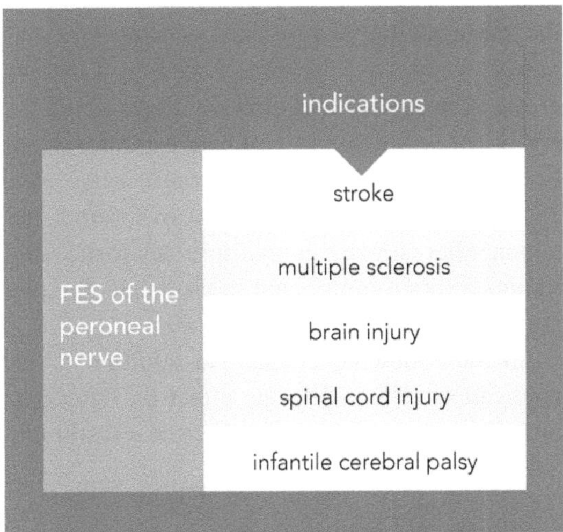


## 7.3 Effect of Functional Electrical Stimulation on Mobility

The efficiency of FES in improving mobility has been repeatedly reported using gait parameters such as walking speed, distance traveled, cadence, and gait symmetry [20–22].

The effect of FES on walking speed and physiological cost index was investigated in 26 patients with drop foot of different neurological

**1**

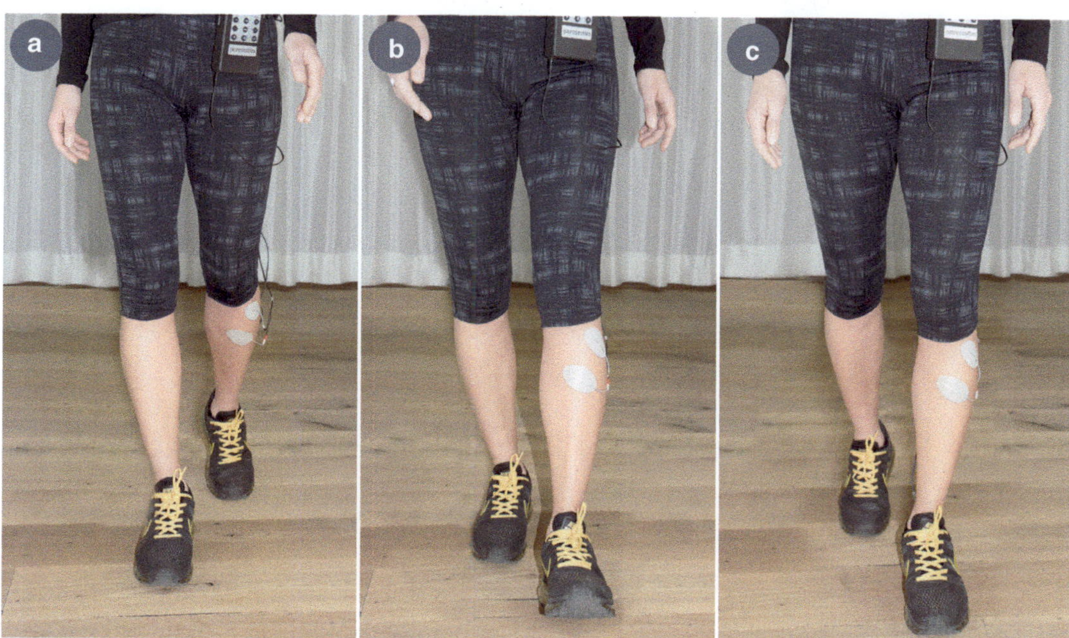

**2**

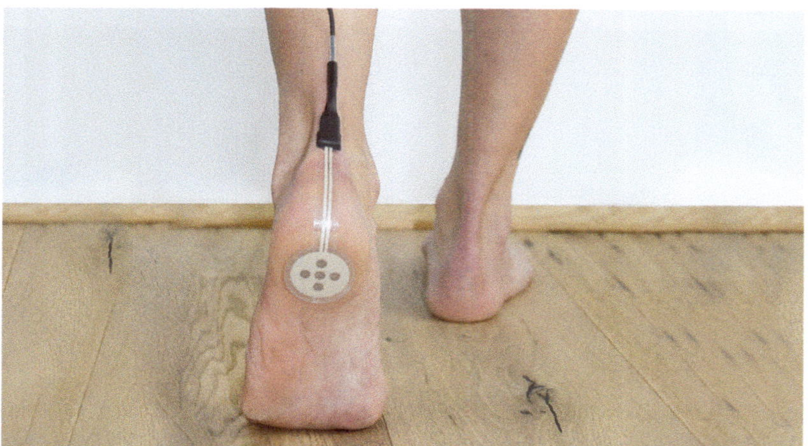

**Fig. 7.1** (1) Application of the electrode over the peroneal nerve and the anterior tibialis muscle, shown in the initial swing phase (**a**), in the middle swing phase (**b**) and in the terminal swing phase (**c**); (2) foot switch is applied to the heel of the affected leg

etiologies: twelve stroke patients, six patients with traumatic spinal cord injury, two patients with traumatic brain injury, two patients with multiple sclerosis, two patients with brain tumor, one patient with hereditary spastic paraparesis, and one patient with infantile cerebral palsy (Stein et al. 2006). After a 3-month intervention period, walking speed and physiological cost index improved significantly both with and without FES.

In another study [19], in addition to gait parameters, the improvement in quality of life in 21 chronic stroke patients and 20 multiple sclerosis patients – induced by FES of the peroneal nerve – was examined. To document changes in quality of life, the Psychological Impact of Assistive Devices Scale was used. After an 18-week intervention period, the following results were obtained: in both intervention groups – stroke patients and patients with mul-

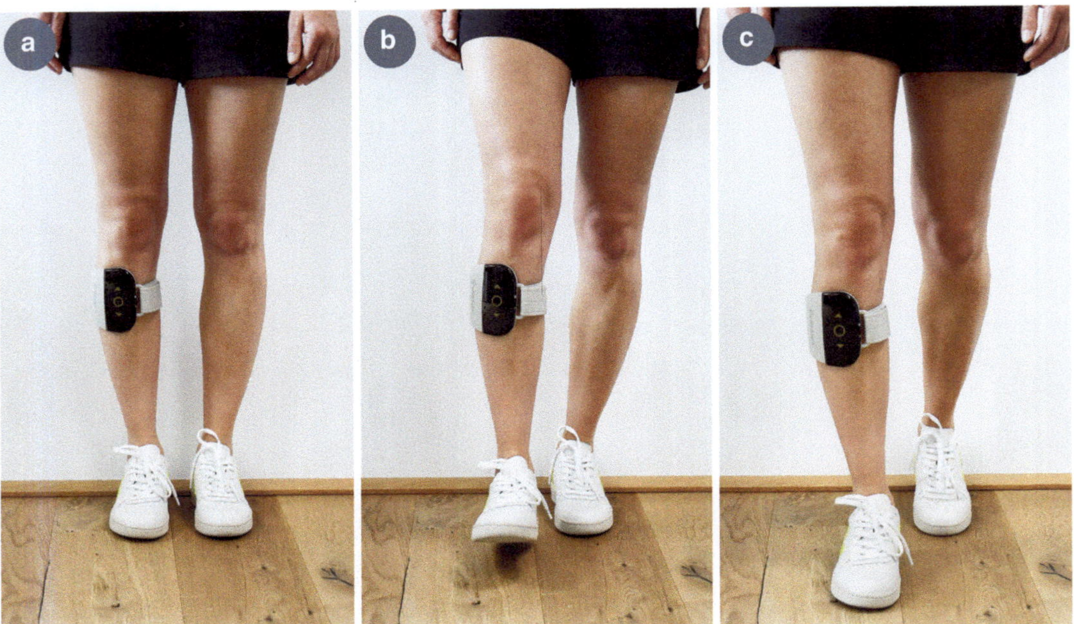


**Fig. 7.2** A myoelectric orthosis-stimulates the peroneal nerve to lift the foot during the swing phase, utilizing a tilt sensor and accelerometer technology; shown in the stance phase (**a**), in the middle swing phase (**b**) and in the terminal swing phase (**c**)

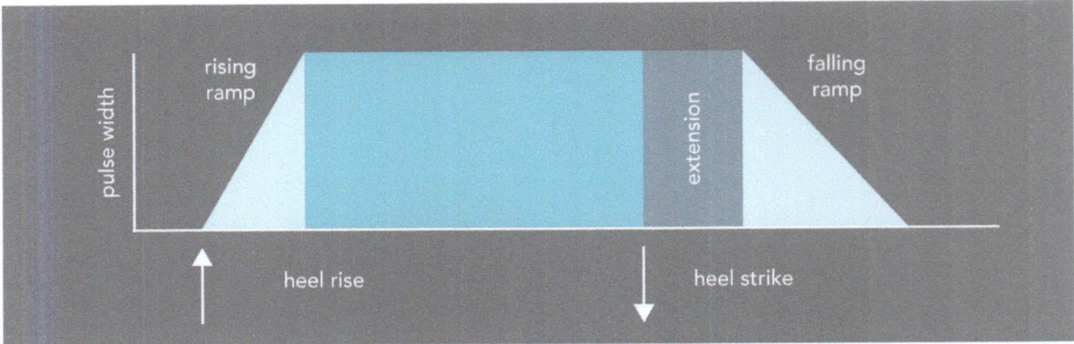


**Fig. 7.3** Stimulation envelop for functional electrical stimulation: pulse width determines the extent of muscle contraction, the rising ramp allows the pulse width to swell slowly, the extension time prevents the foot from falling abruptly after heel striking at the end of the swing phase, and the falling ramp slowly reduces the pulse width to zero

**Table 7.2** Stimulation parameters: μsec microseconds, Hz Hertz

| FES of the peroneal nerve | |
| --- | --- |
| pulse shape | biphasic/rectangular |
| pulse width | 220-300 μsec |
| frequency | 20-60 Hz |

tiple sclerosis – there was a significant increase in walking speed and a significant improvement in the domains of competence, adaptability, and self-esteem of the Psychological Impact of Assistive Devices Scale. Interestingly, the improvement in the domains of competence and adaptability was significantly greater in stroke patients compared with the multiple sclerosis group. Although FES leads to a significant improvement in quality of life, a correlation between objectively measured gait parameters and improvement in quality of life due to FES of the peroneal nerve could not be demonstrated.

The effect of FES combined with conventional therapy in chronic stroke patients (more than 3 months after acute event) was investigated in a prospective controlled intervention study [23]. Twenty-seven patients received the combination of FES with conventional therapy while twenty-four patients received conventional therapy without FES over an intervention period of 12 weeks. A significant improvement in spasticity, muscle strength, and Fugl-Meyer score of the affected leg could be observed after 12 weeks of intervention in the FES group compared to the control group. In addition to a significant increase in walking speed, a significant reduction in falls was further verified, which has a substantial relevance for everyday life.

In a randomized controlled trial of 102 chronic stroke patients (drop out of eight stroke patients), gait training plus FES was compared to standard therapy (ST) [18]. The primary aim of this study was to identify possible mechanisms responsible for the improvement in functional mobility. In both the FES group (54 patients) and the ST group (48 patients), the aforementioned interventions were performed on an outpatient clinic basis for 12 weeks. The 12-week intervention period consisted of a 5-week functional training phase (two 1-hour therapy sessions per week) and a 7-week post functional training phase (three additional one-hour therapy sessions during the remaining 7 weeks). During the functional training phase, patients were trained to use their treatment devices (FES or orthosis) for mobility at home, if necessarily with the prescribed walking device such as walking stick, etc. The content of the therapy sessions on device use was standardized across treatment groups. The effect of each condition, FES versus ST, was compared using kinematic and kinetic parameters of gait. Measurements were taken at the following time points: at the beginning of the intervention (t1), at the end of the 12-week intervention (t2), and at 12 weeks (t3) and 24 weeks (t4) after the end of the intervention. For all investigations including quantitative gait analysis (QGA), patients in the FES group did not wear a stimulator. In the ST treatment group, orthoses were allowed if already prescribed. In principle,

orthoses were not prescribed for patients with mild weakness in forefoot elevation, orthoses were only prescribed for patients with significant weakness in forefoot elevation. A total of 86% of the 48 stroke patients in the ST group had orthoses prescribed in advance. Major findings to be stressed from this study are: both gait training with FES of the peroneal nerve and standard therapy resulted in improvements in hip flexion at the onset of swing and plantar flexion at the ankle during push-off, leading to significantly improved gait speed, cadence, and stride length. However, there were no differences between the two treatment groups. Interestingly, both treatment groups recorded a decrease in ankle dorsiflexion during the swing phase. For the authors, the clinical implications of this finding are unclear. A survey of all cited studies with single-channel stimulator is given in Table 7.3.

As mentioned above, in addition to dorsiflexion of the foot, hip and knee flexion may also be weakened during the swing phase. This will ultimately lead to a circumduction of the affected leg. In addition to the FES of the peroneal nerve, the quadriceps or biceps femoris muscle is further stimulated to support hip flexion and knee flexion, thus actively supporting the swing phase during walking. In this case, a dual-channel stimulator has to be applied.

The "orthotic effect" is basically understood as the prompt improvement of walking, directly induced by the FES, compared to walking without FES. A significantly higher walking speed under dual-channel stimulation (peroneal nerve plus biceps femoris or quadriceps muscles) compared with single-channel stimulation (peroneal nerve) was detectable objectively [24].

In another study, kinematic parameters of the lower extremity were examined in 16 chronic stroke patients after an intervention period of 6 weeks with dual-channel FES over the peroneal nerve and biceps femoris muscle [25]. Kinematic parameters were derived at baseline and after 6 weeks of intervention under the following conditions: Single-channel FES of the peroneal nerve versus dual-channel FES of the peroneal nerve and biceps femoris versus no FES. In nine patients with hip extension weakness, additional

**Table 7.3** Survey of the cited studies with single-channel stimulation

| authors | study | probands & intervention | duration of intervention | primary outcome | secondary otcome |
|---|---|---|---|---|---|
| Stein et al. 2006 | cohort | 26 P-FES | 3 months | significant increased walking speed | significant increased physiological cost index |
| Barret and Taylor 2010 | cohort | 21 P-FES-S 20 P-FES MS | 18 weeks | significant improvement in all domains of PIADS | stroke patients superior to MS patients |
| Sabut et al. 2011 | PC study | 27 P-FES-S 24 KT | 12 weeks | significant increased walking speed and reduced falls | significant improvement of spasticity, muscle strength and of FM-Scores |
| Scheffler et al. 2015 | RCT study | 54 P-FES-S 48 ST | 12 weeks | significant improvement of walking speed, cadence & stride length in both groups | no difference between the groups |

biceps stimulation improved hip extension during the terminal stance phase. In seven patients with hyperextension in the knee, additional biceps stimulation resulted in a reduction of knee hyperextension during the stance phase and thus improved gait efficiency [25].

In a further study, 36 chronic stroke patients were investigated to what extent stroke patients with different walking speeds will benefit to the same extent from dual-channel FES [26]. Depending on walking speed, stroke patients were assigned to three different functional gait categories. Walking speed was investigated in a 2-min walking test with and without dual-channel FES. Testing was performed before the start of the study and after 6 weeks of daily application of the dual-channel FES application. Before analyzing the data, stroke patients were stratified into three functional movement classes according to their initial gait categories. It was found that dual-channel FES enhanced walking speed in all three functional gait categories. Stroke patients with limited ambulation at home improved their walking speed by 63.3%. In contrast, stroke patients with functional walking ability in the public domain improved their walking speed by only 25.5%. The authors concluded that dual-channel FES positively affects walking speed in stroke patients, regardless of initial walking speed. Furthermore, increasing walking speed with dual-channel FES may result in improving a person's walking status to a higher functional category [26]. A survey of cited studies with dual-channel stimulator is listed in Table 7.4.

Alternatively, the nociceptive withdrawal reflex (NWR), elicited by electrical stimulation on the sole of the foot can enhance dorsiflexion of the foot and, in particular, hip and knee flexion during the gait cycle and an improved stance phase on the other leg (Fig. 7.4) and results in a higher walking velocity.

Nociceptive withdrawal reflex-based FES supports gait training in the subacute and chronic post-stroke phase [27, 28].

**Table 7.4**  Survey of the cited studies with dual-channel stimulation

| authors | study | probands & intervention | duration of intervention | primary outcome | secondary otcome |
| --- | --- | --- | --- | --- | --- |
| Springer et al. 2012 | cohort | 45 S P-FES versus P-BF-FES | 6 weeks | walking speed with P-BF-FES significantly higher than with P-FES alone | |
| Springer et al. 2013 | cohort | 16 S P-FES versus P-BF-FES | 6 weeks | walking speed with P-BF-FES significantly higher than with P-FES alone | improved hip extension in the stance leg phase & reduced knee hyperextension under P-BF-FES vs. P-FES |
| Springer et al. 2013 | cohort | 36 S P-BF-FES 3 FGK | 6 weeks | walking speed improved by 63% in the case of limited walking ability when walking outside the home, the walking speed improved by 25.5% | |

Although most of the FES studies have been conducted in chronic stages of neurological disease, it has been shown that FES of the peroneal nerve when applied in the acute stage leads to an improvement in motor function [29]. In a randomized controlled trial in 46 acute stroke patients – an average of 9 days after the stroke onset – daily 30-min FES was performed over a period of 3 weeks compared with placebo stimulation and a control group without stimulation. A total of 84.6% of patients in the FES group were able to walk after the intervention period, compared with only 60% of the placebo-stimulated group and 46.2% of the control group. Against this background, per se FES should not only be used in chronic stroke patients, but FES of the peroneal nerve should be a fixed part of early rehabilitation.

Recently, a systematic review of RCTs and crossover trials was performed to verify whether FES applied to the paretic peroneal nerve, combined or not combined with conventional therapy, could enhance gait speed in stroke individuals with drop foot [30]. The meta-analysis showed positive effects of FES on the peroneal nerve to improve gait speed when combined with physiotherapy while without physiotherapy no significant effect on gait speed was obtained. Nevertheless, the authors noted that because of the high heterogeneity in their analysis, they could not determine the benefits of FES combined with regular activities at home for improving walking speed [30].

## 7.4 Orthotic Effect Versus Therapeutic Effect of Functional Electrical Stimulation

FES of the peroneal nerve is intended to "normalize" gait, increase walking speed, and extend walking distance in patients with distally pronounced leg paresis by activating dorsiflexion in

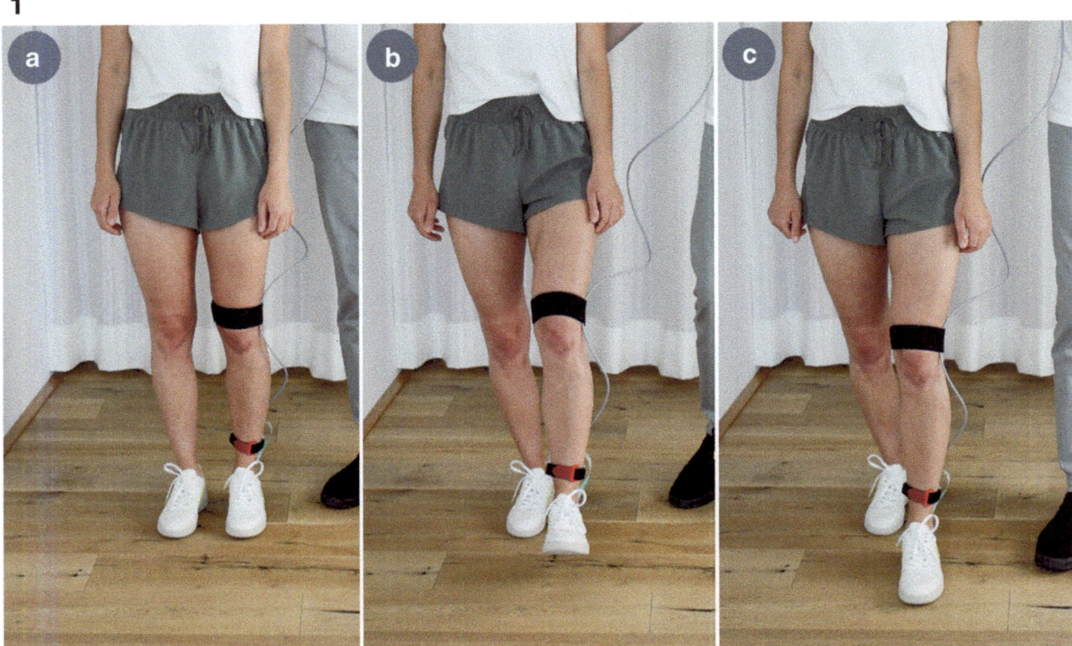

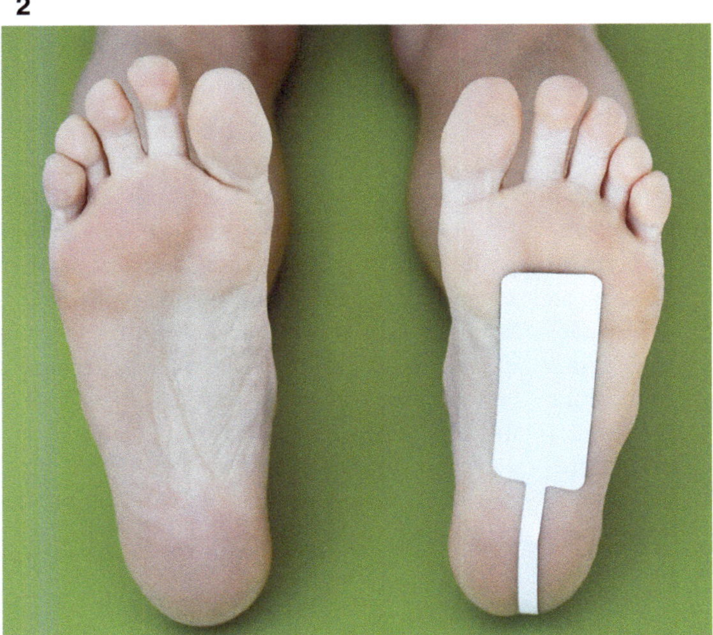

**Fig. 7.4** (1) Application of the electrode for eliciting the nociceptive withdrawal reflex during the gait cycle, in the stance phase (**a**), in the middle swing phase (**b**) and in the terminal swing phase (**c**); (2) the stimulation electrode is applied on the sole of the affected foot

the ankle during the swing phase. The "orthotic effect"is basically understood as the prompt improvement of walking, directly induced by the FES, compared to walking without FES. The "therapeutic effect" is understood as a long-term improvement in walking without FES compared to the initial examination without FES after the application of FES for several weeks [31].

The long-term effect and therefore the therapeutic effect of FES was already demonstrated in

2009 in a total of 16 stroke patients or traumatic brain injury patients [32]. After daily application of FES – for 12 months – all 16 patients improved significantly in walking speed compared to 2 months of daily application of FES and compared to prior to the start of FES. Interestingly, after 12 months of FES, even without FES, there was a significant improvement in all walking tests including walking over obstacles and carpet compared to testing prior to the start of 12 months of daily use of FES – compared to baseline without FES. Therefore, in addition to the quasi "orthotic" effect of the FES, the authors of the study postulate a therapeutic effect and state that the FES per se is superior to the peroneal orthosis in long-term use [32].

A recent study explored the presence of a long-term therapy effect of FES of the peroneal nerve in 133 chronic stroke patients [31]. To objectify a long-term therapy effect, the modified 10-minute-walking-test (10 MWT) was collected before the start of FES and on average after approximately 20 weeks of continuous use of FES. Twenty weeks after the start of the study, FES was still used by 124 patients (93%), with complete data sets finally available for analysis in 104 patients. The most common reason for excluding as many as thirteen patients from the analysis was insufficient length of stay to be able to perform all outcome measures. Nine participants had to be excluded because of cognitive dysfunction, and two because of problems with FES funding. Another two patients dropped out of the study because of pain while walking and two patients because of "inconvenience" caused by the FES. Only one patient discontinued the study because of repeated occurrence of leg spasms under FES. Skin irritation is one of the most common side effects of FES. Thus, minor transient skin irritation occurred in 12% of patients during the study. In all cases, FES could be continued without interruption. As a major finding, the study demonstrated a significant difference in walking speed without FES at baseline compared with walking speed without FES after 20 weeks of daily use of FES, thus demonstrating a treatment effect of FES with long-term use. An immediate initial orthotic effect at baseline and a total orthotic effect after 20 weeks of FES intervention were also significant. The authors interpret the results that the main benefit of FES of the peroneal nerve is the orthotic effect. However, the authors also note that a therapy effect is found with long-term use of FES of the peroneal nerve-especially in less-impaired stroke patients [31]. A survey of the cited studies on the therapy effect is given in Table 7.5.

The therapeutic effect of long-term use of FES is supported by the study of [33]. It was shown on the basis of neurophysiological parameters that after 12 months of daily FES application the maximum voluntary contraction of active dorsal extension increased by 48% in patients after stroke and by 17% in patients with multiple sclerosis, the amplitude of motor evoked potentials over the motor cortex increased by 50% in

**Table 7.5** Orthotic effect versus therapeutic effect of functional electrical stimulation

| authors | study | probands & intervention | duration of intervention | outcome – therapeutic effect |
|---|---|---|---|---|
| Laufer et al. 2009 | cohort | 16 S P-FES | 12 weeks | walking speed without P-FES after 12 months of daily FES significantly higher compared with walking speed without P-FES at baseline |
| Street et al. 2017 | cohort | 104 S P-FES | 20 weeks | walking speed without P-FES after 20 weeks of daily FES significantly higher compared with walking speed without P-FES at baseline |

patients after stroke and by 27% in patients with multiple sclerosis. On the basis of the described results, the authors concluded: regular use of FES induces activation of the areas of motor cortex and residual descending corticospinal pathways. This may also be the explanation for the fact that after one year of daily FES, even without FES, walking speed is higher – in terms of the therapy effect – than before the start of FES [33].

## 7.5 Discussion

In conclusion, continuous single-channel and dual-channel FES leads to an economization of gait, a strengthening of the stimulated muscles, a decrease in spasticity and fall frequency, and an increase in stride length, walking speed, and endurance during walking.

Furthermore, an improvement in quality of life can be observed using long-term FES [19]. Moreover, daily use of FES leads to activation of cortical motor areas and residual efferent neural pathways [33].

Reflecting on the cited studies with single-channel FES, the direct effect of FES of the peroneal nerve in terms of significant increase in walking speed is always present when FES is switched on during end-tests [17, 19, 23, 34]. Only in the study by Scheffler et al. (2015), where the end-tests were performed without FES, a significant improvement in walking speed is shown in both the FES group and the standard therapy group, but no difference in the training effect of both groups [18]. The results found are related exclusively to the study condition performed in the study.

It must also be noted that dual-channel FES is superior to single-channel FES in all studies cited [24–26]. This effect is due to the fact that an isolated distally pronounced leg paresis is rather rarely present, but usually an additional weakness in hip flexion and knee flexion is present.

The differentiation between orthotic effect and therapeutic effect of FES should also be briefly discussed. It should be noted that in order to achieve a therapeutic effect and the associated activation of motor cortex areas and residual efferent corticospinal pathways, a daily long-term use of FES of at least 6 months is conditio sine qua non [31, 32].

Finally—reflecting the results of the application of FES of the peroneal nerve in acute stroke patients [29]—per se FES should not only be applied in chronic stroke patients but should be a part of early rehabilitation in acute stroke patients.

**Summary**
FES should not only be applied to chronic stroke patients, but FES should be an integral part of early rehabilitation in acute stroke patients.

## References

1. Pinter MM, Brainin M. Rehabilitation after stroke in older people. Maturitas. 2012;71(2):104–8.
2. Bohannon RW, Horton MG, Wikholm JB. Importance of four variables of walking to patients with stroke. Int J Rehabil Res. 1991;14:246–50.
3. Dobkin BH. Clinical practice. Rehabilitation after stroke. N Engl J Med. 2005;352(16):1677–84.
4. Jorgensen HS, Nakayama H, Raaschou HO, Olsen TS. Recovery of walking function in stroke patients: the Copenhagen Stroke Study. Arch Phys Med Rehabil. 1995;76(1):27–32.
5. Preston E, Ada L, Dean CM, Stanton R, Waddington G. What is the probability of patients who are nonambulatory after stroke regaining independent walking? A systematic review. Int J Stroke. 2011;6:531–40.
6. Olney SJ, Richards C. Hemiparetic gait following stroke. Part I: Characteristics. Gait Posture. 1996;4:136–48.
7. van de Port IG, Wood-Dauphinee S, Lindeman E, Kwakkel G. Effects of exercise training programs on walking competency after stroke: a systematic review. Am J Phys Med Rehabil. 2007;86:935–51.
8. Dean CM, Richards CL, Malouin F. Task-related circuit training improves performance of locomotor tasks in chronic stroke: a randomized, controlled pilot trial. Arch Phys Med Rehabil. 2000;81:409–17.
9. Laufer Y, Dickstein R, Chefez Y, Marcovitz E. The effect of treadmill training on the ambulation of stroke survivors in the early stages of rehabilitation: a randomized study. J Rehabil Res Dev. 2001;38:69–78.
10. Ada L, Dean CM, Hall JM, Bampton J, Crompton S. A treadmill and overground walking program improves walking in persons residing in the community after stroke: a placebo-controlled, randomized trial. Arch Phys Med Rehabil. 2003;84:1486–91.

11. Eich HJ, Mach H, Werner C, Hesse S. Aerobic treadmill plus Bobath walking training improves walking in subacute stroke: a randomized controlled trial. Clin Rehabil. 2004;18:640–51.

12. Salbach NM, Mayo NE, Wood-Dauphinee S, Hanley JA, Richards CL, Cote R. A task-orientated intervention enhances walking distance and speed in the first year post stroke: a randomized controlled trial. Clin Rehabil. 2004;18:509–19.

13. Pohl M, Werner C, Holzgraefe M, Kroczek G, Mehrholz J, Wingendorf I, Hoölig G, Koch R, Hesse S. Repetitive locomotor training and physiotherapy improve walking and basic activities of daily living after stroke: a single-blind, randomized multicentre trial (DEutsche GAngtrainerStudie, DEGAS). Clin Rehabil. 2007;21:17–27.

14. Martin CL, Phillips BA, Kilpatrick TJ, Butzkueven H, Tubridy N, McDonald E, Galea MP. Gait and balance impairment in early multiple sclerosis in the absence of clinical disability. Mult Scler. 2006;12:620–8.

15. Liberson WT, Holmquest HJ, Scot D, Dow M. Functional electrotherapy: stimulation of the peroneal nerve synchronized with the swing phase of the gait of hemiplegic patients. Arch Phys Med Rehabil. 1961;42:101–5.

16. Stein RB, Everaert DG, Thompson AK, Chong SL, Whittaker M, Robertson J, Kuether G. Long-term therapeutic and orthotic effects of a foot drop stimulator on walking performance in progressive and nonprogressive neurological disorders. Neurorehabil Neural Repair. 2010;24:152–67.

17. Sabut SK, Sikdar C, Mondal R, Kumar R, Mahadevappa M. Restoration of gait and motor recovery by functional elektrical stimulation therapy in persons with stroke. Disabil Rehabil. 2010;32:1594–603.

18. Sheffler LR, Taylor PN, Balley SN, Gunzler DD, Burrke JH, Ijzermann MJ, Chae J. Surface peroneal nerve stimulation in lower limb hemiparesis: effect on quantitative gait parameters. Am J Phys Med Rehabil. 2015;94(5):341–57.

19. Barret C, Taylor P. The effect of the Odstock Drop Foot Stimulator on perceived quality of life for people with stroke and multiple sclerosis. Neuromodulation. 2010;13(1):58–64.

20. Burridge JH, Taylor PN, Hagan SA, Wood DE, Swain ID. The effects of common peroneal stimulation on the effort and speed of walking: a randomized controlled trial with chronic hemiplegic patients. Clin Rehabil. 1997;11(3):201–10.

21. Granat MH, Maxwell DJ, Ferguson AC, Lees KR, Barbenel JC. Peroneal stimulator: evaluation for the correction of spastic drop-foot in hemiplegia. Arch Phys Med Rehabil. 1996;77:19–24.

22. Lamontagne A, Malouin F, Richards CL. Locomotor-specific measure of spasticity of plantarflexor muscles after stroke. Arch Phys Med Rehabil. 2001;82:1696–704.

23. Sabut SK, Sikdar C, Kumar R, Mahadevappa M. Functional electrical stimulation of dorsiflexor muscle: effect on dorsiflexor strength, plantarflexor spasticity, and motor recovery in stroke patients. NeuroRehabilitation. 2011;29:393–400.

24. Springer S, Vatine JJ, Lipson R, Wolf A, Laufer Y. Effects of dual-channel functional electrical stimulation on gait performance in patients with hemiparesis. Sci World J. 2012;2012:530906.

25. Springer S, Vatine JJ, Wolf A, Laufer Y. The effects of dual-channel functional electrical stimulation on stance phase sagital kinematic in patients with hemiparesis. J Electromyogr Kinesil. 2013;23(2):476–82.

26. Springer S, Laufer Y, Becher M, Vatine JJ. Dual-channel functional electrical stimulation improvements in speed-based gait classifications. Clin Interv Aging. 2013;8:271–7.

27. Spaich EG, Svaneorg N, Jorgenson HRM, Andersen OK. Rehabilitation of the hemiparetic gait by nociceptive withdrawal reflex-based functional electrical therapy: a randomized, a single-blinded study. J NeuroEng Rehabil. 2014;11(81):1–10.

28. Salzmann C, Sehle A, Liepert J. Using the flexor reflex in a chronic stroke patient for gait improvement: a case report. Front Neurol. 2021;12:691214.

29. Hausmann J, Sweeney-Reed C, Sobiaray U, Matzke M, Heinze HJ, Voges J, Buentjen L. Functional electrical stimulation through direct 4-channel nerve stimulation to improve gait in multiple sclerosis: a feasibility study. J Neuroeng Rehabil. 2015;12:100.

30. da Cunha MJ, Rech KD, Salazar AP, Pagnussat AS. Functional electrical stimulation of the peroneal nerve improves post-stroke gait speed when combined with physiotherapy. A systematic review and meta-analysis. Ann Phys Rehabil Med. 2021;64(1):101388.

31. Street T, Swain I, Taylor P. Training and orthotic effects related to functional electrical stimulation of the peroneal nerve in stroke. J Rehabil Med. 2017;49:113–9.

32. Laufer Y, Ring H, Sprecher E, Hausdorff JM. Gait in individuals with chronic hemiparesis: one year follow-up of the effect of a neuroprothesis that ameliorates foot drop. H Neurol Phys Ther. 2009;33:104–10.

33. Everaert DG, Thompson AK, Chong SL, Stein RB. Does functional electrical stimulation for foot drop strengthen corticospinal connections? Neurorehabil Neural Repair. 2010;24(2):168–77.

34. Stein RB, Chong S, Everaert DG, Rolf R, Thompson AK, Whittaker M, Robertson J, Fung J, Preuss R, Momose K, Ihashi K. A multicenter trial of a footdrop stimulator controlled by a tilt sensor. Neurorehabil Neural Repair. 2006;20:371–9.

# Electrical Stimulation for Improvement of Function and Muscle Architecture in Lower Motor Neuron Lesions

8

Ines Bersch-Porada

In the last 20 years, electrical stimulation has become increasingly important in cases of damage to the second or lower motoneuron (LMN).). In clinical practice, increased attention is paid to the stimulation of denervated and partially denervated muscles. This development is mainly due to the promising results of the RISE (Research and Innovation Staff Exchange) project. The EU project showed that electrical stimulation of denervated muscles in people with paraplegia increases muscle mass and improves their trophic in the lower extremities [1]. In addition, muscles that had already been structurally altered into fat and connective tissue could be reversed into contractile muscle tissue through electrical stimulation [2, 3]. However, a limiting factor of the previously mentioned effects seems to be prolonged time after spinal cord injury (SCI) or after

damage to the lower motoneuron [4–6]. In animal experiments on rats, the changes in muscle fibre cross-section and the effect of electrical stimulation were investigated depending on the time of application after damage had occurred [7]. It could be shown that the muscle fibre cross-section increased with electrical stimulation due to an immediate start of the stimulation after the injury and that the structure could be normalized again [7].

## 8.1 Denervation

The process of denervation of a muscle can be described in four chronological steps. After a few days, the first fibrillations occur, followed by a loss in the electrically evoked tetanic contraction. After a few months, there is then a dissolution of the contractile structures in the muscle and finally, after years, it ends in a transformation of muscle fibres into fat and connective tissue [8] (Fig. 8.1).

The best results in terms of structural conversion to contractile muscle tissue through direct muscle stimulation were observed in animal studies within 3 years of the onset of spinal paralysis [9]. Nevertheless, muscles could still be

**Supplementary Information** The online version contains supplementary material available at [https://doi.org/10.1007/978-3-030-90123-3_8].

I. Bersch-Porada (✉)
International FES Centre®, Swiss Paraplegic Centre, Nottwil, Switzerland
e-mail: ines.bersch@paraplegie.ch

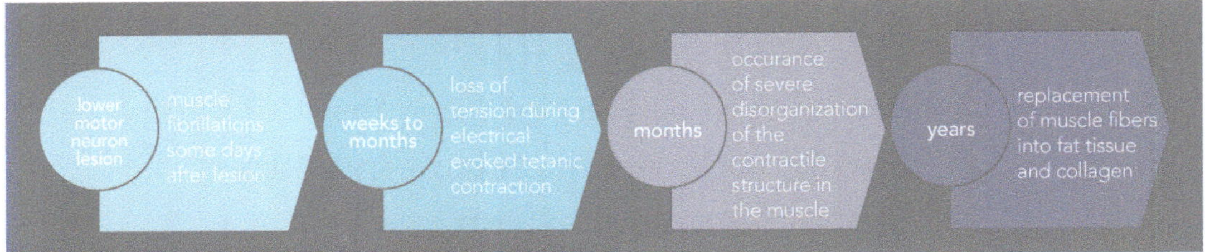


**Fig. 8.1** Chronological sequence of the degeneration process in the muscle

partially converted into contractile structures after 5 years of denervation in a period of 2 years of daily direct muscle stimulation [10, 11]. Denervated muscles do not respond to short stimulation pulses (μs-microseconds) as used for innervated muscles. They require pulses with a longer pulse duration (ms-milliseconds) to achieve a muscle response in terms of a contraction (Table 8.1). 100 ms corresponds to 0.1 μs.

In a stimulation protocol [12], which consisted only of single twitches for the first 12 weeks, a training intensity of five to seven times per week for 30 min was used. The 12 weeks were followed by a short warm-up phase with single twitches, followed by a training phase with tetanic contractions [13]. In chronic SCI, it usually takes several months before a tetanic contraction can be achieved [1]. A tetanic contraction can be elicited with a pulse duration of 40 ms, a pulse pause of 10 ms and bursts ("pulse packages") of 2 s. In many studies, stimulation of the quadriceps muscles, hamstring muscles and the gluteus maximus muscles was performed to enable or train standing and walking for people with low paraplegia. It was found that early electrical stimulation increased the cross-sectional area of denervated muscle fibres and prevented structural degenerative changes [7].

Targets and stimulation parameters are related to the period of time after onset of damage to the

**Table 8.1** Differences in stimulation parameters between upper and lower motoneuron lesion

|  | upper motoneuron | lower motoneuron |
|---|---|---|
| pulse duration (ms/μs) | 250 - 600 μs | 35 - 200 ms |
| frequency (Hz) | 20 - 50 Hz | 0.25 - 22 Hz |
| amplitude (mA) | 20 -140 mA | 10 - 160 mA |
| pulse shape | biphasic rectangular | biphasic rectangular<br>biphasic triangular<br>biphasic trapezoidal |

LMN. Acute/subacute damage is referred to up to 2 years after the onset of the damage, and chronic damage beyond 2 years (Fig. 8.2). This classification depends on the chronological phases of the denervation process.

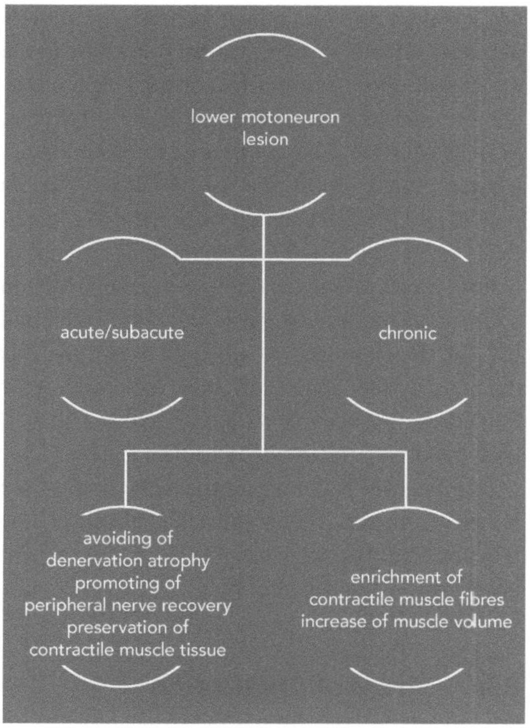

lower motoneuron
lesion

acute/subacute

chronic

avoiding of
denervation atrophy
promoting of
peripheral nerve recovery
preservation of
contractile muscle tissue

enrichment of
contractile muscle fibres
increase of muscle volume

**Fig. 8.2** Treatment goals for lower motoneuron damage in the acute/subacute and chronic phases after SCI

## 8.2 Differentiation Between Lower and Upper Motoneuron Lesion

As a rule, electrical stimulation is carried out via nerves (NMES-neuromuscular electrical stimulation) to elicit action potentials. An electric field is generated under the electrodes that depolarizes the cell membrane of neighbouring nerve cells. If the critical threshold is exceeded, action potentials are transmitted via the neuromuscular junction and a muscle contraction is triggered. Functional electrical stimulation or *FES* is based on the physiological background that nerve fibres can be excited with a shorter pulse duration than muscle fibres. Thus, when stimulating via nerve, the LMN from the anterior horn of the spinal cord to the neuromuscular junctions in the muscle must be intact in order to achieve a muscle contraction [14].

**Summary**
If no muscle contraction occurs through stimulation via nerve, the lower motoneuron must accordingly be affected. In case of partial innervation, no complete muscle contraction is to be expected.

Therefore, electrical stimulation can be used as a diagnostic tool to detect damage to the LMN [15]. When examining muscles of the lower extremities, conventional large to medium-sized electrodes can be used, e.g., on the quadriceps muscle or the calf muscles. Identifying motor points or detecting partial or complete damage to the LMN in the lower limbs is easy because of the individual muscle layers and their only partially overlapping arrangement. In contrast, the muscles of the upper limbs, especially those of the forearm muscles, are arranged in two layers. If a muscle cannot be tested selectively at a motor point due to overlapping muscle layers, a clear statement about differentiation between damage to the LMN and upper motoneuron (UMN) is not possible. There are limitations in this clinical reliable methodology.

The Medical Research Council Scale (MRC) can be used to classify the muscle as innervated, partially innervated and denervated. Here, the MRC scale tests the range of motion through electrical stimulation. A muscle is classified as innervated in the case of $\geq 3$ MRC under testing with electrical stimulation, partially innervated/denervated in the case of <3 MRC and denervated if no muscle contraction can be provoked.

A conventional neurostimulator can be used for testing (Fig. 8.3).

In addition, a pen electrode and a reference electrode are needed. Depending on the size of the target muscle, the head of the pen electrode can be selected larger (Fig. 8.4) or smaller for testing. The stimulation parameters for testing are 250–300 µs pulse duration and 35 Hz. The amplitude is between 20 and 100 mA depending on the muscle architecture and size.

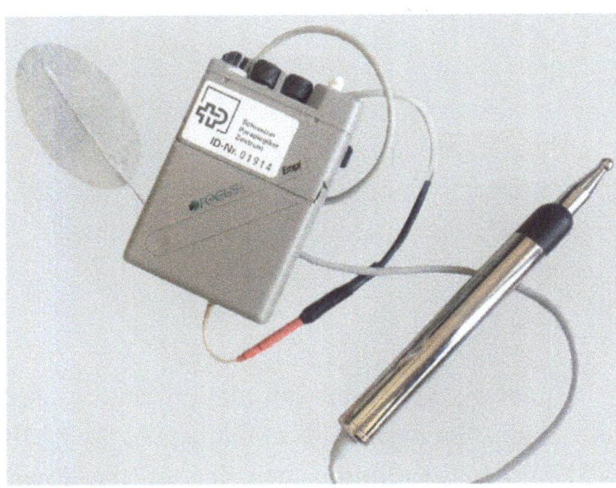

**Fig. 8.3** Neurostimulator with pen electrode (0.5 cm)

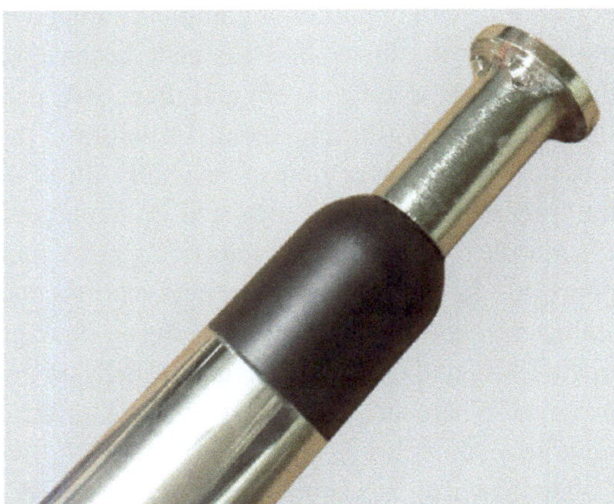

**Fig. 8.4** Pen electrode with larger head (1 cm)

## 8.3 Clinical Appearance

The identification of a denervated muscle, in addition to clinical and neurophysiological diagnostics, also requires knowledge of different neurological diseases and their clinical appearance regarding the motoneuron damage. In addition, the treatment goal has to be defined. Furthermore, appropriate assessments that evaluate the course

of treatment are part of this process. In clinical practice, selective peripheral nerve lesions of the lower and upper extremities, damage to the brachial or lumbar plexus, Guillain Barré syndrome, SCI, peripheral neuropathies and, more rarely, Charcot Marie Tooth disease (CMT) occur. In patients with SCI, it should be noted that often at the level of injury and one segment above and/or below, there might be damage to the LMN in addition to damage to the UMN (Fig. 8.5a and b). The distinction as to whether or not there is damage to the LMN can only be made after 8-10 days, as acutely damaged axons can still transmit action potentials until then [3, 16].

If the LMN is damaged, the reflex arches are no longer intact. This results in areflexia of the reflexes and flaccid paralysis with consequent degenerative muscle atrophy.

## 8.4 Areas of Application

Stimulation has an effect on promoting axonal regeneration and reinnervation after peripheral nerve injury. There is scientific evidence that stimulation after peripheral nerve injury has a positive effect on nerve sprouting and plasticity. Electrical stimulation of the nerve for 1 h postoperatively after nerve suture could increase the release of BDNF (brain-derived neurotrophic factor) and pro-regenerative associated genes [17]. Furthermore, it has been shown to promote the growth rate of sensory and motor axons across the junction [18]. It seems to have a positive influence on the regenerative capacity of the axotomized motor and sensory neurons. In postoperative follow-up, the combination of functional movement exercises in combination with electrical stimulation is effective [19]. The combination of stimulation and exercise showed better early reinnervation than either exercise alone [20].

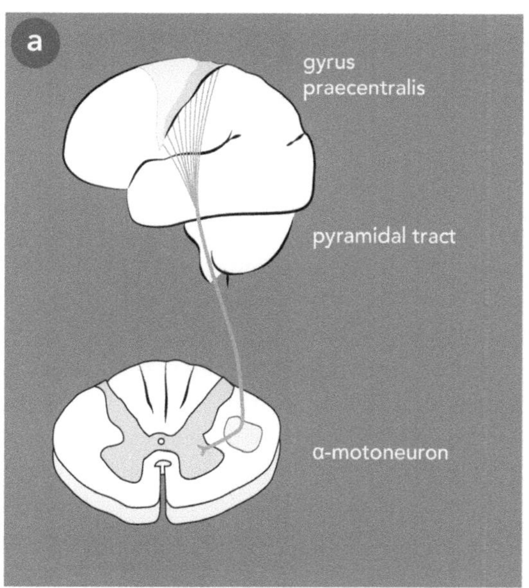


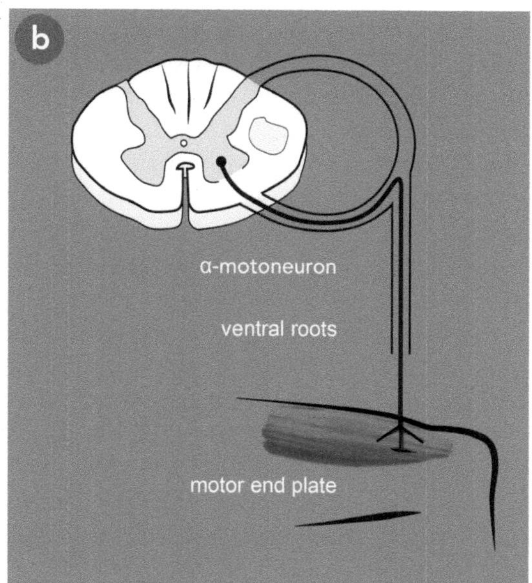


**Fig. 8.5** (**a**) The upper motoneuron reaches from the gyrus praecentralis over the pyramid tracks to the motoric anterior horn cell. (**b**) The lower motoneuron ranges from the anterior horn cell of the spinal cord via the ventral roots of the spinal nerves into the peripheral nerves to the motor end plates of a muscle

**Summary**
Direct muscle stimulation of the target muscle after surgical nerve transfer can be performed to preserve muscle tissue and contractility. To support reinnervation and regeneration, this is recommended in combination with functional exercises and additional stimulation via nerve.

## 8.5 Decrease in the Cross-Sectional Area of a Muscle in Denervation Atrophy

If the LMN is affected, muscle fibre atrophy occurs. The trophic, which is caused by muscle contractions and chemical substances released at the synapse that influence protein synthesis in the muscle, is also disturbed. The muscle fibres that lose innervation change structurally.

They lose 80% to 90% of their mass within a few months. In the course of denervation, there is a loss of muscle filaments, but there is no muscle fibre necrosis. Muscle fibre atrophy is manifested by a decrease in muscle cross-section.

Individuals with paraplegia below TH 12 generally have LMN damage in the skeletal muscles of the lower extremities as a result of a lesion of the cauda equina. The consequences of long-term denervation are a decrease in muscle mass and thickness of the epidermis [10, 21]. Either the loss muscle mass and thickness of the epidermis can be halted and/or restored through the use of direct muscle stimulation, of the muscles affected by the paralysis. The positive influence of muscle stimulation on muscle structure and volume was demonstrated in the RISE project mentioned in the previous chapter. It was observed [13] that the average increase in size of the muscle fibres in the vastus lateralis muscle showed a significant 75% increase from $16.6 \pm 14.3$ ($n = 48$) to $29.1 \pm 23.3$ ($n = 35$) mm after 2 years of regular stimulation. This means that stimulation of the gluteal and ischiocrural muscles can be performed as hypertrophy training. For people with paraplegia below TH12, who have flaccid paralysis and are prone to pronounced denervation atrophy, this type of stimulation is a prevention for pressure injuries at the gluteal muscles. Due to the cushioning effect that can be achieved, the pressure is distributed over a larger area and pressure peaks are reduced, especially under the tuber ossis ischii [22]. The increase in thickness of the epidermis over the course of 2 years of daily electrical stimulation was studied. The effect was seen in an increase from 47.6 μm ± 8.8 μm to 60.8 μm ± 12.7 μm [21]. This observation can be used in the prevention of pressure sores and other skin defects in diabetics and in geriatric treatment.

Denervation atrophies can affect joint mobility and promote contractures. This can be the case when the synergistic interaction of a muscle group is disturbed by damage to the LMN in the antagonists. In the rehabilitation of people with SCI, this can be seen in the clinical phenomenon of the so-called hypertonic biceps brachii muscle in tetraplegia lesion level C6. In this case, the triceps brachii muscle has suffered damage to the LMN due to its segmental innervation level. The biceps brachii muscle is innervated more or less voluntarily. As a result, there is permanent activation of the agonist (biceps brachii muscle) without corresponding reflex activity of the antagonist (triceps brachii muscle), which could counteract shortening of elbow flexors [23, 24]. A similar situation is seen in the forearm with a denervated pronator teres muscle and voluntarily innervated supinator muscle in the form of a supination contracture [15].

Thomas and colleagues studied the excitability of motoneurons after SCI. They found that the intrinsic excitability of the motoneurons can alter the extent and strength of involuntary muscle contractions. Furthermore, they mention that excitability is lower in the centre of the lesion and one to two segments below, and in contrast increases further away from the centre of the lesion [25, 26]. This observation correlates with the explanation that around the centre of the lesion the LMN is damaged and therefore the excitability of the motoneurons is reduced. Another study investigated the excitability in muscle spindles in statically stretched muscles in people with SCI [27]. According to this study, muscle spindles have sensitive receptors that respond to different tensions in skeletal muscles. Activation induced in the longitudinal direction leads to excitation of the Ia and II afferents in the muscle spindle [28]. The excitation of the muscle spindle afferents depends on the resting length of a muscle. It can be increased by three factors. These are pressure and/or traction on the muscle belly, pressure and/or traction on the tendon or by moving the joint in the direction that increases muscle stretch [29].

The assumption is that excessive stretching, e.g., through positioning splints or other therapeutic interventions, stimulates the afferents of the agonist at least temporarily. This effect therefore counteracts the actual intention of maintaining or even increasing mobility.

In the lower extremities, a similar situation can be seen clinically in the development of a pes equinus. Here, the triceps surae muscle as agonist has damage to the UMN and the tibialis anterior muscle as antagonist has damage to the LMN. So far, the latter neuromuscular imbalance has not been scientifically investigated.

The loss of reflex activity of the antagonist supports the overactivity and thus the risk of contracture of the agonist. The consequence would be electrical stimulation of the antagonist to compensate for the synergistic activity.

## 8.6 Preservation of Contractile Muscle Fibres

Direct muscle stimulation can stop the denervation process in the muscle. Furthermore, it is also possible to convert muscle that has already been converted into connective and fatty tissue back into contractile muscle tissue [30]. Stimulation can preserve the number and length of muscle fibres, the cross-sectional area of a muscle, the speed of contraction, and muscle strength [31]. The best results have been demonstrated within the first 3 years after damage to the LMN [7].

> **Summary**
> Electrical stimulation results in a structural and functional restoration of a muscle without voluntary control. Whether this makes sense as a therapeutic goal in treatment depends on the question and proposed treatment goal. There are reasons that justify the procedure. One example was the prevention of pressure injuries in people with flaccid paralysis using stimulation as hypertrophy training as described above.

Another indication may be the structural preservation of a muscle before a planned nerve transfer or suture. This includes the group of people with brachial plexus damage or people with tetraplegia who will receive improved functions in the arm and/or hand by nerve transfer. In the latter group, it is important that the recipient muscle does not show a degeneration [32]. Often, damage to the LMN in the recipient muscle is a contraindication to the planned procedure. However, if the recipient muscle is partially or completely denervated, early stimulation of the muscle can prevent the structural transformation of the muscle into connective and adipose tissue and thus ensure optimal conditions for gaining function after surgery [15]. This could make nerve transfer possible for a larger group of affected individuals.

Structural preservation of muscle, or the reversion of muscle that has been altered by connective and adipose tissue, also represents a change in elasticity and can have a positive effect on functions, even though there has been no improvement in motor control. A clinical example is the loss of voluntary motor control in the calf muscles. As a compensation during walking the muscles of the long and short toe flexors are used to replace the missing force during terminal stance. After some time, this leads to a clawed toe position, which can present problems in shoe fitting, among other things. Pressure points can occur at the level of the interphalangeal joints of the foot. If the calf muscles are stimulated so that contractile muscle tissue develops, the elasticity in the muscle changes and thus the terminal stance in gait. Over time, the toes come into an extended position and the risk of pressure points decreases. Walking is described by those affected as "more stable." The prerequisite, however, is that there have not already been capsular contractures in the toe joints. This described clinical observation justifies stimulation even without voluntary motor improvement. It requires good compliance on the part of the affected person, as it must be continued permanently in order to maintain the result. This applies to any type of stimulation where no neurological recovery is expected.

## 8.7 Effect on the Bone Structure

The mechanical properties of a bone depend on the mineral density of a bone, the trabecular structure, and the organic composition.

The cortical areas of the bones of the lower limbs are located in the medial part of the tibia and femur, and the trabecular bone is located in the distal femur and proximal tibia.

Within the first few years after SCI, bone mineral density decreases by about 45% in the femur and 56% in the tibia. In addition, the incidence of fractures in people with SCI is twice as high as in able-bodied. The most frequent fractures in SCI population occur in the distal femur and proximal tibia.

Mechanical bone loads as well as muscle contractions are important factors for the maintenance of bone density. Stimulation of denervated muscles has a positive effect on bone stiffness [33]. If possible, stimulation should take place in a loaded position.

## 8.8 Stimulation of Denervated Muscles to Support Reinnervation During Neurological Recovery

The effect of stimulation on reinnervation regarding motor learning has not been proven scientifically. However, clinical observations indicate a positive effect. In a retrospective data analysis, the AIS (ASIA Impairment Scale) was collected at the beginning of the additive stimulation to conventional treatment and at the end of the treatment period (Table 8.2). The end of the treatment period was determined by the desired improvement, the "expected outcome," and explains the different treatment volumes of the patients.

SCI is classified according to the American Spinal Injury Association (ASIA). The ASIA Impairment Scale (AIS) is divided into A-E. It is used to categorize sensory and motor deficits in people with spinal paralysis and consists of a five-point scale and the classification of A-E.

All 15 patients shown in table (Table 8.3) had a traumatic SCI and received stimulation in the acute/subacute phase after injury. The data from 15 patients give a representative picture of stimulation being used for motor learning and reinnervation.

All stimulated patients improved by at least one value in the AIS classification during the time in which the stimulation was carried out. Of course, it cannot be concluded here that the stimulation alone is responsible for the improvement. However, the clinical evidence shows that it should be used as part of a complementary therapy program.

**Table 8.2** ASIA Impairment Scale (AIS)

| | |
|---|---|
| A | No sensory or motor function is preserved in the sacral segments S4-S5. (complete) |
| B | Sensory but not motor function is preserved below the neurological level and includes the sacral segments S4-S5. (incomplete) |
| C | Motor function is preserved below the neurological level, and more than half of the key muscles below the neurological level have a muscle grade less than 3 (grades 0-2 motor exam guide). (incomplete) |
| D | Motor function is preserved below the neuerological level, and at least half of the key muscles below the neurological level have a muscle grade greater than 3 or equal to 3 (motor exam guide). (incomplete) |
| E | Sensory and motor function are normal. (normal) |

**Table 8.3** Unpublished data presented at the annual congress of the International Functional Electrical Stimulation Society (IFESS) 2018 at the Swiss Paraplegic Centre

| patient ID | gender | age | AIS initial | AIS final | level of lesion | stimulated muscles | time between lesion and stimulation (month) | number of treatment |
|---|---|---|---|---|---|---|---|---|
| 1 | m | 64 | C | D | L1 | gluteal muscles, hamstrings | 1 | 17 |
| 2 | m | 52 | A | C | L3 | gluteal muscles, hamstrings | 5 | 36 |
| 3 | w | 28 | A | B | T10/L1 | gluteal muscles, hamstrings | 3 | 43 |
| 4 | m | 42 | B | D | T12 | gluteal muscles, hamstrings | 3 | 43 |
| 5 | w | 18 | C | D | T12/L2 | gluteal muscles, hamstrings | 3 | 55 |
| 6 | m | 30 | B | D | T10/T12 | gluteal muscles, hamstrings | 1 | 24 |
| 7 | m | 65 | A | C | T77 | gluteal muscles, hamstrings | 3 | 35 |
| 8 | w | 59 | B | C | T9/T11 | gluteal muscles, hamstrings | 1 | 27 |
| 9 | w | 80 | C | D | L1 | tibialis anterior | 5 | 15 |
| 10 | m | 19 | C | D | C4/C5 | delta muscle | 13 | 7 |
| 11 | w | 80 | C | D | L1 | quadriceps | 5 | 15 |
| 12 | m | 64 | C | D | C4 | finger, hand extensors | 1 | 32 |
| 13 | m | 29 | C | D | L1 | gluteal muscles, hamstrings | 1 | 22 |
| 14 | m | 59 | B | C | L3 | gluteal muscles, hamstrings | 2 | 7 |
| 15 | m | 75 | C | D | C4 | finger, hand extensors | 6 | 22 |

Abbreviations: *AIS* ASIA impairment scale, *m* male, *w* female, *L* lumbar, *T* thoracic, *C* cervical

In contrast to the existing literature, in clinical practice the quadriceps muscle is rarely stimulated in AIS A patients [8, 13, 34, 35]. This could be the reason for the relatively poor functional outcome in terms of standing or walking ability of a motor-complete paraplegic patient (T12-L1) when only the ventral located muscle group is stimulated. The patient's desire to learn to walk or stand again is very often based on the comparison of how it was before injury. In addition, walking is often associated with a certain walking speed and the requirement to use at least one hand to carry objects. Clinical experience has shown that this group of patients considers themselves less disabled in daily activities with a wheelchair. Motor incomplete patients (AIS C or D) or patients with a lesion below L2 notice more stability in standing and walking due to structural changes [33] and in some cases an increase in voluntary muscle activity [7] after stimulation of the hamstrings and gluteal muscles.

## 8.9 Stimulation Parameters and Stimulation Schedule

Depending on the time after damage to the LMN, patients can be classified into the acute, subacute, or chronic phase after lesion. The acute and subacute phase covers the period from the damage to 2 years afterwards. After 2 years, the damage can be described as chronic [1, 10, 36].

The schedule of the stimulation and the choice of stimulation parameters depend on the duration of the damage. At best, stimulation begins in the acute and subacute phase after lesion to the LMN. As a rule, a slight structural change in the muscle can be expected here. After a short stimulation warm-up phase, the stimulation training phase can be started, and a tetanic contraction provoked. The warm-up phase consists of single twitches and serves to increase the excitability of the muscle fibres. It is also a good preparation for the skin for the subsequent intense stimulation, which involves a high current application. A warm-up phase of 3 min is recommended. This should be done before each application and does not change in time or parameters. The subsequent training phase lasts 30 min (Table 8.4). It is not always possible to start with the entire 30-min stimulation time at the beginning. This depends on one hand on the individual tolerance of the stimulation and on the other hand on the fatigability of the stimulated muscle. Both must be assessed during the initial test. How and with which intensity (amplitude) the stimulation is tolerated varies individually. Both stimulation time and stimulation intensity can be increased after repeated application. Based on clinical experience, the stimulation time can be increased by 5 min every 2–3 days with daily application. The intensity (amplitude) depends on the muscle size. Clinically, the goal should be to see a definite contraction of the entire muscle. If this is not tolerated after repeated stimulation, the pulse shape can be changed from rectangular to triangular. Ultimately, a stimulation treatment should last 33 min per muscle group. This contains a 3-min warm-up program and a 30-min training program.

A muscle response cannot be expected directly in the chronic phase after damage to the LMN. The warm-up program consists of single twitches with an even lower frequency (0.86 Hz). The subsequent training program also consists of single twitches with a frequency of 2 Hz (Table 8.5). The latter represents the training until a tetanic muscle contraction is achieved. When a tetanic contraction can be provoked, varies individually and depends on the extent of muscle degeneration. Based on clinical experience, it can take up to 18 months before a tetanic contraction can be seen (Fig. 8.6). Here, a high compliance and discipline is required from both the therapists and the affected person to carry out the stimulation, at best daily, at least five times a week. This should be done at home under regular supervision and follow up visits by the therapist. Often, an assistant is needed to help to fix the electrodes and/or operate the stimulation device. Depending on the number of muscles to be stimulated (33 min per muscle), a preparation and release time of 10–15 min must be added.

**Table 8.4** Recommended stimulation parameters for the acute/subacute phase after lower motoneuron damage

| pulse shape | pulse duration (ms) | pause (ms) | burst on (sec) | burst off (sec) | stimulation time (min) | frequency |
| --- | --- | --- | --- | --- | --- | --- |
| rectangular | 200 | 500 | 11 | 11 | 3 | 1.42 Hz |
| rectangular | 40 | 10 | 2 | 2 | 5-30 | 20 Hz |
| rectangular | 35 | 10 | 2 | 2 | 5-30 | 22 Hz |

**Abbreviations:** *ms* **milliseconds,** *sec* **seconds,** *min* **minutes,** *Hz* **hertz (frequency of stimulation)**

**Table 8.5** Recommended stimulation parameters for the chronic phase after lower motoneuron damage

| pulse shape | pulse duration (ms) | pause (ms) | burst on (sec) | burst off (sec) | stimulation time (min) | frequency |
| --- | --- | --- | --- | --- | --- | --- |
| rectangular | 150 | 1000 | 11 | 11 | 3 | 0.86 Hz |
| rectangular | 100 | 400 | 4 | 4 | 5-30 | 2 Hz |
| rectangular | 40 | 10 | 2 | 2 | 5-30 | 20 Hz |

**Abbreviations:** *ms* **milliseconds,** *sec* **seconds,** *min* **minutes,** *Hz* **hertz (frequency of stimulation)**

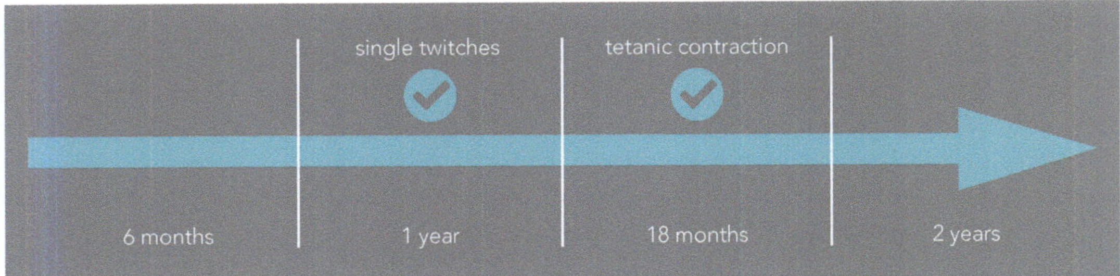


**Fig. 8.6** Timeline of chronic lower motoneuron damage to achieve a tetanic contraction

## 8.10 Electrodes

With direct muscle stimulation, high current intensities are applied due to the long pulse duration. It is mandatory to work either with safety electrodes and salt-free gel or sponge pouches with appropriate electrodes. When using gel, the gel should be spread generously over the entire electrode surface. It is critical to ensure that there is also enough gel on the edges of the electrode. The sponge pouches for the electrodes are soaked with water and lightly squeezed. They must be well wet but should not drip. Specially approved self-adhesive electrodes may only be used for pulse widths up to 200 ms. The subsequent skin check must be carried out in all cases.

## 8.11 Skin Irritations

A reddening of the area after stimulation, which subsides after 2 h, is to be expected, as the stimulation has a blood circulation-stimulating effect. This is to be evaluated as positive regarding the trophic properties of the skin. However, if red spots appear under the electrodes after stimulation or if only the edge of the electrode is sharply marked, an undesirable skin irritation can be assumed. If blisters form on the red spots after 1–2 h, a burn must be assumed. It is not allowed to continue the stimulation. The reason for the burn must be determined. Furthermore, it should

be noted that stimulation never should be applied on skin defects.

Regular renewal of safety electrodes, sponge pouches, and associated electrodes and self-adhesive electrodes is necessary. The manufacturer's recommendations and guidelines must be observed.

▶ **Under the safety aspects mentioned above, direct muscle stimulation can be carried out without hesitation and poses no danger if used properly.**

## 8.12 Practical Examples of Stimulation of Denervated Muscles

The following examples are a selection of treatment options and give an overview of how and under which conditions denervated muscles can be stimulated.

### 8.12.1 Stimulation of the Gluteal Muscles

**Indication:**
Hypertrophy training.
Prevention of pressure sores and skin injuries.

**Starting position:**
Prone position.

**Electrodes:**

Safety electrodes with salt-free gel or sponge pouches of the same size with corresponding electrodes for insertion.

**Fixation:**

For testing, it is recommended to hold the electrodes manually. The stimulus response, if weak, can be well assessed by palpation. Afterwards, the electrodes can be fixed with fixation foil or elastic bands. It is essential to ensure that the electrode is in full contact and evenly covered with gel.

**Treatment volume:**

Once a day, five to seven times a week 30–45 min (Fig. 8.7).

Stimulation parameters (Table 8.6).

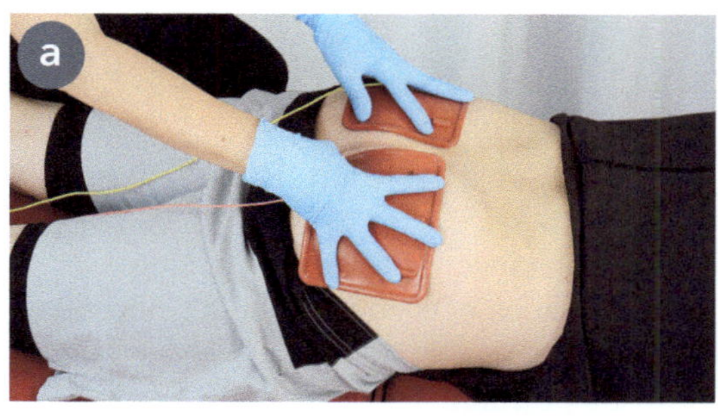
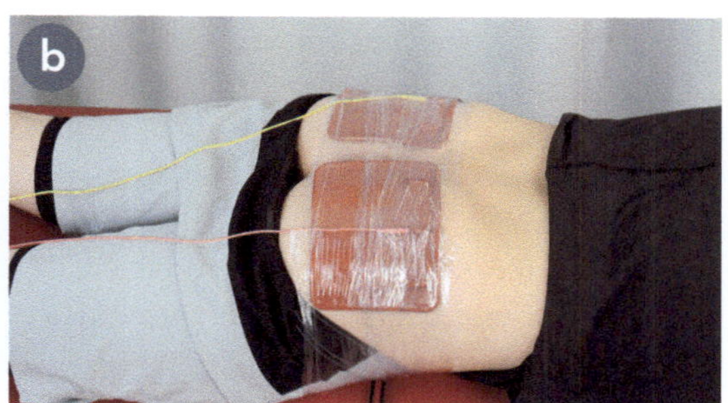

**Fig. 8.7** Stimulation of the gluteal muscles with safety electrodes. (**a**) Manual fixation of the safety electrodes during the test for stimulation. The correct position of the electrodes is determined. (**b**) Securing the safety electrodes with fixation foil, after determining the correct position

**Table 8.6** Stimulation protocol in acute and chronic phase after injury

| acute/subacute lesion | pulse duration (ms) | pause (ms) | burst on (sec) | burst off (sec) |
|---|---|---|---|---|
| warm-up | 200 | 500 | 11 | 11 |
| treatment | 35 | 10 | 2 | 2 |

| chronic lesion | pulse duration (ms) | pause (ms) | burst on (sec) | burst off (sec) |
|---|---|---|---|---|
| warm-up | 150 | 1000 | 11 | 11 |
| treatment | 100 | 400 | 4 | 4 |
| treatment | 40 | 10 | 2 | 2 |

## 8.12.2 Stimulation of the Gluteal and Hamstrings' Muscles

**Indication:**
Hypertrophy training.
  Prevention of pressure sores and skin injuries.
  Support of reinnervation/motor learning.

**Starting position:**
Prone position.
  Stand in, e.g., standing frame.
  Parallel bars.

**Electrodes:**
Safety electrodes with salt-free gel or sponge pouches of the same size with corresponding electrodes for insertion. The size of the electrode is chosen according to the patient's constitution. The proximal electrode is placed on the gluteal muscles and the distal on the hamstrings. Figure 8.8 shows the two possibilities. In practice, one electrode size is used bilaterally.

**Switch:**
If available, an external switch can be used to trigger the stimulation in trained patients. This is recommended when stimulation is used during gait-specific exercises in the parallel bar.

**Fixation:**
Fixing foil or elastic bands can be used to attach the electrodes. It is essential to ensure that the electrode has full contact and is evenly covered with gel.

**Treatment volume:**
Once a day, five to seven times a week 30–45 min.
  Twice a day for 20 min for reinnervation/motor learning.
  Stimulation parameters (Table 8.7).

## 8.12.3 Stimulation of the Foot Extensors

**Indication:**
Support of reinnervation/motor learning.
  Preservation of contractile muscle fibres.

**Starting position:**
Seated, with leg hanging free.
  Seated with foot placed on the floor.

**Electrodes:**
Sponge pockets with corresponding electrodes to insert. The placement of the electrodes depends on the muscles to be stimulated. Placement towards the edge of the tibia reaches the tibialis anterior muscle, further laterally the peroneal muscles are reached. Placement in between results in stimulation of both muscle groups.

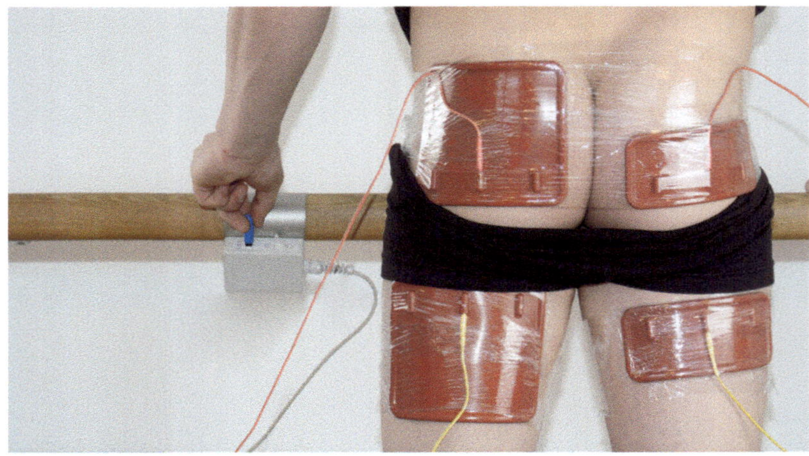

**Fig. 8.8** (**a**) Larger sized electrodes to stimulate the glutaeus muscle and the hamstrings; (**b**) Smaller sized electrodes to stimulate the glutaeus muscle and the hamstrings; the size of the electrodes depends on the anatomical shape of the patient

**Table 8.7** Stimulation protocol in acute and chronic phase after injury

| acute/subacute lesion | pulse duration (ms) | pause (ms) | burst on (sec) | burst off (sec) |
|---|---|---|---|---|
| warm-up | 200 | 500 | 11 | 11 |
| treatment | 35 | 10 | 2 | 2 |

| chronic lesion | pulse duration (ms) | pause (ms) | burst on (sec) | burst off (sec) |
|---|---|---|---|---|
| warm-up | 150 | 1000 | 11 | 11 |
| treatment | 100 | 400 | 4 | 4 |
| treatment | 35-40 | 10 | 2 | 2 |

**Fixation:**

For testing, it is recommended to hold the electrodes manually. The stimulus response, if weak, can be well assessed by palpation. Afterwards, the electrodes can be attached with fixation foil or elastic bands. It is important to ensure that the electrodes are in full contact with the skin.

**Treatment volume:**

Once a day, five to seven times a week for 30 min to maintain contractility.

Twice a day for 20 min for reinnervation/motor learning (Figs. 8.9 and 8.10).

Stimulation parameters (Table 8.8).

### 8.12.4 Stimulation of the Triceps Surae Muscle

**Indication:**

Support of reinnervation/motor learning.

Preservation of contractile muscle fibres (e.g., to prevent and/or reduce claw toes in case of weakness or paresis of the calf muscle).

**Starting position:**

Seated with foot placed on the floor; this starting position is recommended in the chronic phase when no tetanic contraction can yet be provoked.

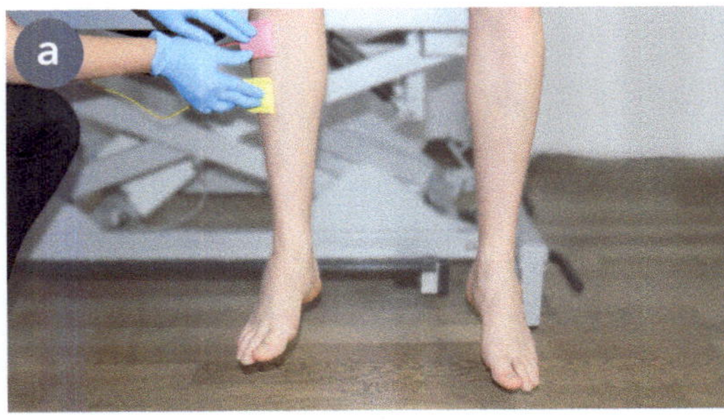 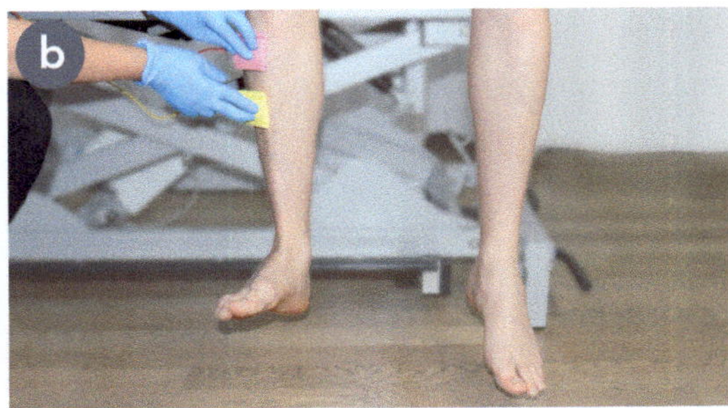

**Fig. 8.9** Stimulation of the tibialis anterior muscle. (**a**) without stimulation in the relaxed position (**b**) with stimulation, anticipated stimulation response is illustrated

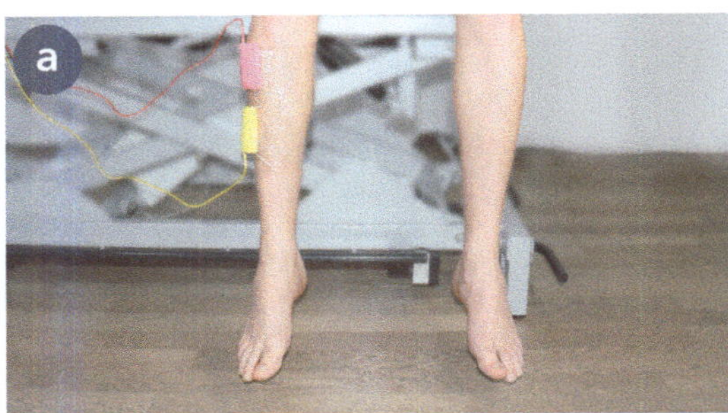 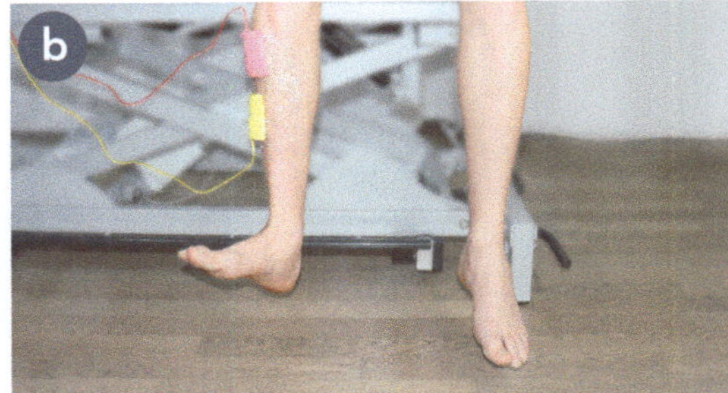

**Fig. 8.10** Stimulation of the peroneal muscles. (**a**) without stimulation in the relaxed position (**b**) with stimulation, anticipated stimulation response is illustrated

**Stand:**
During the terminal stance of gait-specific exercises, if necessary, with switch to trigger stimulation at the desired time.

**Electrodes:**
Sponge pouches with corresponding electrodes for insertion.

**Fixation:**
The electrodes can be attached with fixing foil or elastic bands. It is essential to ensure that the electrodes are in full contact with the skin.

**Treatment volume:**
Once a day, five to seven times a week for 30 min to maintain contractility.

Twice a day for 20 min for reinnervation/motor Learning (Fig. 8.11).

Stimulation parameters (Table 8.9).

### 8.12.5 Stimulation of the Deltoid Muscle

**Indication:**
Support of reinnervation/motor learning.

Preservation of contractile muscle fibres (e.g., for subluxation prophylaxis or preoperatively before reconstructive surgery).

**Starting position:**
Seated with 30° abducted arm/arms and 90–100° flexed elbow.

**Electrodes:**
Self-adhesive electrodes or sponge pouches with corresponding electrodes for insertion. The choice of adhesive electrodes or sponge pouches depends on the stimulation parameters.

**Table 8.8** Stimulation protocol in acute and chronic phase after injury

| acute/subacute lesion | pulse duration (ms) | pause (ms) | burst on (sec) | burst off (sec) |
| --- | --- | --- | --- | --- |
| warm-up | 200 | 500 | 11 | 11 |
| treatment | 35 | 10 | 2 | 2 |

| chronic lesion | pulse duration (ms) | pause (ms) | burst on (sec) | burst off (sec) |
| --- | --- | --- | --- | --- |
| warm-up | 150 | 1000 | 11 | 11 |
| treatment | 100 | 400 | 4 | 4 |
| treatment | 35 | 10 | 2 | 2 |

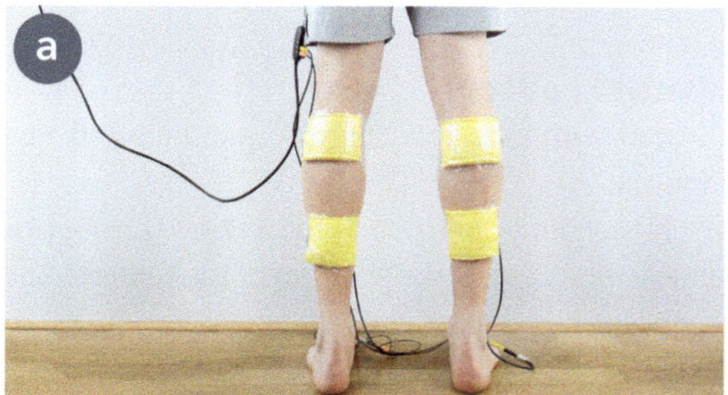
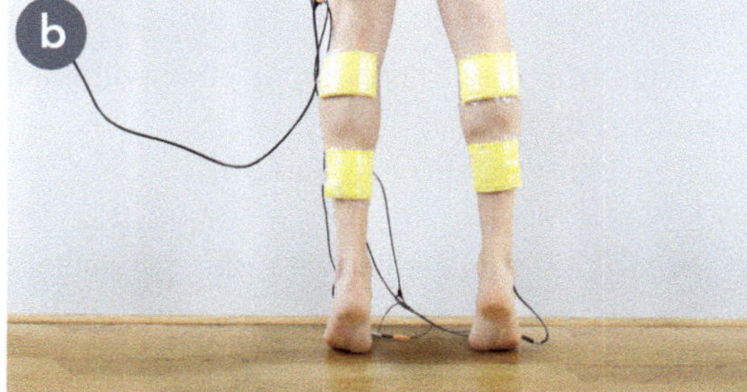


**Fig. 8.11** Stimulation of the triceps surae muscle in activity. (**a**) without stimulation in the relaxed position (**b**) with stimulation, anticipated stimulation response is illustrated

**Fixation:**

When using sponge electrodes, fixation foil or elastic bands can be used to attach the electrodes. It is essential to ensure that the electrodes are in full contact with the skin. In practice, this is not easy in the area of the upper arm. It is often advisable to work with adhesive electrodes.

**Treatment volume:**

Once a day, five to seven times a week for 30 min to maintain contractility.

**Table 8.9** Stimulation protocol in acute and chronic phase after injury

| acute/subacute lesion | pulse duration (ms) | pause (ms) | burst on (sec) | burst off (sec) |
|---|---|---|---|---|
| warm-up | 200 | 500 | 11 | 11 |
| treatment | 35 | 10 | 2 | 2 |

| chronic lesion | pulse duration (ms) | pause (ms) | burst on (sec) | burst off (sec) |
|---|---|---|---|---|
| warm-up | 150 | 1000 | 11 | 11 |
| treatment | 100 | 400 | 4 | 4 |
| treatment | 35 | 10 | 2 | 2 |

Twice a day for 20 min for reinnervation/motor learning (Fig. 8.12).

Stimulation parameters (Table 8.10).

▶ **Note** The application with the parameters described above includes a triangular pulse. The treatment example mainly refers to the acute/subacute phase after damage to the LMN.

### 8.12.6 Stimulation of the Elbow Flexors

**Indication:**

Support of reinnervation/motor learning.

Preservation of contractile muscle fibres (e.g., preoperatively before reconstructive surgery).

**Starting position:**

Seated with arm abducted 30° and elbow flexed approx. 80°.

Depending on which of the flexors is to be primarily stimulated, the position of the forearm and the electrode placement changes. When stimulating the biceps brachii muscle, the forearm is supinated, and the electrodes are placed on both heads of the muscle. When stimulating the brachialis muscle, the forearm is pronated, and the electrodes are placed medial to the short head of the biceps brachii muscle. Selective stimulation of the brachialis muscle is difficult. The pronatory movement of the forearm during stimulation serves as a clinical assessment of whether this is largely successful. With constant pronation under elbow flexion, a more or less selective excitation of the brachialis muscle can be expected.

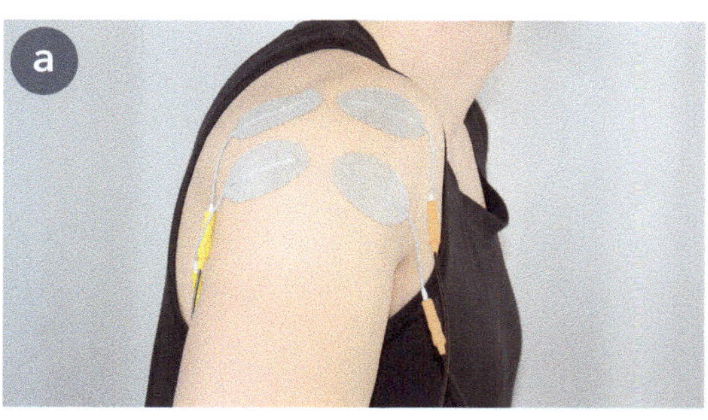
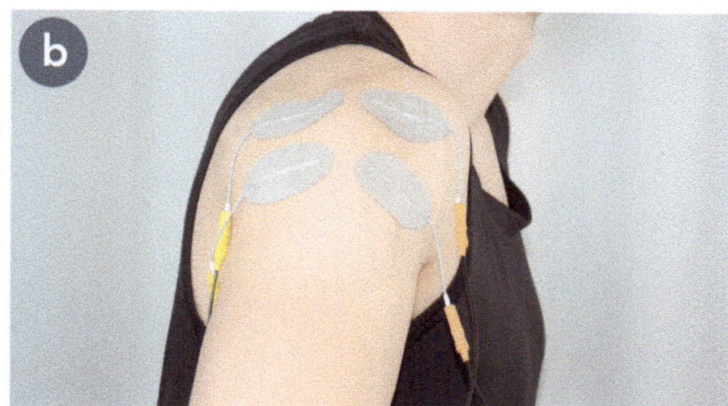

**Fig. 8.12** Stimulation of the deltoid muscle in all parts. (**a**) without stimulation in the relaxed position (**b**) with stimulation, anticipated stimulation response is illustrated

**Table 8.10** Stimulation protocol in acute/subacute phase after injury

| acute/subacute lesion | pulse duration (ms) | pulse interval (ms) | plateau (sec) |
|---|---|---|---|
| parameter | 10 | 30 | 3 |

**Electrodes:**

Self-adhesive electrodes or sponge pouches with corresponding electrodes for insertion. The choice of adhesive electrodes or sponge pouches depends on the stimulation parameters.

**Fixation:**

When using sponge electrodes, fixation foil or elastic bands can be used to attach the electrodes. It is essential to ensure that the electrodes are in full contact with the skin.

**Treatment volume:**

Once a day, five to seven times a week for 30 min to maintain contractility.

Twice a day for 20 min for reinnervation/motor learning (Fig. 8.13).

Stimulation parameters (Table 8.11).

▶ **Note** The application with the parameters described above includes a triangular pulse shape. The treatment example mainly refers to the acute/subacute phase after lesion to the lower motoneuron.

### 8.12.7 Four-Channel Stimulation of Denervated Arm Muscles

In the treatment example, all parts of the deltoid muscle, the triceps brachii, and the brachioradialis muscle are stimulated at the same time.

**Indication:**

Support of reinnervation/motor learning.

Preservation of contractile muscle fibres (e.g., in brachial plexus lesions preoperatively).

**Starting position:**

Seated with arm abducted 30° and elbow flexed approximate 80°.

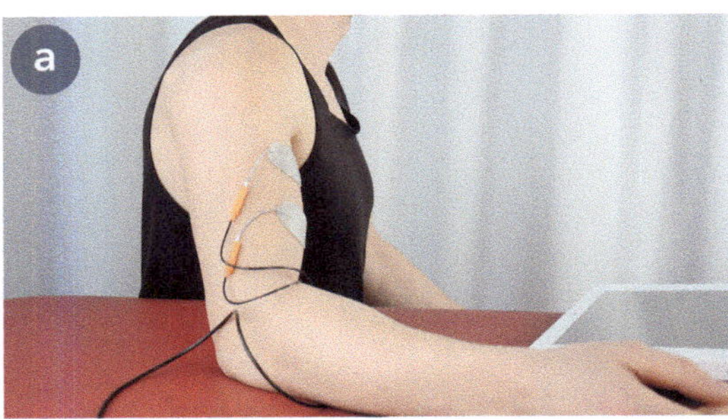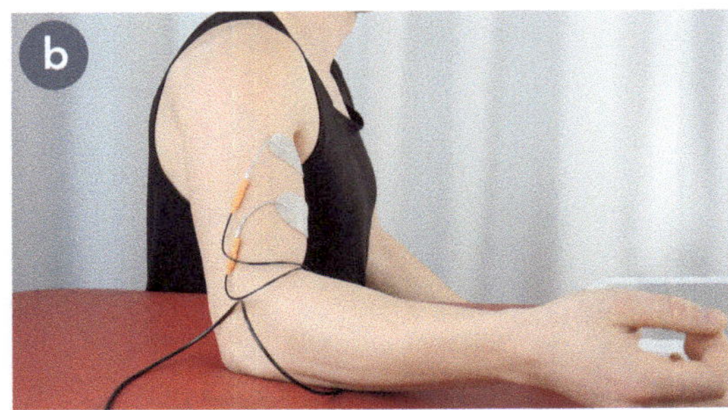

**Fig. 8.13** Stimulation of the biceps brachii. (**a**) without stimulation in the relaxed position (**b**) with stimulation, anticipated stimulation response is illustrated

**Table 8.11** Stimulation protocol in acute/subacute phase after injury

| acute/subacute lesion | pulse duration (ms) | pulse interval (ms) | plateau (sec) |
| --- | --- | --- | --- |
| parameter | 10 | 30 | 3 |

**Electrodes:**
Self-adhesive electrodes or sponge pouches with corresponding electrodes. The choice of adhesive electrodes or sponge pouches depends on the stimulation parameters.

**Fixation:**
When using sponge electrodes, fixation foil or elastic bands can be used to fix the electrodes. It is essential to ensure that the electrodes are in full contact with the skin. Here, attaching the sponge electrodes in the area of the delta is a challenge so that they do not lose contact under the resulting movement due to the muscle contraction.

**Treatment volume:**
Once a day, five to seven times a week for 30 min to maintain contractility.

Twice a day for 20 min for reinnervation/motor learning (Fig. 8.14).

Stimulation parameters (Table 8.12).

▶ **Note** The application with the parameters described above includes a triangular pulse shape. The treatment example mainly refers to the acute/subacute phase after damage to the LMN.

### 8.12.8 Stimulation of the Triceps Brachii Muscle in Function

**Indication:**
Support of reinnervation/motor learning.

Preservation of contractile muscle fibres (e.g., preoperatively before reconstructive surgery).

**Starting position:**
Seated with arms extended. The hands are placed next to the body so that the elbow extension can be executed under stimulation.

**Electrodes:**
Self-adhesive electrodes or sponge pouches with corresponding electrodes. The choice of self-adhesive electrodes or sponge pouches depends on the stimulation parameters.

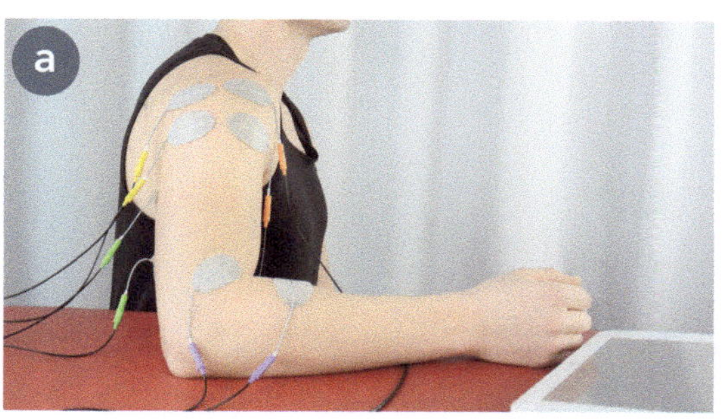

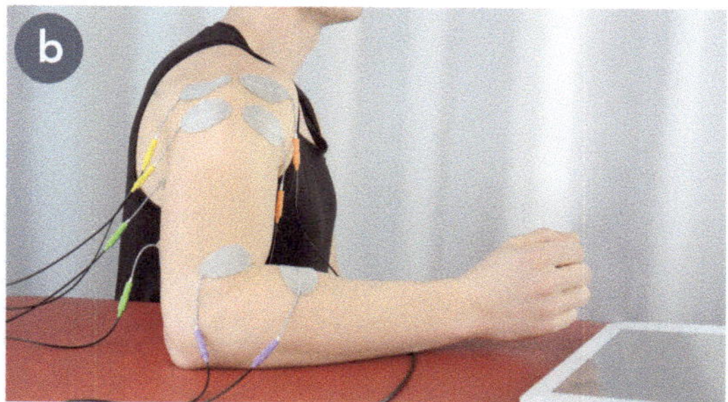


**Fig. 8.14** Stimulation of the deltoid muscle in all parts, the triceps brachii and the brachioradialis muscle. (**a**) without stimulation in the relaxed position (**b**) with stimulation, anticipated stimulation response is illustrated

**Table 8.12** Stimulation protocol in acute/subacute phase after injury

| acute/subacute lesion | pulse duration (ms) | pulse interval (ms) | plateau (sec) |
|---|---|---|---|
| parameter | 10 | 30 | 3 |

**Fixation:**

When using sponge electrodes, fixation foil or elastic bands can be used to attach the electrodes. It is essential to ensure that the electrodes are in full contact with the skin.

**Treatment volume:**

Once a day, five to seven times a week for 30 min to maintain contractility.

Twice a day for 20 min for reinnervation/motor learning (Fig. 8.15).

Stimulation parameters (Table 8.13).

▶ **Note** The application with the parameters described above includes a triangular pulse shape. The treatment example mainly refers to the acute/subacute phase after damage to the LMN.

### 8.12.9 Stimulation of the Intrinsic Hand Muscles

**Indication:**

Support of reinnervation/motor learning.

Preservation of contractile muscle fibres (e.g., in preparation for reconstructive hand surgery).

The intrinsic hand muscles are crucial for grasping. The group of dorsal Mm. interossei

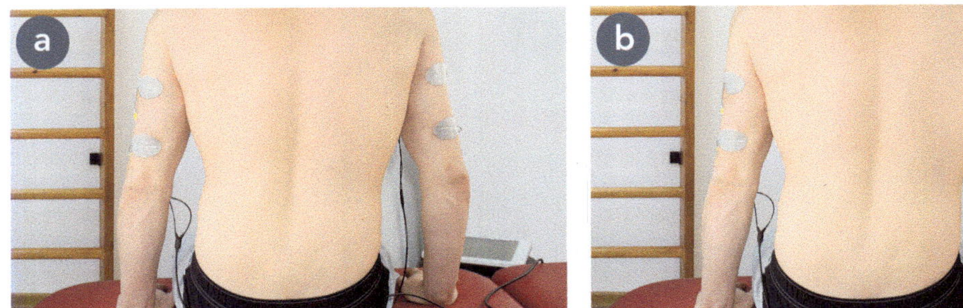


**Fig. 8.15** Stimulation of the triceps brachii muscle in function. (**a**) without stimulation in the relaxed position (**b**) with stimulation, anticipated stimulation response is illustrated

**Table 8.13** Stimulation protocol in acute/subacute phase after injury

| acute/subacute lesion | pulse duration (ms) | pulse interval (ms) | plateau (sec) |
|---|---|---|---|
| parameter | 10 | 30 | 3 |

ensures the correct sequence of finger joint flexion. Loss of elasticity or degeneration results in a clawed hand during grasping. Sufficient mobility in the metacarpophalangeal joints ensures a closed fist.

**Starting position:**
Seated.

**Electrodes:**
Sponge pouches with corresponding electrodes.

**Fixation:**
When using sponge electrodes, fixation foil, or elastic bands can be used to attach the electrodes. It is essential to ensure that the electrodes are in full contact with the skin.

**Treatment volume:**
Once a day, five to seven times a week for 30 min to maintain contractility.

Twice a day for 20 min for reinnervation/motor learning.

The following sequence of pictures shows from different perspectives the application of the electrodes as well as the possibility of fixation with a foil (Figs. 8.16, 8.17, and 8.18).

Stimulation parameters (Table 8.14).

▶ **Note** The primary indication for this treatment is in the acute and subacute phase after damage to the LMN. Whether stimulation in the chronic phase leads to a shortening of the intrinsic muscles and an increase in mobility and elasticity has not yet been scientifically proven.

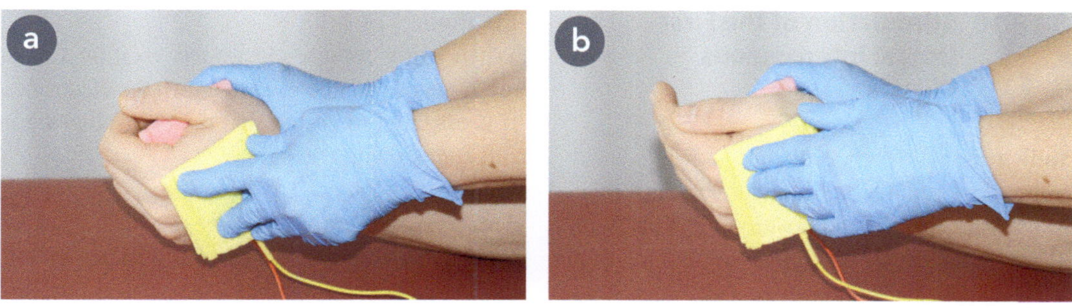

**Fig. 8.16** Stimulation of the intrinsic muscles (**a**) without stimulation (**b**) with stimulation

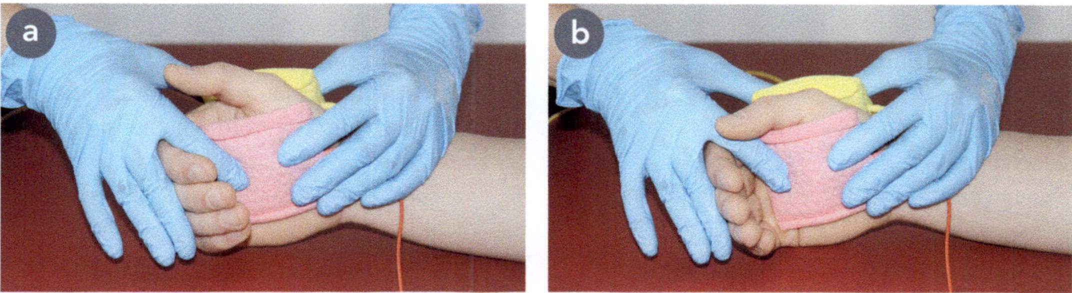

**Fig. 8.17** Stimulation of the intrinsic muscles (**a**) without stimulation (**b**) with stimulation

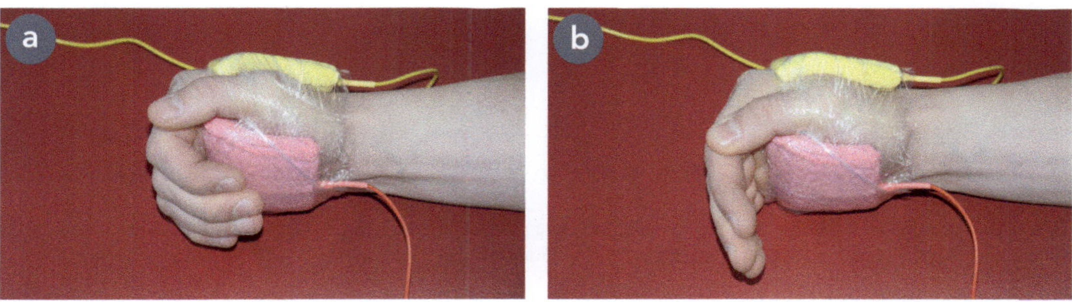

**Fig. 8.18** Stimulation of the intrinsic muscles (**a**) without stimulation (**b**) with stimulation

**Table 8.14** Stimulation protocol in acute/subacute phase after injury

| acute/subacute lesion | pulse duration (ms) | pause (ms) | bursts on (sec) | bursts off (sec) |
|---|---|---|---|---|
| warm-up | 200 | 500 | 11 | 11 |
| treatment | 35 | 10 | 2 | 2 |

## 8.12.10 Stimulation of the First Dorsal Interosseous Muscle

**Indication:**

Support of reinnervation/motor learning related to the lateral grasp and positioning of the thumb at the level of the interphalangeal joint of the index finger.

Preservation of contractile muscle fibres (e.g., in preparation for reconstructive hand surgery).

**Starting position:**

Seated.

**Electrodes:**

Sponge pouches with corresponding electrodes.

**Fixation:**

When using sponge electrodes, fixation foil or elastic bands can be used to attach the electrodes. It is essential to ensure that the electrodes are in full contact with the skin.

**Treatment volume:**

Once a day, five to seven times a week for 30 min to maintain contractility.

Twice a day for 20 min for reinnervation/motor learning (Fig. 8.19).

Stimulation parameters (Table 8.15).

▶ **Note** The primary indication of this treatment is in the acute and subacute phase after damage to the lower motoneuron. Whether stimulation in the chronic phase results in an increase in mobility and elasticity has not yet been scientifically proven.

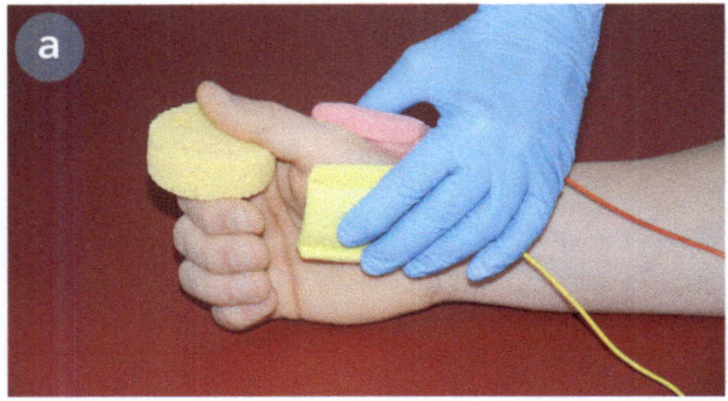
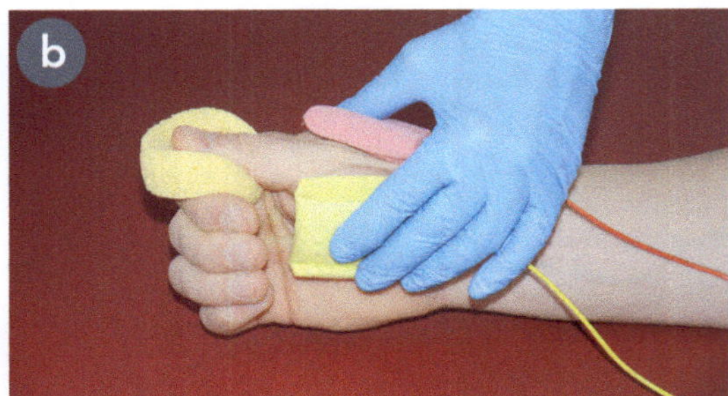

**Fig. 8.19** Stimulation of the interosseus dorsalis I muscle performing the lateral grasp. (**a**) without stimulation in the relaxed position (**b**) with stimulation, anticipated stimulation response is illustrated

**Table 8.15** Stimulation protocol in acute/subacute phase after injury

| acute/subacute lesion | pulse duration (ms) | pause (ms) | bursts on (sec) | bursts off (sec) |
|---|---|---|---|---|
| warm-up | 200 | 500 | 11 | 11 |
| treatment | 35 | 10 | 2 | 2 |

### 8.12.11 Stimulation of the Extensor Carpi Radialis Muscle

**Indication:**
Support of reinnervation/motor learning.

Preservation of contractile muscle fibres (e.g., in preparation for reconstructive hand surgery).

**Starting position:**
Seated.

**Electrodes:**
Sponge pouches with corresponding electrodes to insert. In the area of the forearm, the existing two layers of muscles have to be taken into account. Stimulating selective movement or individual muscles is therefore difficult and not always possible selectively. Small electrodes are helpful as well as precise placement of them.

**Fixation:**
When using sponge electrodes, the electrodes can be fixed with fixing foil or elastic bands. For testing, it is recommended to hold the electrodes manually. The stimulus response, if weak, can be well assessed by palpation.

Often the electrodes must be held manually without applying much pressure. Full contact of the electrodes must be ensured.

**Treatment volume:**
Once a day, five to seven times a week for 30 min to maintain contractility.

Twice a day for 20 min for reinnervation/motor learning (Figs. 8.20 and 8.21).

Stimulation parameters (Table 8.16).

▶ **Note** Currently, the primary indication for this treatment is in the acute and subacute phase after damage to the LMN.

▶ In rare cases, the pressure exerted by the foil or bands is too high and the antagonists are activated ("spill over").

### 8.12.12 Stimulation of the Extensor Digitorum Communis Muscle

**Indication:**
Support of reinnervation/motor learning.

Preservation of contractile muscle fibres (e.g., in preparation for reconstructive hand surgery).

**Starting position:**
Seated.

**Electrodes:**
Sponge pouches with corresponding electrodes to insert. In the area of the forearm, the muscles are organized in two layers. Especially the muscle group of M. extensor carpi radialis, M. extensor carpi ulnaris, and M. extensor digitorum communis is difficult to stimulate selectively. It is critical to find the best possible position of the electrodes to obtain the best selectivity of the

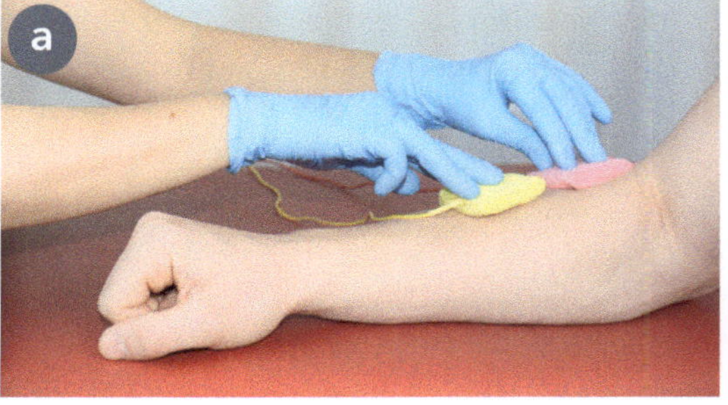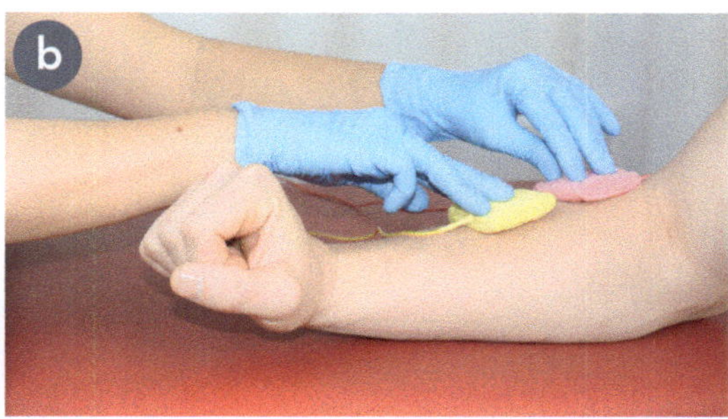

**Fig. 8.20** Stimulation of the extensor carpi radialis (**a**) without stimulation (**b**) with stimulation with manual fixation of the electrodes

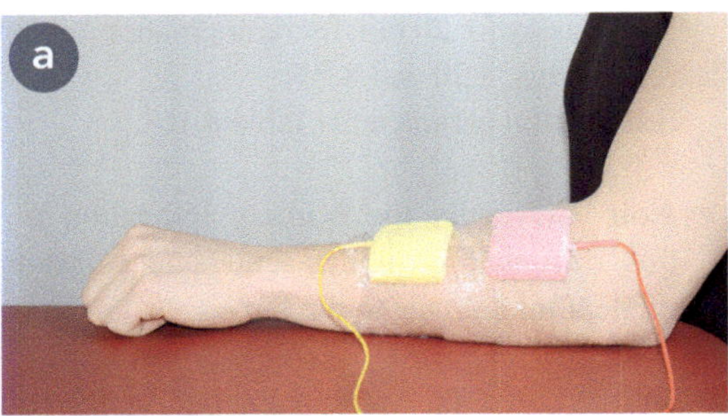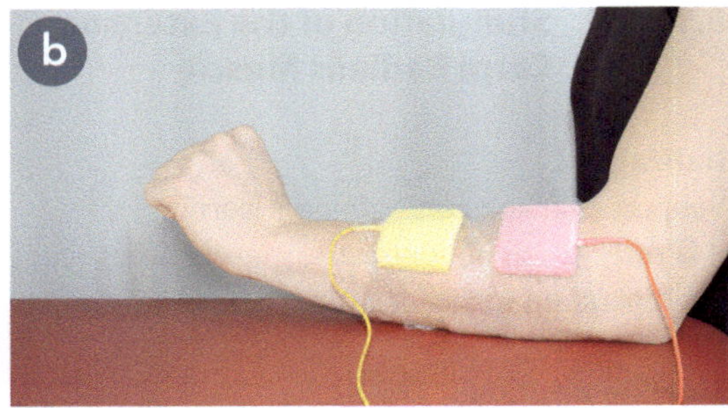

**Fig. 8.21** Stimulation of the extensor carpi radialis (**a**) without stimulation (**b**) with stimulation

**Table 8.16** Stimulation protocol in acute/subacute phase after injury

| acute/subacute lesion | pulse duration (ms) | pause (ms) | bursts on (sec) | bursts off (sec) |
|---|---|---|---|---|
| warm-up | 200 | 500 | 11 | 11 |
| treatment | 35 | 10 | 2 | 2 |

expected movement. Small electrodes are helpful as well as precise placement of the electrodes.

**Fixation:**

When using sponge electrodes, the electrodes can be attached with foil or elastic bands. For testing, it is recommended to hold the electrodes manually. The stimulus response, if weak, can be well assessed by palpation. In rare cases, the pressure exerted by the foil or elastic bands is too high and consequently the antagonists are activated ("spill over").

**Treatment volume:**

Once a day, five to seven times a week for 30 min to maintain contractility.

Twice a day for 20 min for reinnervation/motor learning (Figs. 8.22 and 8.23).

Stimulation parameters (Table 8.17).

▶ **Note:** Currently, the primary indication for this treatment is in the acute and subacute phase after damage to the lower motoneuron.

### 8.12.13 Stimulation of the Extensor Carpi Ulnaris Muscle in Function

**Indication:**
Support of reinnervation/motor learning.

Preservation of contractile muscle fibres (e.g., in preparation for reconstructive hand surgery).

Balancing of wrist extension even in the chronic phase after damage to the LMN.

**Starting position:**
Seated.

**Electrodes:**
Sponge pouches with corresponding electrodes. The extensor carpi ulnaris muscle is the easiest

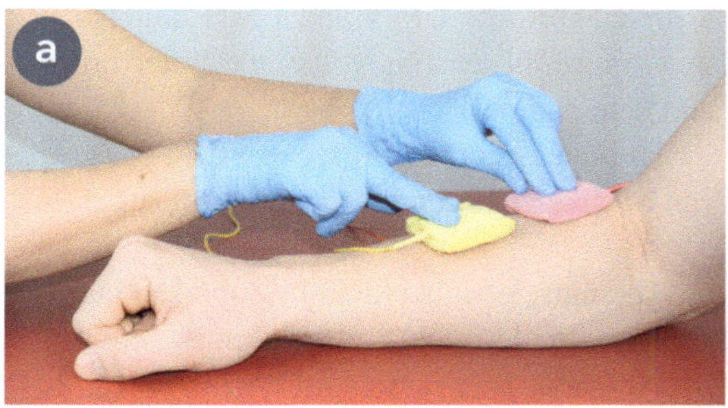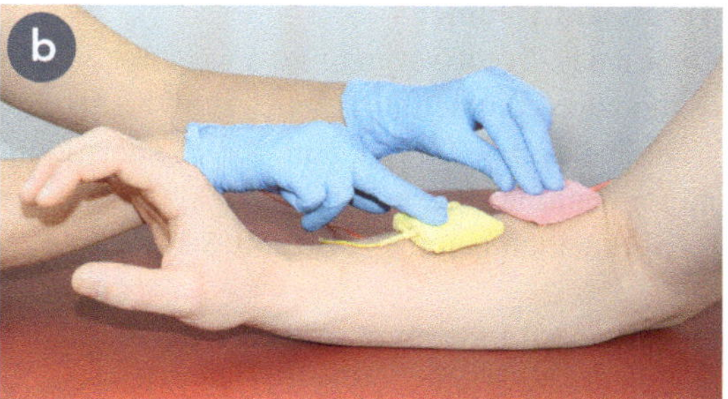

**Fig. 8.22** Stimulation of the extensor digitorum communis (**a**) without stimulation (**b**) with stimulation with manual fixation of the electrodes

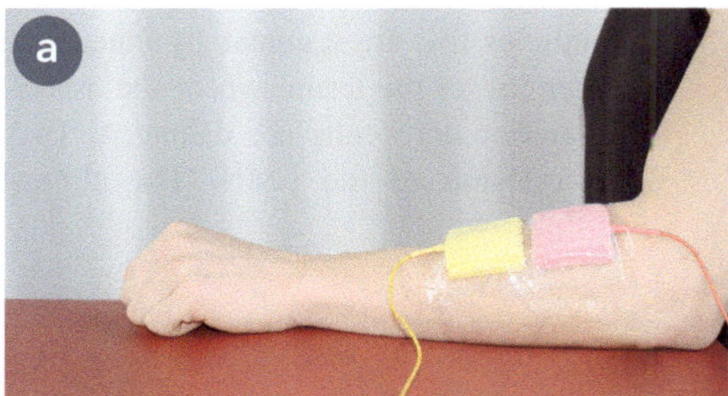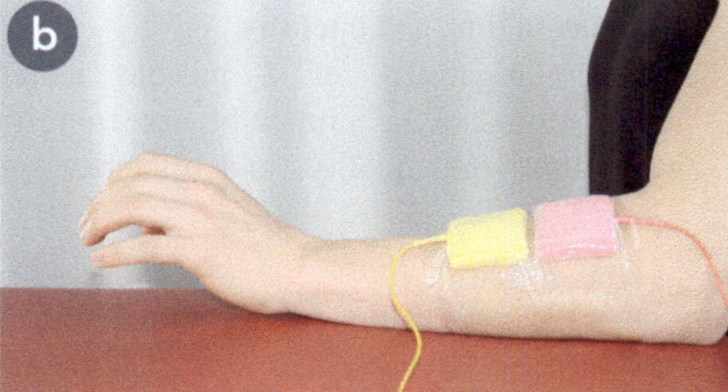

**Fig. 8.23** Stimulation of the extensor digitorum communis (**a**) without stimulation (**b**) with stimulation

**Table 8.17** Stimulation protocol in acute/subacute phase after injury

| acute/subacute lesion | pulse duration (ms) | pause (ms) | bursts on (sec) | bursts off (sec) |
|---|---|---|---|---|
| warm-up | 200 | 500 | 11 | 11 |
| treatment | 35 | 10 | 2 | 2 |

one to stimulate selectively in the group of the wrist and finger extensors. However, stimulating selective movement or individual muscles remains difficult. Small electrodes are helpful as well as precise placement.

**Fixation:**
When using sponge electrodes, fixation foil, or elastic bands can be used to attach the electrodes.

**Treatment volume:**
Once a day, five to seven times a week for 30 min to maintain contractility.

Twice a day for 20 min for reinnervation/motor learning (Fig. 8.24).

Stimulation parameters (Table 8.18).

▶ **Note:** All forearm muscles can be stimulated against resistance. Whether this is used is determined by both the goal and the structural situation of the muscle. If resistance is used, a denervated muscle must have a certain level of training. This can be achieved with increasing stimulation time and intensity.

The fatigability of a muscle under stimulation can be clinically assessed by evaluating the quality and quantity of muscle contraction. The quality of the range of motion during stimulation is observed and documented. If the range of motion decreases, fatigue can be clinically assumed.

## 8.13 Partially Innervated/Partially Denervated Muscles

Muscles are partially innervated when they have a mixed form of UMN and LMN damage or a mixed form of existing voluntary motor function and denervation.

This can occur in the case of SCI. Four groups can be divided around the area of injury.

1. The muscles innervated by supralesional segments underlying to the voluntary control of the brain.
2. The muscles innervated by infralesional segments and characterized by increased reflex activity and muscle weakness. They are not controlled voluntarily.
3. The muscles that are segmentally innervated in the centre of the lesion where the associated anterior horn cells are damaged. They show a lesion of the LMN. The clinical

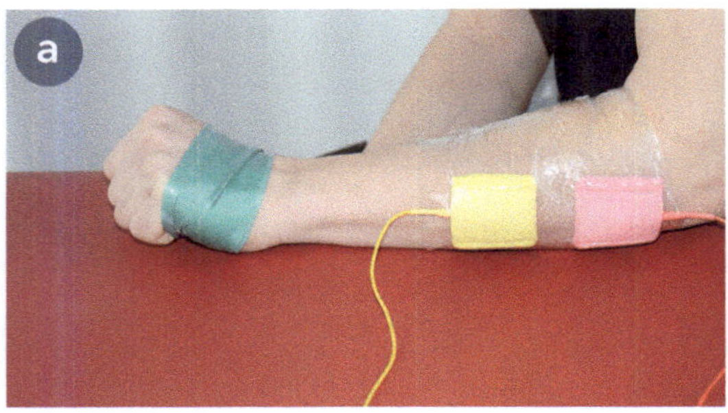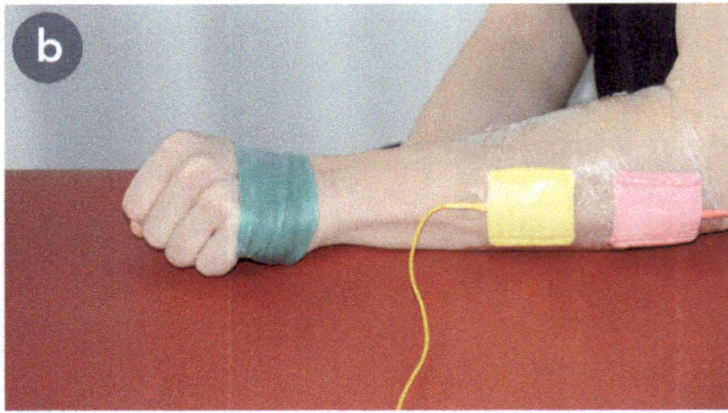

**Fig. 8.24** Stimulation of the extensor carpi ulnaris muscle against resistance (**a**) without stimulation (**b**) with stimulation

**Table 8.18** Stimulation protocol in the acute and chronic phase after injury

| acute/subacute lesion | pulse duration (ms) | pause (ms) | bursts on (sec) | bursts off (sec) |
|---|---|---|---|---|
| warm-up | 200 | 500 | 11 | 11 |
| treatment | 35 | 10 | 2 | 2 |

| chronic lesion | pulse duration (ms) | pause (ms) | bursts on (sec) | bursts off (sec) |
|---|---|---|---|---|
| warm-up | 150 | 1000 | 11 | 11 |
| treatment | 100 | 400 | 4 | 4 |
| treatment | 40 | 10 | 2 | 2 |

appearance of these muscles is similar to that of a peripheral nerve lesion. There is flaccid paralysis with signs of denervation and degeneration.

4. The muscles innervated near the centre of the lesion (one segment above or below). These may show partial denervation respectively innervation.

In addition to the population of people with SCI, patients with, e.g., lumbar nerve root compression, Guillain-Barré syndrome or CMT disease may show partially innervated muscles. Here, might be a mixture of existing voluntary motor function and denervation in a muscle or muscle group. The first-mentioned manifestation of nerve root compression, caused by protrusion or prolapse of an intervertebral disc, is clinically the most common appearance. Affected persons show clinically a drop foot. An early combination of electrical stimulation, exercises and techniques to maintain and enhance function are recommended. A useful combination with electrical stimulation via muscle and/or nerve is the principle of irradiation. If the treatment volume cannot be implemented daily in outpatient treatment, the delivery of a stimulation device for domestic use is an option (see also Chap. 12). In this way, the stimulation can be conducted in the recommended frequency to provide the best possible stimulus to the peripheral and central nervous system.

**Noteworthy**
When selecting the stimulation parameter, the first decision to be made is whether the stimulation can be conducted via nerve or muscle.

> It should be taken into account that partially denervated muscle fibres do not respond to stimulation via nerve. Nerve fibres are excitable from 50 μs (0.05 ms) pulse duration, while muscle fibres require longer pulse durations over 10 ms. Partially voluntary innervated muscle fibres cannot replace and compensate for all muscle function, including strength, volume, and coordination.

There are several treatment approaches that can be followed. The target muscle can be stimulated with direct muscle stimulation as well as via nerve. Ideally, this is done in one treatment session. This means 30 min of stimulation via nerve followed by 30 min of direct muscle stimulation.

It is also possible to alternate between direct muscle stimulation in one treatment session and nerve stimulation in the next. Ideally, this should be done in daily alternation.

If the muscle is partially innervated, it can be actively trained with conventional treatment methods and the denervated parts with direct muscle stimulation.

Successful treatment depends on the time after a lesion and its extent and can take weeks to years. Possible recovery can be expected in the acute and subacute phases after the lesion. Regular reassessments of the innervation status of the stimulated muscles are required. This may change over time. It also requires timely adjustment of stimulation parameters. To some extent, structural but non-functional changes in a muscle can lead to improvement. Changes in muscle structure can support residual function.

## References


1. Mödlin M, Forstner C, Hofer C, Mayr W, Richter W, Carraro U, et al. Electrical stimulation of denervated muscles: first results of a clinical study. Artif Org. 2005;29(3):203–6.
2. Helgason T, Gargiulo P, Jóhannesdóttir F, Ingvarsson P, Knútsdóttir S, Gudmundsdóttir V, et al. Monitoring muscle growth and tissue changes induced by electrical stimulation of denervated degenerated muscles with CT and stereolithographic 3D modeling. Artif Org. 2005;29(6):440–3.
3. Carraro U, Rossini K, Mayr W, Kern H. Muscle fiber regeneration in human permanent lower motoneuron denervation: relevance to safety and effectiveness of FES-training, which induces muscle recovery in SCI subjects. Artif Org. 2005;29(3):187–91.
4. Kern H, Carraro U. Home-based functional electrical stimulation for long-term denervated human muscle: history, basics, results and perspectives of the Vienna rehabilitation strategy. Eur J Transl Myol. 2014;24(1):3296.
5. Kern H, Boncompagni S, Rossini K, Mayr W, Fanò G, Zanin ME, et al. Long-term denervation in humans causes degeneration of both contractile and excitation-contraction coupling apparatus, which is reversible by functional electrical stimulation (FES): a role for myofiber regeneration? J Neuropathol Exp Neurol. 2004;63(9):919–31.
6. Kesar T, Chou L-W, Binder-Macleod SA. Effects of stimulation frequency versus pulse duration modulation on muscle fatigue. J Electromyogr Kinesiol. 2008;18(4):662–71.
7. Koh ES, Kim HC, Lim J-Y. The effects of electromyostimulation application timing on denervated skeletal muscle atrophy. Muscle Nerve. 2017;56(6):E154–61.
8. Kern H, Boncompagni S, Rossini K, Mayr W, Fanó G, Zanin ME, et al. Long-term denervation in humans causes degeneration of both contractile and excitation-contraction coupling apparatus, which is reversible by functional electrical stimulation (FES): a role for myofiber regeneration? J Neuropathol Exp Neurol. 2004;3:919–31.
9. Ashley Z, Salmons S, Boncompagni S, Protasi F, Russold M, Lanmuller H, et al. Effects of chronic electrical stimulation on long-term denervated muscles of the rabbit hind limb. J Muscle Res Cell M. 2007;28(4–5):203–17.
10. Kern H, Hofer C, Loefler S, Zampieri S, Gargiulo P, Baba A, et al. Atrophy, ultra-structural disorders, severe atrophy and degeneration of denervated human muscle in SCI and aging. Implications for their recovery by functional electrical stimulation, updated 2017. Neurol Res. 2017;39(7):660–6.
11. Carraro U, Kern H, Gava P, Hofer C, Loefler S, Gargiulo P, et al. Recovery from muscle weakness by exercise and FES: lessons from masters, active or sedentary seniors and SCI patients. Aging Clin Exp Res. 2017;29(4):579–90.
12. Kern H, Stramare R, Martino L, Zanato R, Gargiulo P, Carraro U. Permanent LMN denervation of human skeletal muscle and recovery by h-b FES: management and monitoring. Eur J Transl Myol. 2010;20(3):91–104.

13. Kern H, Carraro U, Adami N, Biral D, Hofer C, Forstner C, et al. Home-based functional electrical stimulation rescues permanently denervated muscles in paraplegic patients with complete lower motor neuron lesion. Neurorehabilit Neural Repair. 2010;24(8):709–21.

14. Peckham PH, MORTIMER JT, Marsolais EB. Alteration in the force and fatigability of skeletal muscle in quadriplegic humans following exercise induced by chronic electrical stimulation. Clin Orthop Relat Res. 1976;1976(114):326–34.

15. Bersch I, Koch-Borner S, Fridén J. Motor point topography of fundamental grip actuators in tetraplegia - implications in nerve transfer surgery. J Neurotrauma. 2020;37(3):441–7.

16. Salmons S, Ashley Z, Sutherland H, Russold MF, Li F, Jarvis JC. Functional electrical stimulation of denervated muscles: basic issues. Artif Org. 2005;29(3):199–202.

17. Gordon T, Amirjani N, Edwards DC, Chan KM. Brief post-surgical electrical stimulation accelerates axon regeneration and muscle reinnervation without affecting the functional measures in carpal tunnel syndrome patients. Exp Neurol. 2010;223(1):192–202.

18. Brushart TM, Jari R, Verge V, Rohde C, Gordon T. Electrical stimulation restores the specificity of sensory axon regeneration. Exp Neurol. 2005;194(1):221–9.

19. Gordon T, English AW. Strategies to promote peripheral nerve regeneration: electrical stimulation and/or exercise. Eur J Neurosci. 2016;43(3):336–50.

20. Asensio-Pinilla E, Udina E, Jaramillo J, Navarro X. Electrical stimulation combined with exercise increase axonal regeneration after peripheral nerve injury. Exp Neurol. 2009;219(1):258–65.

21. Albertin G, Hofer C, Zampieri S, Vogelauer M, Löfler S, Ravara B, et al. In complete SCI patients, long-term functional electrical stimulation of permanent denervated muscles increases epidermis thickness. Neurol Res. 2018;40(4):277–82.

22. Smit CAJ, Haverkamp GLG, de Groot S, Stolwijk-Swuste JM, Janssen TWJ. Effects of electrical stimulation-induced gluteal versus gluteal and hamstring muscles activation on sitting pressure distribution in persons with a spinal cord injury. Spinal Cord. 2012;50(8):590–4.

23. Bryden AM, Kilgore KL, Lind BB, Yu DT. Triceps denervation as a predictor of elbow flexion contractures in C5 and C6 tetraplegia. Arch Phys Med Rehabil. 2004;85(11):1880–5.

24. Mulcahey MJ, Smith BT, Betz RR. Evaluation of the lower motor neuron integrity of upper extremity muscles in high level spinal cord injury. Spinal Cord. 1999;37(8):585–91.

25. Thomas CK, Häger CK, Klein CS. Increases in human motoneuron excitability after cervical spinal cord injury depend on the level of injury. J Neurophysiol. 2017;117(2):684–91.

26. Zijdewind I, Gant K, Bakels R, Thomas CK. Do additional inputs change maximal voluntary motor unit firing rates after spinal cord injury? Neurorehabilit Neural Repair. 2012;26(1):58–67.

27. Macefield VG. Discharge rates and discharge variability of muscle spindle afferents in human chronic spinal cord injury. Clin Neurophysiol Pract. 2013;124(1):114–9.

28. Hulliger M, Matthews PB, Noth J. Static and dynamic fusimotor action on the response of ia fibres to low frequency sinusoidal stretching of widely ranging amplitude. J Physiol. 1977;267(3):811–38.

29. Burke D, Gandevia SC, Macefield G. Responses to passive movement of receptors in joint, skin and muscle of the human hand. J Physiol. 1988;402:347–61.

30. Kern H, McKay WB, Dimitrijevic MM, Dimitrijevic MR. Motor control in the human spinal cord and the repair of cord function. Curr Pharm Des. 2005;11(11):1429–39.

31. Lømo T, Westgaard RH, Hennig R, Gundersen K. The response of denervated muscle to long-term electrical stimulation. Eur J Transl Myol. 2014;24(1)

32. Fox IK, Miller AK, Curtin CM. Nerve and tendon transfer surgery in cervical spinal cord injury: individualized choices to optimize function. Top Spinal Cord Inj Rehabil. 2018;24(3):275–87.

33. Gargiulo P, Helgason T, Reynisson PJ, Helgason B, Kern H, Mayr W, et al. Monitoring of muscle and bone recovery in spinal cord injury patients treated with electrical stimulation using three-dimensional imaging and segmentation techniques: methodological assessment. Artifi Org. 2011;35(3):275–81.

34. Boncompagni S, Kern H, Rossini K, Hofer C, Mayr W, Carraro U, et al. Structural differentiation of skeletal muscle fibers in the absence of innervation in humans. Proc Natl Acad Sci U S A. 2007;104(49):19339–44.

35. Stickler Y, Martinek J, Hofer C, Rattay F. A finite element model of the electrically stimulated human thigh: changes due to denervation and training. Artif Org. 2008;32(8):620–4.

36. Mayr W, Hofer C, Bijak M, Rafolt D, Unger E, Reichel M, et al. Functional electrical stimulation (FES) of denervated muscles: existing and prospective technological solutions. Basic Appl Myol. 2003;6:287–90.

# Sensory Afferent Stimulation

Kerstin Schwenker and Stefan M. Golaszewski

## 9.1 Introduction

Sensory afferent stimulation is a method of non-invasive brain stimulation (NIBS) that induces neuromodulation especially at the synaptic level in the area of the sensorimotor cortex [1–3]. In sensory afferent electrical stimulation (SAES), electrical stimuli are used in continuous series or in time-structured stimulation patterns, which trigger peripheral action potentials in afferent nerve fibers, which lead to an increased sensory afferent input into the sensorimotor centers in the brain. SAES is currently developing into a promising adjuvant intervention in the field of NIBS in combination with conventional sensorimotor therapy in a temporal correlation to improve the outcome in neurorehabilitation.

**Stefan M. Golaszewski** was deceased at the time of publication.

K. Schwenker (✉)
Department of Neurology, University Hospital Salzburg, Spinal Cord Injury and Tissue Regeneration Center Salzburg, Paracelsus Medical University, Salzburg, Austria
e-mail: kerstin.schwenker@pmu.ac.at

S. M. Golaszewski
Salzburg, Austria

## 9.2 Sensory Afferent Stimulation

### 9.2.1 Neurobiology of Sensory Afferent Stimulation

Synapses can be highly plastic and change the strength of their synaptic transmission due to an "intrinsic" change in their own activity or a change in the synaptic input from other nerve cells "extrinsically". Intrinsic and extrinsic synaptic plasticity are considered to be the basic neurobiological mechanisms for memory, learning, and restitution of lost functions.

The model of long-term potentiation (LTP) and long-term depression (LTD) (② and ③ in Fig. 9.1) describes an extrinsic change in the strength of a synaptic transmission [4]. Sensory afferent stimulations induce neuromodulatory effects in the area of short-term plasticity (STP, ① in Fig. 9.1) and structural neuroplasticity with sprouting of new synapses (synaptic sprouting, ④ in Fig. 9.1) and the formation of new anatomical connections (wiring) in the nervous system. Due to the increased sensory afferent input in SAES (① lightning symbol ⚡ in Fig. 9.1), more glutamate is released from the presynaptic vesicles into the synaptic cleft. This happens with almost complete opening of the AMPA (α-amino-3-hydroxy-5-methyl-4-isoxazolepropionic acid) receptors, which leads to a strong $Na^+$ influx into the cell with a strong depolarization of the cell membrane. Through glutamate binding to the

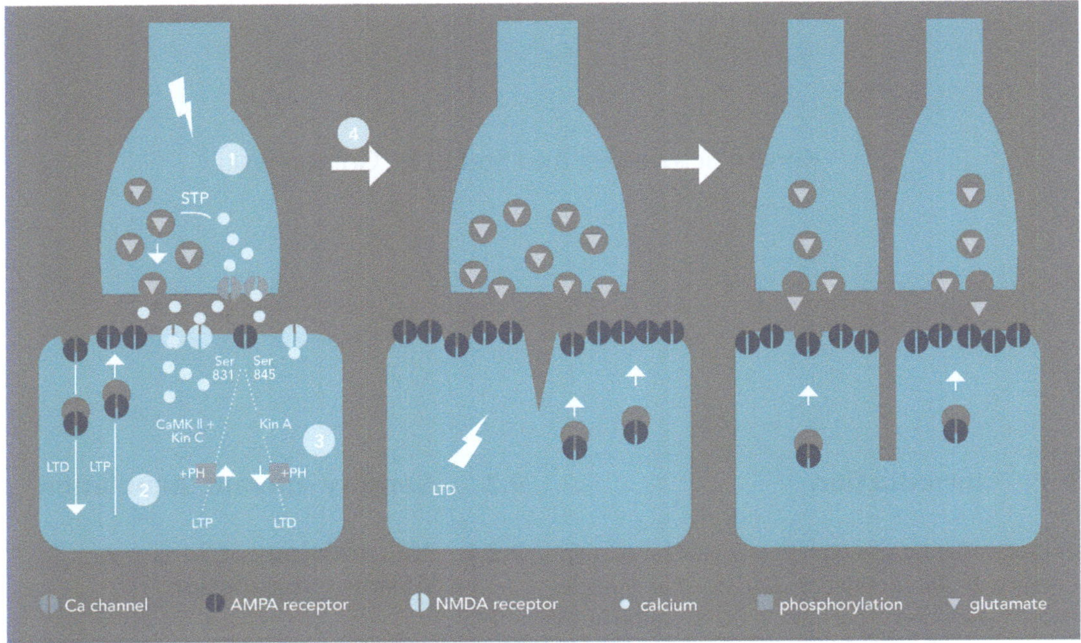


**Fig. 9.1** Increased sensory-afferent input ($\frac{1}{2}$) induces neuroplasticity in the short-term (①), the long-term (② and ③), and the structural areas (④). Depending on the type of sensory-afferent stimulation, the synaptic transmission can be increased (LTP, long-term potentiation) or reduced (LTD, long-term depression). With LTD, the mechanisms of the LTP can be reversed again (②, ③, and ④)

NMDA (*N*-methyl-D-aspartate, NMDA) receptor and strong depolarization of the cell membrane, the $Mg^{2+}$ ions, which block the NMDA receptor, can also diffuse out, causing it to become a massive $Ca^{2+}$ influx at the NMDA receptor into the cell which leads to a number of intracellular signaling pathways with enzyme induction. Depending on the type of sensory afferent input, LTP increases and LTD decreases synaptic transmission. In LTP there is also an increased incorporation of AMPA receptors into the postsynaptic membrane and activation of calcium/calmodulin-dependent kinase II (CaMK II), which with kinase C (Kin C) leads to a phosphorylation (+PH) of the subunit GluR1 of the AMPA receptor of the amino acid Serine 831 (Ser 831). This increases the conductivity of the AMPA receptor (↑), combined with a massive influx of ions into the cell, which maintains LTP (② in Fig. 9.1). Together with kinase A, there is a phosphorylation (+PH) of the amino acid Serine 845 (Ser 845) of GluR1, which reduces the synaptic transmission (↓) and initiates the LTD (③ in Fig. 9.1).

The LTP further increases the density of the AMPA receptors in the postsynaptic membrane, which leads to a splitting of the postsynaptic membrane with the formation of new synapses (④ in Fig. 9.1). In this way, new neuronal networks can be built up permanently, combined with new behavioral skills or with the restitution of lost functions. Depending on the type of sensory afferent stimulation, a LTD can also be induced, which counteracts the LTP and can reverse it (e.g., downregulation of the LTP upregulated AMPA receptors in the postsynaptic membrane, ④ in Fig. 9.1) [5].

With a single stimulation lasting at least 30 min, the duration of the neuromodulatory effects is in the range of a few hours [6–8], whereby with prolongation and repetition of the stimulation a sustainable prolongation of the effects is possible. The optimal parameters and stimulation patterns for the stimulation are not yet exactly known [9]. In addition to the frequency, the stimulation intensity seems to have the greatest influence on neuromodulation [8].

The stimulation depolarizes afferent proprioceptive and exteroceptive nerve fibers of group Ia (thick afferents of the muscle spindles), Ib (thick afferents of the tendon receptors and Golgi organs), and group II (slowly and quickly adapting afferents of the mechanoreceptors of the skin and the γ-fibers of the muscle spindle) with short latency [10–12]. The afferent signals are further forwarded in the posterior funicles and in the spinocerebellar tract of the spinal cord to the brain stem, to the ventroposterolateral nucleus of the thalamus with projection to the contra- and ipsilateral sensorimotor cortex in the Brodmann areas (BA) 3a, 2, 1 and 4 and to the cerebellum [13–15]. In addition to the direct afferents, BA 4 (primary motor cortex, M1) also receives projections from BA 3a, 2 and 1 [16] as well as transcallosal projections from the contralateral cerebral cortex [17–19]. In their small intrinsic muscles, the hand and foot have a high density of muscle spindles [20, 21], joint receptors, and Golgi tendon organs [10, 22,

23], which is why these muscles are an abundant source of proprioceptive inputs for the spinal cord and brain. Proprio- and exteroceptive afferents are the basis for the perception of kinesthetics in the brain [24].

**Summary**
In sensory afferent stimulation, nerve fibers of deep and fine surface sensitivity are stimulated with the induction of short-term, long-term, and structural neuroplasticity in the brain.

## 9.2.2 Sensory Afferent Electrical Stimulation

In SAES, action potentials are triggered below the stimulating cathode by extra- and intracellular ion currents with depolarization of the cell membrane (Fig. 9.2).

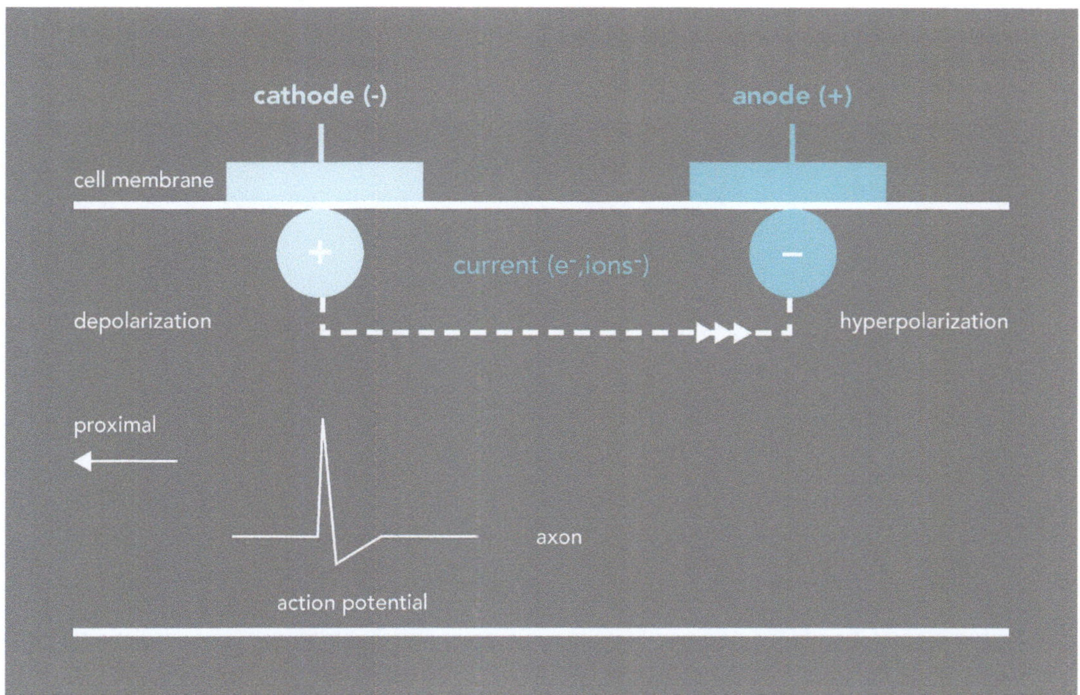


**Fig. 9.2** With SAES (sensory afferent electrical stimulation), the current flows from the cathode in all spatial directions in the extracellular space (ECS) and thus also vertically through the cell membrane, in order to continue to flow intracellularly along the electric field lines (arrows) to the anode, from where it flows again vertically through the cell membrane into the ECS. Negative charges (electrons, e-, and negatively charged ions, "−") are shifted along the course of the peripheral nerve fibers primarily intracellularly towards the anode (arrows) with local hyperpolarization of the membrane, positive charges (positively charged ions, "+") toward the cathode with local depolarization of the membrane. The action potentials for the sensory afferent input into the brain are then triggered under the cathode

Ordinary self-adhesive electrodes are used, like in nerve or neuromuscular stimulation. A more increased sensory afferent input can also be induced with anodes in the form of an electrode glove (mesh glove, MG) (Fig. 9.3) or an electrode sock (mesh sock, MS), which is due to the stimulated size of the skin area to bring about a particularly strong neuromodulatory input in the sensorimotor cortex.

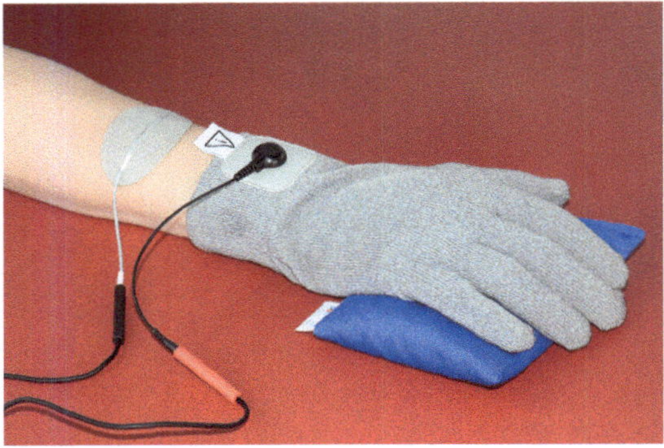

**Fig. 9.3** With mesh glove stimulation, the afferent action potentials are triggered in the three hand nerves (N. radialis, medianus et ulnaris) under the dorsal and palmar cathode on the forearm

MG or MS are connected to a two-channel electrical stimulation device and function as anode, carbon surface electrodes over the tendons of the flexors and extensors on the forearm or lower leg as cathodes (Fig. 9.3). The current is applied in a pulsed manner. The pulse shape is rectangular or trapezoidal and mono- or biphasic with a frequency of 50 Hz and a pulse width of 300 µs. The stimulation is carried out for 30–60 min (Fig. 9.4).

Neuromodulatory effects through SAES can be demonstrated in fMRI (functional Magnetic Resonance Imaging) with a finger-to-thumb tap paradigm (Test Motor Task, TMT) with a self-selected frequency of approximately 2 Hz in a pre−/post-design [6, 25]. With TMT, brain activity in the form of the so-called BOLD effect (Blood Oxygenation Level Dependent, BOLD) is detected in the contra- and ipsilateral hemisphere in the pre- and postcentral gyrus, in the superior frontal gyrus and in both halves of the cerebellum with a dominance ipsilateral to the tapping hand. After 30 min of SAES, finger-to-thumb tapping (Conditioned Motor Task 1, CMT1) shows an increase in brain activity in both hemispheres in

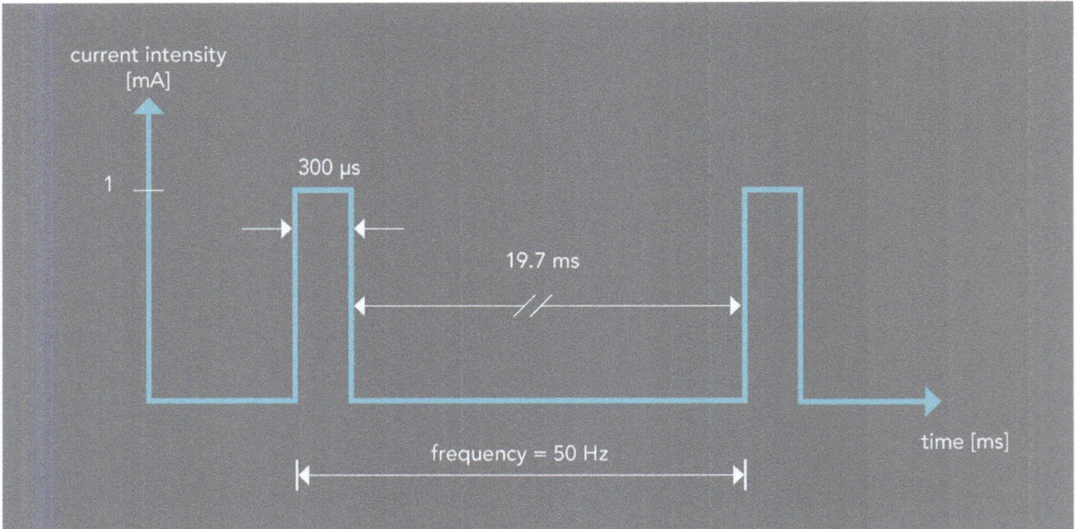


**Fig. 9.4** Current pulse with SAES (sensory afferent electrical stimulation): rectangular pulse with a width of 300 µs and a frequency of 50 Hz. The duration of the stimulation is at least 30 min at a sensitive level (at approx. 5 mA, depending on skin resistance), which already results in inducing neuroplasticity in the long-term range (LTP, long-term potentiation; LTD, long-term depression). At the motor level, the current intensities are higher (up to approx. 10 mA, depending on skin resistance). Due to its higher effectiveness, SAES also uses protocols with a shorter stimulation duration (10–30 min) at the motor level. The frequencies vary between 1 and 50 Hz, the pulse width between 100 and 1000 µs, depending on the level of stimulation (Table 9.1)

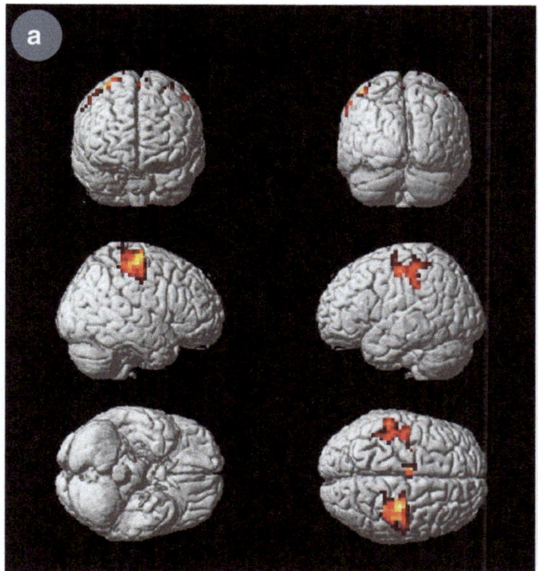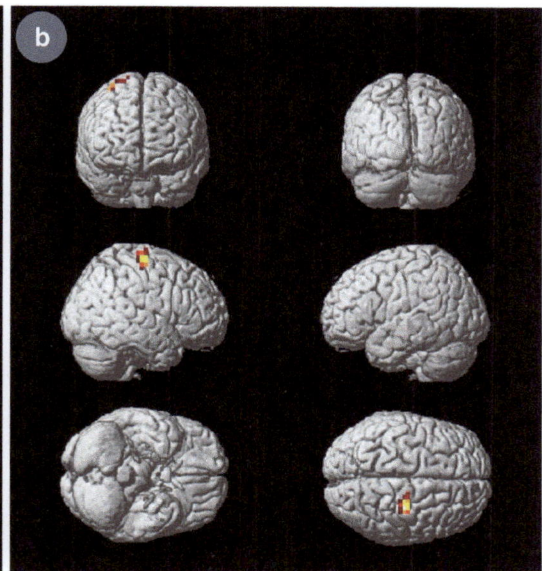

**Fig. 9.5** (**a**) Subtraction analysis (CMT1–TMT) in fMRI (functional magnetic resonance imaging): Conditioned Motor Task at T1 (CMT1)-Test Motor Task (TMT) at T0 shows an increase in the BOLD (Blood Oxygenation Level Dependent) response during CMT1 in the contralateral hemisphere within SM1 (sensorimotor cortex), within the premotor cortex (PM), in the inferior parietal lobule (IPL) and in the ipsilateral hemisphere within SM1, PM, IPL, SMA (supplementary motor area) and the cingulate gyrus (CG). (**b**) Subtraction analysis (CMT2–TMT): Conditioned Motor Task at T2 (CMT2)-Test Motor Task (TMT) at T0 two hours after the end of the afferent electrical stimulation. The increase in the BOLD response in the sensorimotor cortex in CMT1 has almost fallen back to the BOLD level in TMT, except for a residual increased level contralateral to the stimulated hand in SM1 (sensorimotor cortex)

the pre- and postcentral brain regions as well as in the superior frontal gyrus (supplementary motor area, SMA) and in the middle frontal gyrus. Fig. 9.5a shows the subtraction image of the BOLD response for the CMT1 after 30 min of SAES minus the BOLD response for the TMT before the SAES. The "net BOLD effect" corresponds to the increase in brain activity induced by the SAES when finger-to-thumb tapping after the SAES, which is still visible two hours after the end of the SAES contralateral in the area of the sensorimotor cortex (SM1) of the active hand, but has otherwise already subsided (Fig. 9.5b).

At the motor neuronal level, the net BOLD effect corresponds to an increased level of activity of the motor cortex, as has been demonstrated in Transcranial Magnetic Stimulation (TMS) studies and with intracortical recordings in monkeys [3, 7, 26]. Accordingly, SAES can shift intracortical excitability parameters such as short interval intracortical inhibition (SICI) or intracortical facilitation (ICF) in the direction of disinhibition of the motor cortex (Fig. 9.6).

The sham stimulation without current flow showed no disinhibition, the subsensitive SAES with 50 Hz an incipient and the SAES with 120% of the sensitive level and 50 Hz showed a clear shift in the excitability parameters in the direction of disinhibition of the motor cortex. Another interesting result of these studies is that the SAES already shows visible rhythmic muscle contractions at the motor level and at a frequency of 2 Hz similarly good neuromodulatory effects in the motor cortex as the SAES at the sensitive level. The lower frequency is apparently compensated for by an increased current intensity (Fig. 9.6). A strong correlation between spatially localized BOLD response and local field potentials could also be demonstrated [26]. SAES evidently induces an increased local field potential (LFP) in the sensorimotor cortex for at least a few minutes, which has already been demonstrated with

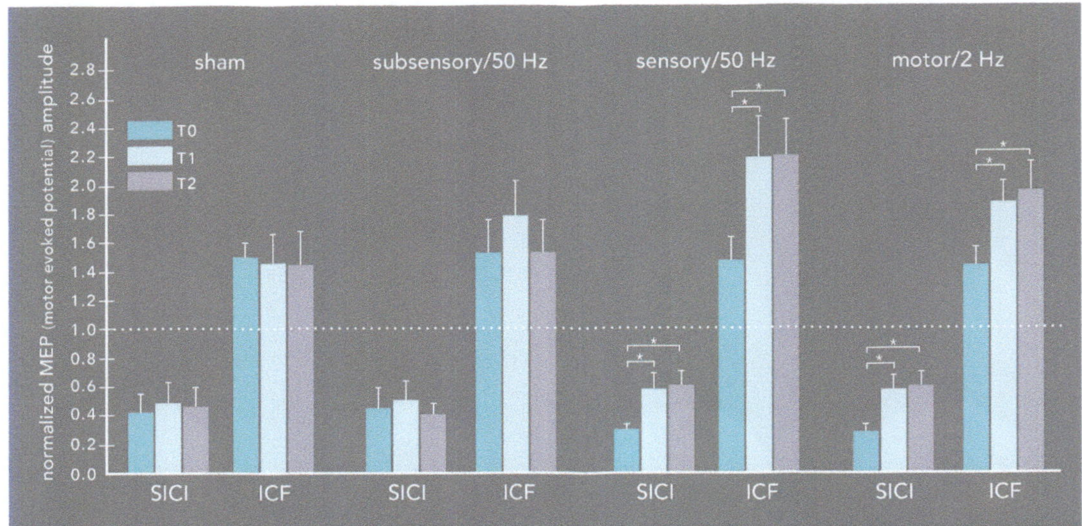

**Fig. 9.6** TMS stimulation with paired TMS (transcranial magnetic stimulation) pulses: before (T0), after (T1), and one hour after (T2) mesh glove (MG) stimulation with sensory afferent stimulation at 50 Hz ("Subsensory" = 80% of the sensitive threshold, "Sensory" = 120% of the sensitive threshold) and 2 Hz ("Motor" = motor level). The values for short intracortical inhibition (SICI) and intra-cortical facilitation (ICF) are normalized for each condition to their corresponding values for single pulse stimulation and then plotted as a mean value (SEM, standard error of the mean). The asterisk (*) indicates a significant difference ($p < 0.05$) compared to T0. A significant decrease in SICI and a significant increase in ICF can be seen at T1 and T2

somatosensory evoked potentials (SSEP) [15]. Augmented LFPs change the intracortical excitability of the motor cortex in the direction of disinhibition and facilitation with stronger recruitment of the motor neurons involved in finger-to-thumb tapping with additional functional gain, as could be shown in stroke patients treated with SAES in combination with daily motor therapy for three months compared to those treated only with motor therapy [27–29]. The SAES induces this increased motor neuron recruitment by transforming pre-existing silent synapses into functional synapses via an increased presynaptic release of glutamate, the reduction of inhibition by γ-aminobutyric acid (GABA), and the upregulation of postsynaptic AMPA receptors with unmasking of latent intracortical horizontal connections (Fig. 9.1) [30–32].

During a SAES of at least 30 min, the LTP is already involved, since the neuromodulation can still be detected after two hours (Fig. 9.5b). During a SAES of less than 30 min, only longer-lasting forms of STP such as post-tetanic potentiation or augmentation are observed (Fig. 9.1). During augmentation, there is an increase in the release of transmitters from the presynaptic vesicles in the range of seconds; in post-tetanic potentiation, the increase in transmitter release continues for a few minutes after the repetitive electrical stimulus has ceased [33]. So far, it is not known at what duration of the SAES the LTP begins. To date, it is also not known to what extent the neuromodulatory effects can be further enhanced upon SAES >30 min. However, there is consensus that the sustainability of the SAES can be increased by increasing the duration of stimulation and by increasing the number of sessions. There are currently no recommendations for the duration of stimulation and the number of sessions based on a good level of evidence. In numerous clinical studies, the duration of the SAES is three to six weeks with daily sessions of 30–60 min in length.

Depending on the skin resistance, the current strength for the sensitive threshold is between 2

**Table 9.1** Recommended parameters of SAES (sensory afferent electrical stimulation) in therapy

| level | current | pulse width | frequency | pulse shape | duration |
| --- | --- | --- | --- | --- | --- |
| motoric | 6-10 mA | 100-300 μs | 1-5 Hz | mono-/ biphasic, rectangle, (trapezoid) | 10-30 min |
| sensitive | 2-5 mA | 250-1000 μs | 10-50 Hz | mono-/ biphasic, rectangle, (trapezoid) | 30-60 min |

and 4 mA. In therapy, for supra-threshold stimulation at a sensitive level, the current strength is set to 120% of the sensitive threshold for a duration of 30–60 min at a frequency between 10 and 50 Hz [7]. At this level, electromyography does not yet show any muscle contractions. For stimulation at the motor level in therapy, the current intensity is increased until slight contractions of the small hand muscles are visible, which is reached at approximately 6–10 mA, depending on the skin resistance. A frequency between 1 and 5 Hz is chosen to avoid tetanic contractions of the muscles. The stimulation is carried out over a period of 10–30 min. The SAES then changes to a peripheral neuromuscular stimulation as in the peripheral functional electrical stimulation (FES) (Table 9.1). Fig. 9.6 shows that SAES at a sensitive level with 50 Hz increases the excitability of the motor cortex similarly effective as peripheral neuromuscular stimulation with 2 Hz.

**Summary**

The SAES with 50 Hz at a sensitive level increases the excitability of the motor cortex similarly effective as peripheral neuromuscular stimulation with 2 Hz.

## 9.3 SAES in Neurorehabilitation

### 9.3.1 Sensorimotor Paresis After Stroke

SAES has been known to induce cortical neuroplasticity for several decades. It offers the possibility of non-invasive neuromodulation in stroke patients with sensorimotor paresis in the subacute and chronic phase [9]. The acute phase has not yet been adequately investigated, in particular the question of the connection between SAES and an increased release of excitotoxic amino acids in the acute phase of the stroke. In patients after a stroke with a chronic sensorimotor paresis of the upper or lower extremity without further improvement through conventional sensorimotor therapy, the SAES has shown an improvement in the sensorimotor performance of the affected extremity [27, 28, 34]. In particular, there was a positive effect on a spastically increased tone of the affected extremity. The SAES was performed for half an hour every day for three months. As the neuromodulatory effect of a 30-min SAES treatment lasts for up to two hours [6, 7], the opportunity arises to combine it with a subsequent sensorimotor therapy. Thereby, the SAES should be applied within one hour prior to sensorimotor therapy.

In a recently published meta-analysis it was found that the SAES in combination with neurological standard rehabilitation in this temporal correlation in the chronic phase after stroke could improve significantly the maximum torque of the affected hand during dorsiflexion and also the performance in the Timed up and go test [35]. The Ashworth score for spasticity was reduced, but not significantly. Overall, it was possible to conclude in this meta-analysis that SAES can improve impaired motor functions of the lower extremity in the early phase and impaired motor functions of the upper and lower extremity in the chronic phase, without significant effects on spasticity. In particular, longer periods of SAES combined with sensorimotor therapy over several weeks showed positive effects on impaired sensorimotor functions.

So far, six randomized, controlled (RCT) studies have dealt with SAES in the rehabilitation of stroke patients with sensorimotor paresis of the upper extremity:

Yozbatiran et al. (2006) [36] examined motor exercises of the upper extremity with and without SAES with kinesthesia and position detection tests, a hand function test, and a hand movement scale before and after treatment. There was no significant difference between the groups after the treatment with regard to the hand movement scores and the kinesthesia and position detection tests. In the SAES group, however, there was a significant improvement in hand function after the treatment [36].

McDonnell et al. (2007) [37] combined the SAES with task-specific training ("grip lift" task), which showed significant improvements compared to the control group.

Conforto et al. (2010) [38] combined the SAES of the hand with two different stimulation intensities 1 and 2 (1 < 2) in patients with subacute stroke before motor training. The stimulation intensity 1 showed a greater improvement in the Jebsen-Taylor test after the first month of stimulation with a decrease in the difference two and three months after the intervention with no difference in the other motor function tests [38].

Fleming et al. (2015) [39] examined task-specific training in combination with SAES with

regard to the function of the upper extremities and the arm use in patients in the chronic stage after stroke. Immediately after the intervention, there was great improvement in the ARAT scores, which was no longer detectable three and six months after the intervention [39].

Since several randomized controlled studies have so far demonstrated a benefit of SAES in stroke patients with sensorimotor paresis, which was also confirmed in a meta-analysis [35], a recommendation at evidence level A can be given for the use of SAES in sensorimotor rehabilitation after a stroke for the lower extremity in the subacute phase and for the upper and lower extremity in the chronic phase.

**Summary**
With regard to the adjuvant use of SAES in sensorimotor therapy after stroke, a recommendation at evidence level A can be given for the upper and lower extremity in the chronic phase and for the lower extremity in the subacute phase.

### 9.3.2 Therapy of Neglect

The SAES is also used in neglect therapy. So far, various modalities of sensory afferent inputs (optokinetic, vibration of the neck muscles, vestibular and magnetic stimuli, SAES) have been investigated, which showed an impressive reduction in neglect [40, 41]. Sensory afferent input of various modalities (e.g., proprio-/exteroceptive, visual, vestibular, auditory) into the brain is achieved through multimodal integration in sensory afferent centers of a higher order (especially in the parietal lobe in the superior parietal lobule, SPL, and in the inferior parietal lobule, IPL) converted into information for voluntary, purposeful motor actions. In particular, proprioceptive, exteroceptive, premotor, and visual information converge in SPL and IPL when grasping with the hand. In the case of multimodal integration, the IPL is mainly involved in the transformation of retinal signals from targeted objects into a motor action pattern for voluntary, visually controlled,

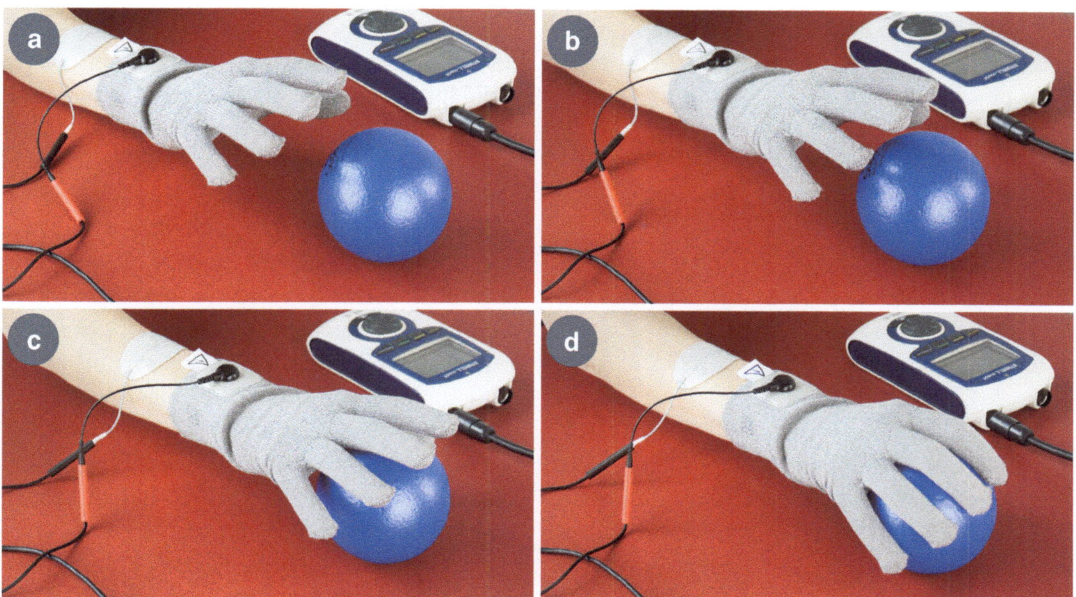

**Fig. 9.7** Visually controlled, targeted gripping of a ball while applying SAES (sensory afferent electrical stimulation) with the mesh glove. (**a**) start movement, (**b**) reaching the object, (**c**) gripping the object, (**d**) manipulate the object. A task-oriented context of SAES may bring an additional therapeutic effect in neglect, in sensorimotor paresis or for motor learning. However, this has not yet been scientifically proven in randomized, controlled studies

targeted movements in relation to the targeted object and is of great importance for eye-hand coordination (e.g., grasping a ball with the hand; Fig. 9.7) [42, 43].

The information running to the brain for voluntary, visually controlled, targeted movements is primarily transmitted by the Ia and Ib nerve fibers, which are primarily excited in the SAES. The bilaterally increased activity in the IPL demonstrated in the fMRI in the conditioned motor task immediately after the SAES indicates an increased bilateral afferent sensory input in the IPL by the SAES (Figs. 9.5a and 9.7) [6]. Daily 30-min SAES treatments for stroke patients for three months also led to a clinical improvement in neglect, as has already been demonstrated in several studies [28, 44, 45].

With peripheral FES, peripheral nerves and the muscles innervated by them are stimulated at the same time, triggering muscle contractions, which is why this additional intensive stimulation of muscle spindles, Golgi tendon, and joint receptors in comparison to SAES provides an additional sensory afferent input or boost to the brain and especially to the higher-order sensory afferent centers with a possibly greater effect than with the SAES. However, a direct comparison between SAES and peripheral FES with regard to the benefit in unilateral neglect has not yet been carried out. Nevertheless, a recently published randomized controlled study in patients in the acute phase after stroke with multimodal, unilateral neglect clearly demonstrates the benefit of peripheral FES on the affected side, the benefit of a combination of peripheral FES with conventional therapy of prism adjustment for neglect was greater than with peripheral FES or prism adjustment alone. The treatments were carried out 50 min a day, five times a week for a total of three weeks [46]. Since no larger randomized studies exist for the SAES in neglect, but several clinical studies speak for the benefit of the SAES in neglect, a recommendation at evidence level B can be given for the use of the SAES in the treatment of neglect.

**Summary**

A recommendation at evidence level B can currently be given for the adjuvant use of SAES in the treatment of neglect.

## 9.4 Discussion

The SAES induces a modulation in the nervous system in the area of short-term and long-term as well as structural neuroplasticity; this through an increased proprioceptive and exteroceptive input into the nervous system with the consequence of increased activity of the motor cortex [17]. Many studies suggest that this plasticity is mainly induced at the level of the synapses in the area of the sensorimotor cortex. With the adjuvant use of SAES in neurorehabilitation in combination with subsequent motor therapy, the overall outcome can be improved compared to motor therapy alone, as randomized, controlled studies have shown. The strongest modulation with the SAES can be achieved with a current intensity at the motor level depending on the skin resistance with 6–10 mA at a low frequency (2 Hz) with a similarly good effect of an SAES with a current intensity at a sensitive level depending on the skin resistance with 2–5 mA and a frequency of 50 Hz, although there is currently no optimized stimulation protocol with regard to the stimulation parameters. The modulatory effects last up to two hours after at least 30 min of stimulation. The current study situation suggests that an increase in the duration of the stimulation and an increase in the number of sessions can prolong the sustainability of the modulatory effects. Furthermore, there is a consensus that a pulsed current application is superior to a continuous one, although the optimal pulse shape is still unclear. Furthermore, there is still a lack of clarity regarding the pulse rate. The further optimization of the SAES stimulation protocols for therapy will be decisive for further application in neurorehabilitation. Also, there is still no data on the benefit of time-complex, structured stimulation protocols, which could further increase the neuromodulatory effect of the SAES and thus better support a long-term rehabilitation process for brain and spinal cord damage. In addition, it has not yet been clarified whether the SAES can enhance therapeutic effects in a task-oriented context (Fig. 9.7). In particular, there is currently the question of whether the SAES can promote motor learning in a task-oriented context. In a study published in 2014, an improvement in performance compared to the group with sham stimulation in a nine-hole peg test during a SAES with a mesh glove was described even one week after initial training [47]. In addition, there is currently a lack of comparative studies between the SAES and other methods of non-invasive brain stimulation to promote neuroplasticity such as the FES, the repetitive transcranial magnetic stimulation (rTMS), or the transcranial direct current stimulation (tDCS).

In the future, it will be important to further optimize the current stimulation protocols for the SAES and to combine these in an appropriate manner with the conventional methods of neurorehabilitation to optimally promote the rehabilitation process in the brain and spinal cord. In addition, a combination of the SAES with other methods of non-invasive brain stimulation, such as the rTMS, and the application in a task-oriented context could further increase the therapeutic potential of the SAES.

Finally, Table 9.1 gives recommendations based on the current study situation for setting the parameters of the SAES in therapy.

## References

1. Christova M, Golaszewski S, Ischebeck A, Kunz A, Rafolt D, Nardone R, et al. Mechanical flutter stimulation induces a lasting response in the sensorimotor cortex as revealed with BOLD fMRI. Hum Brain Mapp. 2013;34(11):2767–74.
2. Gallasch E, Christova M, Kunz A, Rafolt D, Golaszewski S. Modulation of sensorimotor cortex by repetitive peripheral magnetic stimulation. Front Hum Neurosci. 2015;9:407.
3. Golaszewski SM, Bergmann J, Christova M, Kunz AB, Kronbichler M, Rafolt D, et al. Modulation

of motor cortex excitability by different levels of whole-hand afferent electrical stimulation. Clin Neurophysiol. 2012;123(1):193–9.

4. Keller A, Pavlides C, Asanuma H. Long-term potentiation in the cat somatosensory cortex. Neuroreport. 1990;1(1):49–52.

5. Ghirardi M, Montarolo PG, Kandel ER. A novel intermediate stage in the transition between short- and long-term facilitation in the sensory to motor neuron synapse of aplysia. Neuron. 1995;14(2):413–20.

6. Golaszewski SM, Siedentopf CM, Koppelstaetter F, Rhomberg P, Guendisch GM, Schlager A, et al. Modulatory effects on human sensorimotor cortex by whole-hand afferent electrical stimulation. Neurology. 2004;62(12):2262–9.

7. Golaszewski SM, Bergmann J, Christova M, Nardone R, Kronbichler M, Rafolt D, et al. Increased motor cortical excitability after whole-hand electrical stimulation: a TMS study. Clin Neurophysiol. 2010;121(2):248–54.

8. Christova M, Rafolt D, Golaszewski S, Gallasch E. Outlasting corticomotor excitability changes induced by 25 Hz whole-hand mechanical stimulation. Eur J Appl Physiol. 2011;111(12):3051–9.

9. Chipchase LS, Schabrun SM, Hodges PW. Peripheral electrical stimulation to induce cortical plasticity: a systematic review of stimulus parameters. Clin Neurophysiol. 2011;122(3):456–63.

10. Burne JA, Lippold OC. Reflex inhibition following electrical stimulation over muscle tendons in man. Brain. 1996;119(Pt 4):1107–14.

11. Goldman H. Improvement of double simultaneous stimulation perception in hemiplegic patients. Arch Phys Med Rehabil. 1966;47(10):681–7.

12. Levin MF, Hui-Chan CW. Relief of hemiparetic spasticity by TENS is associated with improvement in reflex and voluntary motor functions. Electroencephalogr Clin Neurophysiol. 1992;85(2):131–42.

13. Bodegard A, Geyer S, Herath P, Grefkes C, Zilles K, Roland PE. Somatosensory areas engaged during discrimination of steady pressure, spring strength, and kinesthesia. Hum Brain Mapp. 2003;20(2):103–15.

14. McIntyre AK, Proske U, Rawson JA. Cortical projection of afferent information from tendon organs in the cat. J Physiol. 1984;354:395–406.

15. Wiesendanger M, Miles TS. Ascending pathway of low-threshold muscle afferents to the cerebral cortex and its possible role in motor control. Physiol Rev. 1982;62(4 Pt 1):1234–70.

16. Porter R, Lemon R. Corticospinal function and voluntary movement. Oxford: Clarendon Press; 1993.

17. Butefisch CM, Netz J, Wessling M, Seitz RJ, Homberg V. Remote changes in cortical excitability after stroke. Brain. 2003;126(Pt 2):470–81.

18. Liepert J, Hamzei F, Weiller C. Motor cortex disinhibition of the unaffected hemisphere after acute stroke. Muscle Nerve. 2000;23(11):1761–3.

19. Ruben J, Schwiemann J, Deuchert M, Meyer R, Krause T, Curio G, et al. Somatotopic organization of human secondary somatosensory cortex. Cereb Cortex. 2001;11(5):463–73.

20. Prochazka A. Proprioceptive feedback and movement regulation. New York: American Physiological Society; 1996.

21. Rothwell J. Control of human voluntary movement. London: Chapman & Hall; 1994.

22. Jami L. Golgi tendon organs in mammalian skeletal muscle: functional properties and central actions. Physiol Rev. 1992;72(3):623–66.

23. Lafleur J, Zytnicki D, Horcholle-Bossavit G, Jami L. Depolarization of Ib afferent axons in the cat spinal cord during homonymous muscle contraction. J Physiol. 1992;445:345–54.

24. Gandevia SC. Kinesthesia: roles for afferent signals and motor commands. Handbook of physiology: American Physiological Society, New York; 1996.

25. Golaszewski S, Kremser C, Wagner M, Felber S, Aichner F, Dimitrijevic MM. Functional magnetic resonance imaging of the human motor cortex before and after whole-hand afferent electrical stimulation. Scand J Rehabil Med. 1999;31(3):165–73.

26. Logothetis NK, Pauls J, Augath M, Trinath T, Oeltermann A. Neurophysiological investigation of the basis of the fMRI signal. Nature. 2001;412(6843):150–7.

27. Peurala SH, Pitkanen K, Sivenius J, Tarkka IM. Cutaneous electrical stimulation may enhance sensorimotor recovery in chronic stroke. Clin Rehabil. 2002;16(7):709–16.

28. Dimitrijevic MM, Stokic DS, Wawro AW, Wun CC. Modification of motor control of wrist extension by mesh-glove electrical afferent stimulation in stroke patients. Arch Phys Med Rehabil. 1996;77(3):252–8.

29. Golaszewski S. Whole hand afferent electrical stimulation to improve motor hand function in subacute poststroke patients. EJN. 2015.

30. Aimonetti JM, Nielsen JB. Changes in intracortical excitability induced by stimulation of wrist afferents in man. J Physiol. 2001;534(Pt 3):891–902.

31. Donoghue JP. Plasticity of adult sensorimotor representations. Curr Opin Neurobiol. 1995;5(6):749–54.

32. Jacobs KM, Donoghue JP. Reshaping the cortical motor map by unmasking latent intracortical connections. Science. 1991;251(4996):944–7.

33. Markram H, Tsodyks M. Redistribution of synaptic efficacy between neocortical pyramidal neurons. Nature. 1996;382(6594):807–10.

34. Ridding MC, McKay DR, Thompson PD, Miles TS. Changes in corticomotor representations induced by prolonged peripheral nerve stimulation in humans. Clin Neurophysiol. 2001;112(8):1461–9.

35. Sharififar S, Shuster JJ, Bishop MD. Adding electrical stimulation during standard rehabilitation after stroke to improve motor function. A systematic review and meta-analysis. Ann Phys Rehabil Med. 2018;61(5):339–44.

36. Yozbatiran N, Donmez B, Kayak N, Bozan O. Electrical stimulation of wrist and fingers for sen-

sory and functional recovery in acute hemiplegia. Clin Rehabil. 2006;20(1):4–11.

37. McDonnell MN, Hillier SL, Miles TS, Thompson PD, Ridding MC. Influence of combined afferent stimulation and task-specific training following stroke: a pilot randomized controlled trial. Neurorehabil Neural Repair. 2007;21(5):435–43.

38. Conforto AB, Ferreiro KN, Tomasi C, dos Santos RL, Moreira VL, Marie SK, et al. Effects of somatosensory stimulation on motor function after subacute stroke. Neurorehabil Neural Repair. 2010;24(3):263–72.

39. Fleming MK, Sorinola IO, Roberts-Lewis SF, Wolfe CD, Wellwood I, Newham DJ. The effect of combined somatosensory stimulation and task-specific training on upper limb function in chronic stroke: a double-blind randomized controlled trial. Neurorehabil Neural Repair. 2015;29(2):143–52.

40. Kerkhoff G. Modulation and rehabilitation of spatial neglect by sensory stimulation. Prog Brain Res. 2003;142:257–71.

41. Kerkhoff G, Heldmann B, Struppler A, Havel P, Jahn T. The effects of magnetic stimulation and attentional cueing on tactile extinction. Cortex. 2001;37(5):719–23.

42. Rizzolatti G, Fogassi L, Gallese V. Parietal cortex: from sight to action. Curr Opin Neurobiol. 1997;7(4):562–7.

43. Sakata H, Taira M, Kusunoki M, Murata A, Tanaka Y. The TINS Lecture. The parietal association cortex in depth perception and visual control of hand action. Trends Neurosci. 1997;20(8):350–7.

44. Dimitrijevic MM, Soroker N. Mesh-glove. 2. Modulation of residual upper limb motor control after stroke with whole-hand electric stimulation. Scand J Rehabil Med. 1994;26(4):187–90.

45. Rossmueller J. Mein Rollstuhl ist ein Einrad. Neurologische Rehabilitation 2007;06 Dez-07 Jaen.

46. Choi HS, Kim DJ, Yang YA. The effect of a complex intervention program for unilateral neglect in patients with acute-phase stroke: a randomized controlled trial. Osong Public Health Res Perspect. 2019;10(5):265–73.

47. Christova M, Rafolt D, Golaszewski S, Nardone R, Gallasch E. Electrical stimulation during skill training with a therapeutic glove enhances the induction of cortical plasticity and has a positive effect on motor memory. Behav Brain Res. 2014;270:171–8.

# Functional Electrical Stimulation in Facial Rehabilitation

**10**

Christina A. Repitsch and Gerd F. Volk

## 10.1 N. facialis

Peripheral facial palsy (FP) can be a form of facial paralysis (complete denervation) or facial paresis (incomplete denervation or weakness) on mostly only one side of the face that results from a lesion to the facial nerve. Every year, 7–40 per 100,000 people suffer from idiopathic facial palsy, which is one of the most common cranial nerve lesions leading to facial muscle dysfunction [1]. While the diagnosis includes numerous medical consequences, one must also consider the social consequences it entails. FP is caused by different etiological factors and can lead to functional deficits in eating, speaking, nasal breathing, eye closure as well as verbal and nonverbal communication, which will be further described in Chap. 10.6. These functional tasks necessary for daily self-care can also be defined as "activities of daily living (ADLs)". An inability to perform these fundamental activities may lead to poor quality of life. The complex interaction of facial muscles enables us to express emotions, such as happiness, sadness, anger, fear, and disgust. But what happens when this is no longer possible? When eating in public becomes an unpleasant experience, physical appearance has changed, and muscle weakness reduces intelligibility of speech? Thus far, people affected by FP have often been left to deal with the unavoidable impact of the disease on mental health by themselves. In many cases, this led to social withdrawal and, in a few cases, secondary depressions [2]. The German Society of Neurology [1] outlined recommendations for pharmaceutical treatment in the acute phase. However, there do not exist recommendations for physical or speech and language therapy intervention in the acute, acute-chronic, and chronic phase. Even though interest in this topic has grown in recent years and treatment options are becoming more diverse, the treatment of FP still lacks in many areas a strong evidence-based research base. Due to the complexity of the topic and numerous treatment options, it is essential that the patient is taken care by an interdisciplinary team where treatment options are carefully presented to the patient, while severity and duration of the disease are being considered. This will allow the patient to make an informed choice about treatment options and the team to optimally collaborate with the patient to work together on the rehabilitation process. From a clinical perspective, the process of healing significantly depends on the cause, the location, and severity of the lesion.

Therefore, anatomy, physiology, and pathology as well as everyday impairments will be discussed in the following chapters.


C. A. Repitsch (✉)
Klinikum Klagenfurt am Wörthersee, ENT Department, Klagenfurt, Austria
e-mail: christina.repitsch@kabeg.at

G. F. Volk
ENT Department, Friedrich-Schiller-University Hospital, Jena, Germany
e-mail: fabian.volk@med.uni-jena.de



© The Author(s), under exclusive license to Springer Nature Switzerland AG 2022
T. Schick (ed.), *Functional Electrical Stimulation in Neurorehabilitation*,
https://doi.org/10.1007/978-3-030-90123-3_10

## 10.2 Anatomy

The n. facialis is the seventh cranial nerve (CN VII). The motor facial nucleus emerges from the pons, lateral to the cerebellopontine angle [3]. In this area, the cranial nerve forms an inner angle, surrounding the abducens nerve. After building the inner angle, fibers of the facial nerve merge with fibers of the vestibulo-cochlear nerve and extend into the bony structure of the skull base. The fibers then pass through the porus acusticus internus of the temporal bone, into the immediate vicinity of the inner and middle ear. These fibers carry afferent and efferent signals from the cranial nerves. At the foramen stylomastoideum, the n. facialis exists the bony structure of the petrosal bone and extends to the glandula parotidea, where it divides into further branches, supplying the occipital, neck, and face muscles.

The main trunks are:

- Posterior auricular nerve: supplies sensory muscles of the inner and outer ear and the occipital muscle.
- Ramus stylohyoideus: leads to the m. stylohyoideus.
- Ramus digastricus: supplies the posterior digastric muscle.
- Plexus parotideus: is the generic term for the nerve plexus between the inner and outer parotic leaf, which supplies the facial muscles and is usually distinguished in five branches.
  - Ramus temporalis,
  - Ramus zygomatici,
  - Ramus buccales,
  - Ramus marginalis mandibule: along the margin of the lower jaw,
  - Ramus colli: supplies the platysma.

In addition, the n. intermedius proceeds with the n. vestibulocochlearis and the n. facialis. This so-called intermediate nerve carries afferent and efferent fibers to supply the nasal and lacrimal secretions, salivary glands and the sense of taste. Damage in the early course of the n. facialis can therefore be associated with a tear secretion disorder, a taste disorder, or a salivary gland secretion disorder.

## 10.3 Causes for FP

A variety of causes can lead to the development of FP. In general, differentiation is made between cryptogenic and symptomatic causes [4]. In case of cryptogenic FP, also known as idiopathic peripheral FP or Bell's palsy, the cause is by definition unknown.

If there is evidence of damage (e.g., iatrogenic, tumor-related, virus-associated) it can be considered symptomatic FP. While the cause of acute paresis continues to remain unclear in more than half of the cases, idiopathic FP has a higher chance of spontaneous recovery.

The most common causes that lead to FP are [5]

- Birth trauma or genetic.
- Neurological diseases.
- Infections.
- Iatrogenic.
- Metabolic.
- Toxic.
- Neoplastic.
- Idiopathic.

## 10.4 Pathology

The disease is characterized by limited mobility of the facial muscles of one side, reduced facial expressions and gestures, difficulty eating and/or drinking, and reduced articulatory movements. A common complaint of those affected is an incomplete closure of the eyelid, which often results in eye dryness and redness and may also lead to permanent corneal damage.

While unilateral cranial nerve lesions are more commonly observed, a bilateral facial nerve paresis may also occur (e.g., with an onset of meningeal neuroborreliosis). Depending on the location of nerve damage, the following deficits may occur (Table 10.1) [4]:

- A nerve lesion distal to the stylomastoid foramen leads to a purely motor paresis of the facial muscles. If the lesion is severe, all facial muscles may be affected, which may be noted by incomplete eyelid closure and the inability to wrinkle skin, located on the forehead.

**Table 10.1** Differences between central and peripheral facial nerve palsy

| distinction central versus peripheral facial nerve paresis | |
| --- | --- |
| central facial nerve paresis | peripheral facial nerve paresis |
| pulling up the m. occipitofrontalis venter frontalis of both sides is possible | pulling up the m. occipitofrontalis venter frontalis muscle is not possible on the affected side |
| eyelid closure is possible | usually the entire facial muscles are paralyzed |
| deficits especially in the area of the mouth | incomplete eyelid closure |

- A lesion to the nerve in the bony structure of the skull base may cause a paralysis of the whole mimic musculature. Depending on the location of the lesion, a lacrimal and/or salivary gland disorder, a taste disorder, and hyperacusis may be observed.
- A lesion to the facial nucleus or the fascicle in the brainstem predominantly causes motor deficits. Deficits may include an incomplete closure of the affected eyelid and inability to wrinkle skin located on the forehead. Lacrimal and salivary secretory functions as well as the sensation of taste typically remain preserved as responsible nerve fibers extend in the petrous bone, together with fibers of the n. facialis.
- A lesion above the facial nucleus (so-called "central facial nerve palsy") may result in a perioral palsy. Due to bilateral supply of the upper facial muscles, eye closure and forehead elevation typically remain intact.

## 10.5 Incomplete vs. Complete Facial Palsy

The terms complete and/or incomplete FP are not synonymous of central and peripheral FP, rather they refer the degree of facial expression loss. There exist various definitions of complete and incomplete FP. When all branches of the n. facialis are reduced in the range of motion (i.e., fore-head, eye, cheek, mouth, and neck), some people may refer to it as a complete FP. However, a more stringent definition of complete FP requires a complete failure of all facial muscle movement. The better-defined neurological pair of terms of paresis and paralysis means something similar: In a paresis, there still should be a residual function of the nerve, while all axons are interrupted by a paralysis. This state of paralysis can be diagnosed by conducting a needle electromyogram of all innervated muscles in question. A further differentiated method for diagnosing a FP is the frequently used House-Brackmann scale (HBS) (Table 10.2).

▶ **Complete vs. Incomplete FP** Complete peripheral facial nerve palsy: The patient presents with the most severe of FP and would be rated as grade 6 on HBS.

Incomplete peripheral FP: FP can be classified after a spontaneous remission and with moderately severe symptoms f.e. as grade 3 on the HBS.

## 10.6 Daily Impairment

An overview about daily impairment and loss of ADLs [6]:

- Impaired facial expression: restricted nonverbal communication.

**Table 10.2** House Brackman scale

| House-Brackmann scale | | | | | |
| degree | result at rest | symmetry | eyes | mouth | forhead |
| --- | --- | --- | --- | --- | --- |
| 1 | normal | normal | normal | normal | normal |
| 2 | mild paresis | normal | eyelid closure possible | mild asymmetry | adequate function |
| 3 | moderate paresis | normal | complete eyelid closure only with effort | mildly affected, completely possible with effort | mild to moderate movement potential |
| 4 | moderately severe paresis | normal | incomplete eyelid closure | asymmetry despite maximum effort | no movement potential |
| 5 | severe paresis | asymmetry | incomplete eyelid closure | little movement potential | no movement potential |
| 6 | complete paresis | asymmetry | incomplete eyelid closure | no movement potential | no movement potential |

- Eyes: impaired eyelid closure or reduced blinking leads to drying out of the cornea, inflamed cornea, visual disturbances, pain and lacrimal secretion disorder.
- Ear: possible impairment of the m. stapedius may lead to hyperacusis.
- Eating and drinking: impaired bolus control; difficulty with chewing and bolus formation; food residues in the cheek and associated difficulties removing residues from the cheek, as a consequence of sensory deficits of the mucous membrane of the cheek (cheek biting).
- Teeth: protective function of saliva against caries and other diseases in the oral cavity; diminished saliva production, dry oral mucosa, disturbed movement-patters of the cheek-muscles, so that self-cleaning, but also brushing teeth becomes more difficult.
- Facial pain: even though the n. facilis is purely motoric, it should not be associated with facial pain, it is often reported by patients. An initial ear pain, which often occurs days before the palsy appears, is often related to the local inflammation of the facial canal. Despite the pain, it is important to distinguish between the initial and muscle pain that occurs months after reinnervation, which is likely associated with the sudden overstraining due to the defective reinnervation and as a response to massage and botulinum toxin injections.
- Speech: Reduced orofacial musculature difficulties, such as slurred speech or an altered vocal quality, may arise.

- "Spasms": misguided reinnervation may cause unilateral cramps or uncoordinated muscle twitching. Although the underlying pathology differs from spasticity, this term is often erroneously used.
- Synkinesias/dyskinesias: In the course of the disease synkinesias or dyskinesias may develop. These terms also refer to involuntary muscle movement and can be explained by errors in reinnervation. For example, nerve fibers that were initially responsible for eye closure may now innervate the m. orbicularis oris, and therefore trigger lid-beat synchronous twitching in the corner of the mouth.

## 10.7 Consequences in the Tissue

Even a mild and short-term form of incomplete facial paresis will have an impact on the soft tissue. This minimal form of FP will course an immediate restriction of movement, a rapid decrease of muscle tone, and thereby several indirect effects like a reduced lymph circulation. If in more severe cases of FP axons and their motor end plates are fully destroyed, it is called a paralysis that leads to denervation atrophy and a complete loss of voluntary movement and muscle tone. The denervation of the VII cranial nerve may subsequently lead to a loss of muscle mass, although there are also indications that muscle breakdown in the face is slower than on the great muscles of the extremities. The lack of neural input may lead to a decrease in muscle fiber thickness and a pathological increase in collagen fibers and connective tissue cells, as a long-term consequence. Therefore, muscle fibers are often remodeled, and affected muscles gradually decrease in tone. This loss of muscle mass may be observed as hypotonic tissue and asymmetry of the facial muscles at rest and in motion [7]. However, facial muscles may also behave similar to striated muscle fibers of the extremities that continue to persist despite denervation of the muscle tissue [8]. When these fibers are stimulated using FES, also a severely damaged muscle may be rebuilt. When stimulation is applied early, the muscle ideally retains its size and function, and the remodeling processes in the muscle tissue may be slowed down or even be stopped entirely.

## 10.8 Treatment Options of FES

The FES is currently being established as a treatment for facial paralysis. For a long time, the treatment's potential was not recognized, as side effects were assumed to cause difficulty with facial application. Interestingly, two contradicting side effects of electrical stimulation have been reported: On the one hand, it is repeatedly argued that a FES would prevent or reduce reinnervation. On the other hand, there exists the assertion that FES increases aberrant reinnervation as dys- or/and synkinesis may be noted during FES. Although both claims are repeatedly made, they are not supported by scientific evidence. A recent study investigated this question while treating patients with completely denervated facial muscles. Results show that surface electrical stimulation neither delayed reinnervation nor decreased functional outcomes [9]. A further review of literature on the current state of studies of electrical stimulation in facial paralysis concludes that there is no evidence for a positive effect of FES on acute paresis and only weak evidence in chronic paresis. One explanation for this may be the poor quality of the studies [10].

To overcome this lack of high-quality evidence, a prospective (but not controlled) study is running in Jena. First, results of the stimulation parameters of the first five paralysis patients were published. By surface electrical stimulation a selective m. zygomaticus response in absence of discomfort and unselective contraction of other facial muscle was reproducibly obtained for all the assessed patients. The most effective results with single pulses were observed with pulse width greater or equal to 50 ms. The required amplitude was remarkably lower ($\leq$5 mA vs. up to 15 mA) in freshly diagnosed ($\leq$3 months) than in long-term facial paralysis patients (>5 years). A triangular waveform was more effective than a rectangular waveform, mostly because of the lower discomfort threshold of the latter. Delivery of trains of stimulation showed similar results to the single pulse setting, though lower amplitudes were necessary to achieve the selective m. zygomaticus response [11]. While this shows well, that FES is tolerated in the face, positive effects like increase of muscle tone self-reported by the patients but also objectively visible and measurable are not yet published (Table 10.3).

However, various studies about FES and peripheral nerve damage in other anatomical illustrate regions and on animals, regarding that the FES in case of damage to muscle groups demonstrate a positive effect on muscles. It is believed that after denervation of the muscle a race between breaking down and reinnervation begins. The output then depends on the speed of nerve growth and the rate of atrophy. From animal experiments as well as clinical observations, we know that the facial nerve growth rate is about 1 mm per day. Very close to reality, no data on the rate of muscle

**Table 10.3** Recommendations for the use of FES in the treatment of central or peripheral facial paralysis

| facial nerve paresis | prognosis/course | therapy recommendation |
| --- | --- | --- |
| central | acute ones with good prognosis | *FES* is not required in spontaneous remission. |
| | acute ones with poor prognosis (e.g. major infarcts or neurosurgical operations with damage to the supranuclear facial tract) | Offering *FES* can be useful to counteract muscle atrophy. But if pain occurs during the stimulation, *FES* should be discontinued. |
| | chronical | *FES* can be used to improve muscle atrophy. For further operations (e.g. CFNTPL vs. neuromuscular replacement operation) it must beconsidered, if it could have an positive effect to the outcome of the operation. |
| peripheral | acute with good prognosis (e.g. incomplete idiopathic paresis) | No *FES*, if recovery is expected within weeks. High organizational effort and unclear assumption of costs. Currently there are only a few studies that show minor benefits. |
| | acute ones with a poor prognosis (e.g. after surgical destruction) | Early muscle stimulation in spite of severe impairment. At least with partial failure and bad recovery to stop atrophy. Regardless of this, check the indiactions of nerve reconstruction. |
| | chronically flaccid | If, after severe damage with at least partial denervation of the facial muscles, the muscle tone is reduced, direct muscle stimulation can be used to try to stimulate the denervated muscle fibers and thus trigger contractions. Regardless of this, the indication for surgical nerve reconstruction, possibly with muscle transfer, should be checked. The surface electrical stimulation is perceived as positive by the patients because the muscle tone remains increased for several hours after the electrical stimulation. |
| | chronically synkinetically reinnervated | Using a biofeedback progam is possible, if any kind of muscle movements are deriveable. Those can be combined with *FES*. |
| | after surgical reconstruction | After surgical reconstruction, the option of muscle stimulation should be discussed with the attending surgeon. Several months pass by between the operation and the first reinnervation, so denervation atrophy can be minimized. After stimulation, the muscles are in better condition and the time of rehabilitation can be minimized. |

atrophy has been published. Successful reinnervation after over a year, but also the sonographic evidence of paralytic facial muscles after more than a year of denervation let hypothesize that the muscular atrophy turns out to be a disintegration process without a defined end. There exist first confirmations that the low-frequency FES affects positive axonal sprouting and functional improvement. A possible reason for this may be that that sensory-mechanical stimulation of the muscles through targeted stimulation of the trigeminal afferents and during the de- and reinnervation period could have positive effects on functional reinnervation. Positive effects of mechanical stimulation, even after surgical nerve reconstruction (i.e., neuromuscular replacement surgery) have already been proven successful for rats [12]. The results of this study can be underpinned through a randomized study of human subjects. This study investigated the effectiveness of low-frequency FES in 20 patients whose Bell palsy had not recovered after 5 months. After randomization, 10 patients received low-frequency FES for 4 weeks, five times a week for 30 minutes, and completed movement exercises under supervision. The other 10 patients merely completed the movement exercises. The evaluation by experts through the Sunnybrook Rating Scale as well as the automatic movement measurement both demonstrated significant improvements of voluntary movements, especially the m. zygomaticus [13]. These results suggest that targeting FP using FES may be a benefit for those affected. In the future FES should present an additional treatment to the occupational, the conservative, and surgical treatment of FP. Before treatment options will be discussed, fields of applications of the FES, indications and contraindications will be discussed in further detail.

## 10.9 Indications and Contraindications Plus Advantages of FES

The use of FES as a treatment option for patients with FP should be adapted to the individual needs and the situation of the patient. A requirement for the application of FES in speech and language therapy or physical therapy is a qualified therapist as well as an in-depth education of the patient when dealing with the electrical stimulation device. Because of the possibility to apply FES during home practice, the person affected receives FES more frequently than those who only receive FES during therapy sessions. From a therapeutic and medical standpoint, the following contraindications discouraged patients using FES [14]:

- Type and severity of pain.
- Lack of motivation, mental state, cognitive limitations.
  Acute infections (e.g., herpes zoster) and/or wound healing disorders
- Acute inflammatory processes.
- Tumor diseases in the to be stimulated area (except after R0-Resection).
- Radiotherapy.
- Internal diseases (internal clarification and statement necessary).
- Surgical sutures in the immediate area proximity to electrical stimulation.
- Limited motor skills (device handling), if no assistance by another person (therapist/relative) is possible.
- Titanium plates in the facial area after severe facial injuries.
- Pacemaker/defibrillator (internal clarification and statement by the internist necessary).

**Indications for FES**
- Good compliance and good cognitive skills to understand the device and the training plan.
- High motivation of the patient.

**Advantages of FES**
- FES as a motivational measure.
- Independent application of the FES during home practice.
- The patient receives immediate feedback and can take corrective measures to improve self-perception.
- Controlling the target muscles at least partially possible.
- Delaying or reducing muscle atrophy.
- Shortening the rehabilitation phase.

## 10.10 Further Recommendations for the Application of FES

- In case of poor reinnervation after occurrence of idiopathic FP.
- With poor reinnervation after occurrence and subsidence of all symptoms after herpes zoster induced FP.
- Immediate use after iatrogenic damage (e.g., acoustic neuroma removal, parotidectomy) after consultation with the attending surgeon to preserve denervated muscle fibers.
- FES with initially long biphasic triangular pulses until the nerve fibers sprout out again, so that the muscle cannot degenerate in this phase and convert into fat or connective tissue.
- If there is a surgical restitution of the VII cranial nerve planned, the optimal setting should be discussed in consultation with the surgeons. It is recommended that the patient carries out FES until the surgery, so that the muscle tissue does not convert in connective tissue and the skin trophic stays preserved. It is expected that a cross-face nerve transplant (CFNTPL) or a hypoglossal facial jump resultanastomosis results in reinnervation of the denervated musculature. FES should be offered for at least 6 months or until the first action potentials are observed in needle electromyography.
- With a two-stage CFNTPL, in combination with a free gracilis graft, FES should be offered 7 days postoperatively for at least 3 months to minimize the atrophy of muscle fibers of the gracilis graft.

## 10.11 Electrodes to Use

The muscles of the face are laid out in several layers, and the muscles to be stimulated are very small and often extend directly into the area above. Therefore, targeted stimulation of individual muscles may be difficult. The size of the electrodes is crucial so that the affected muscles are stimulated in a targeted manner. Additionally, it must be noted that activity of mimic muscles often shifts the facial skin. Thus, adequate adhesion of the electrodes is a prerequisite for successful stimulation. When stimulating facial muscles, it is further recommended that electrodes with a diameter of 2.5 cm (Figs. 10.1, 10.2, 10.3 and 10.4) be utilized [15]. The advantage of small self-adhesive electrodes is that insulated potentials of small muscle groups can be derived. The disadvantage is poor adhesion of the electrodes to the skin, most likely due to the special texture of the facial skin. As previously mentioned, the skin of the face shifts and stretches due to the movement of the underlying muscles. To improve the adhesiveness of the electrodes it is recommended to fix them with a kinesio-tape, band-aid, or elastic bands with Velcro. The latter is often used by patients, however mostly perceived as an unpleasant restriction. Using a elastic-tape may also reduce the range of motion of the desired movement. In patients with completely denervated FP or after surgically reanimated FP, so-called "sponge electrodes" (Fig. 10.5) may be suitable, which enable a wider area of muscle stimulation. Lastly, there is the option to use oval self-adhesive electrodes (Fig. 10.6) (6 × 4 cm), which are more convenient to use due to sponge electrodes.

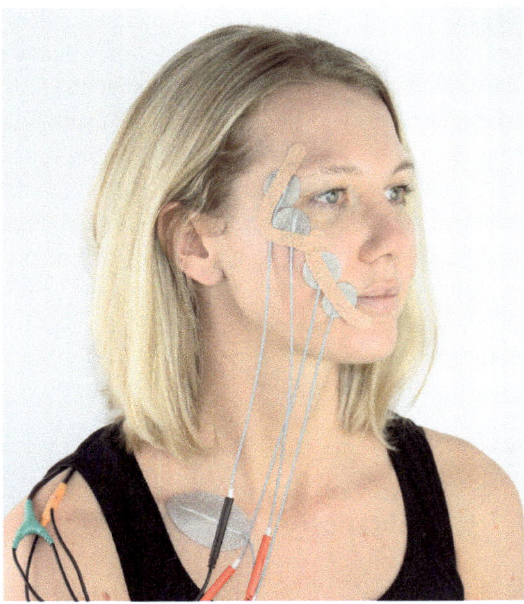

**Fig. 10.1** Possibility of attaching self-adhesive electrodes 2,5 cm

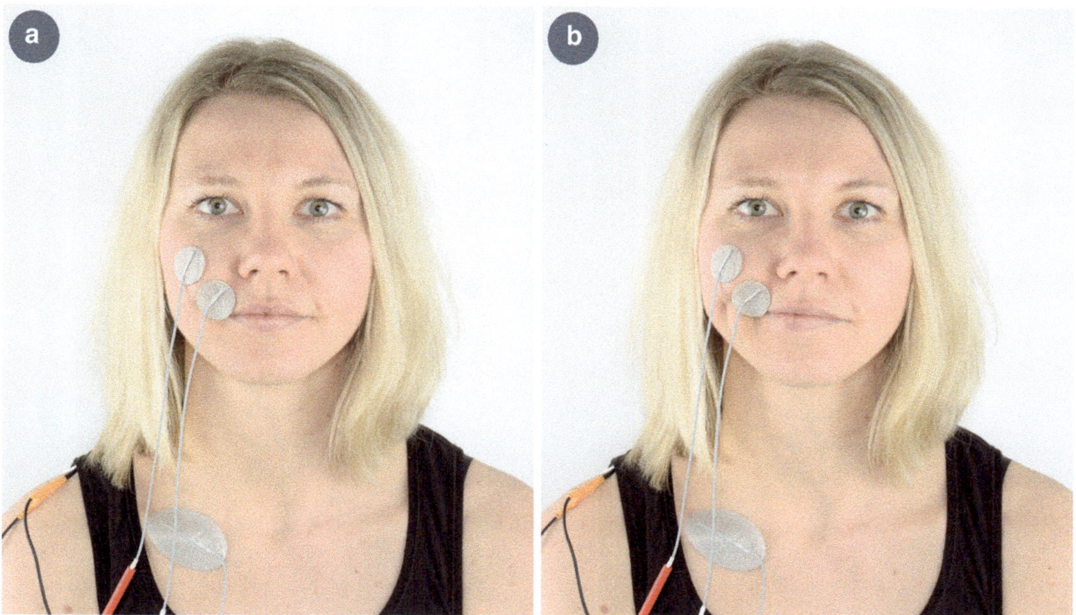

**Fig. 10.2**   Biofeedback stimulation of the Mm. zygomaticii, using self-adhesive electrodes. (**a**) in rest, (**b**) activation of the following muscle

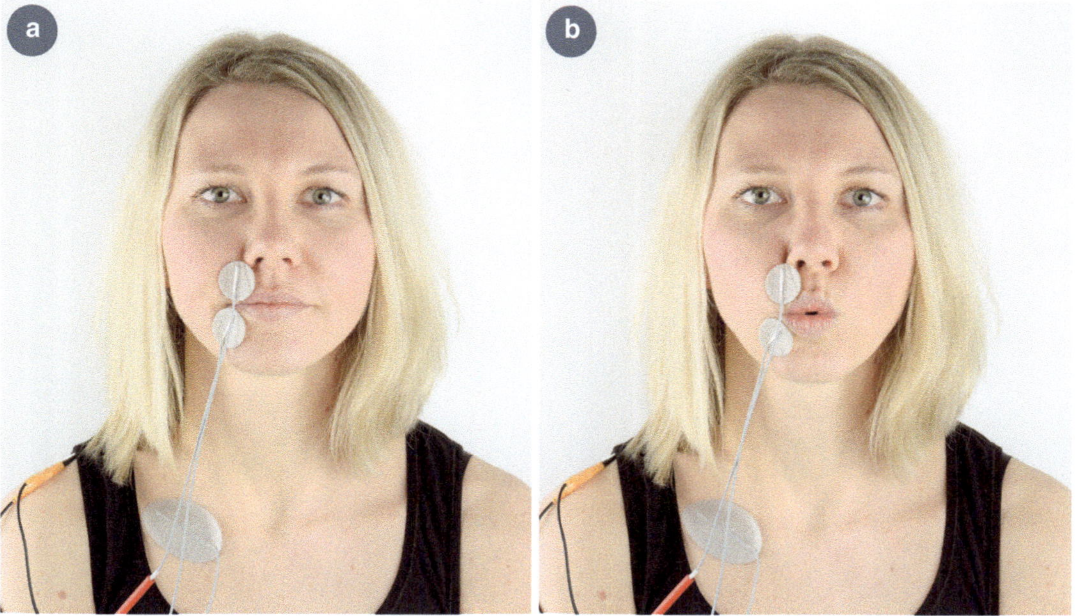

**Fig. 10.3**   Biofeedback stimulation of the m. orbicularis oris, using self-adhesive electrodes. (**a**) in rest, (**b**) activation of the following muscle

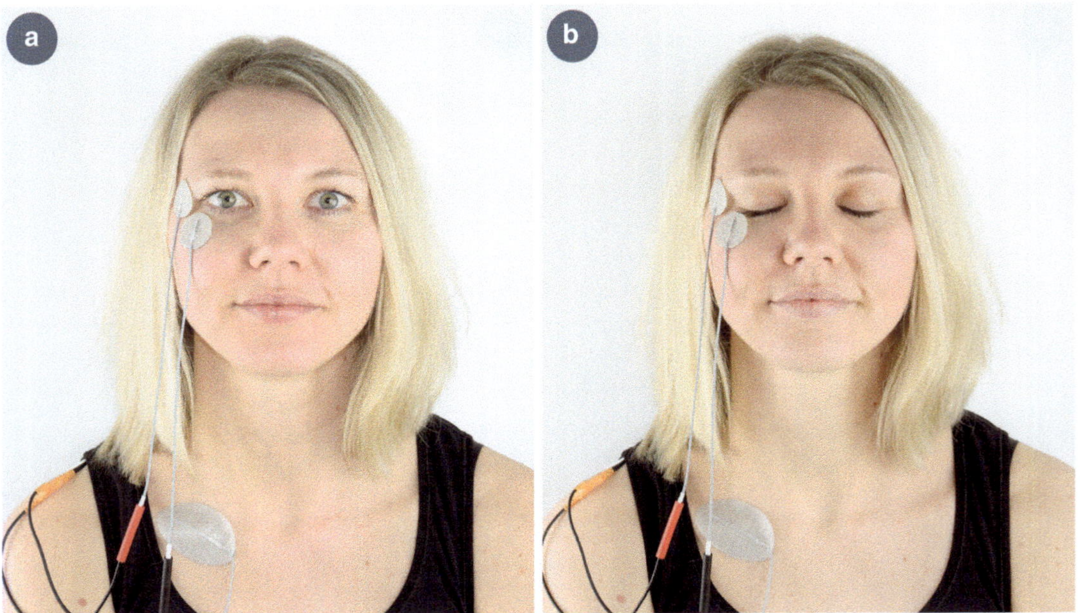

**Fig. 10.4** Biofeedback stimulation of the m. orbicularis oculi, using self-adhesive electrodes. (**a**) in rest, (**b**) activation of the following muscle

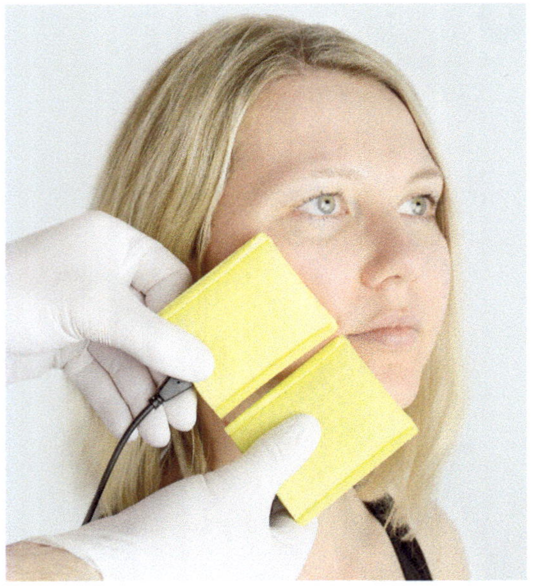

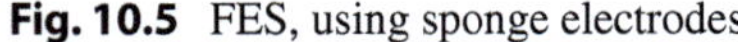

**Fig. 10.5** FES, using sponge electrodes

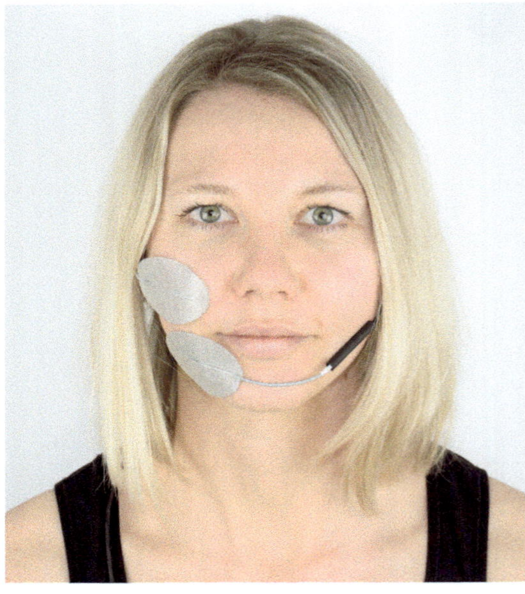

**Fig. 10.6** FES, using self-adhesive electrodes 4 × 6, 4 cm

## 10.12 EMG Biofeedback Incomplete Peripheral FP

As stated in the introduction of this chapter (Sects. 10.8, 10.9, 10.10, and 10.11), there is a variety of options for the treatment of FP [14]. If there is an incomplete or aberrant reinnervation, for example, in peripheral facial palsy, EMG biofeedback programs can be applied. If the patient demonstrates measured action potentials in the muscles when using needle EMG, these programs can be used to build strength and endurance of the muscles. Regular and active practice as possible in home-training is an integral part of the disorder's healing rehabilitation process. The goal is for the patient to independently trigger muscle activity and subsequently be rewarded with electrical stimulation. Biofeedback programs can be used in the following areas:

- Forehead branch area.
- Lateral circular muscles of the eye.
- Cheek area.
- Lateral circular muscles of the mouth.

Using extended options can be used to achieve maximal muscle strength, endurance, and relaxation. In addition, biofeedback aims to improve intermuscular coordination. Therefore, the use of a FES device can have a positive effect on a patient's motivation. The application improves perception of the patient to control facial muscles. Consequently, this leads to an improvement of arbitrary movement activation and control (Fig. 10.7, 10.8, and 10.9). To derive the potential of the target muscles, the round adhesive electrodes with a diameter of <2.5 cm should be used. In the forehead branch area, the oval self-adhesive electrodes with a diameter of 6 × 4 cm can be used. The size of the electrodes should always be tailored to the structural features of the patient.

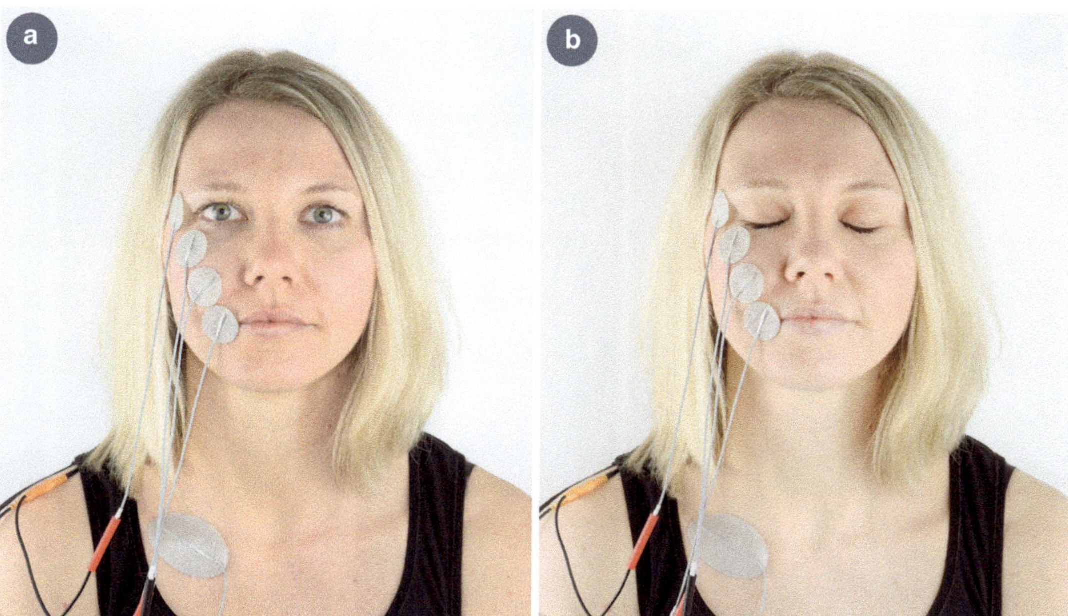

**Fig. 10.7** Biofeedback training (**a** = at rest, **b** = activation of the m. orbicularis oculi, without moving the zygomatici muscles)

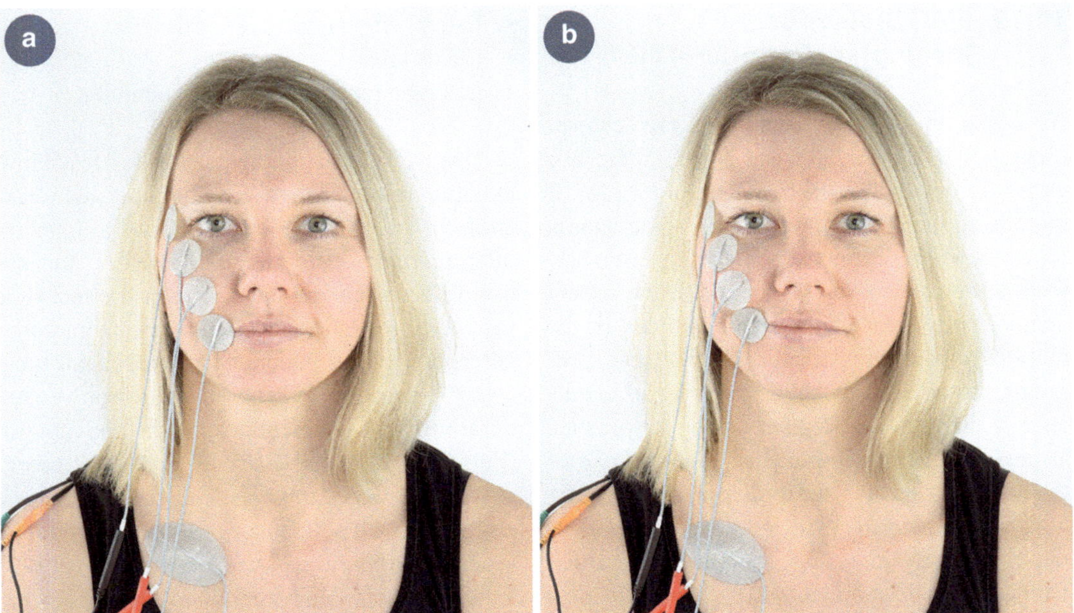

**Fig. 10.8** Biofeedback training (**a** = at rest, **b** = activation of the zygomatici muscles without moving the orbicularis oculi muscle)

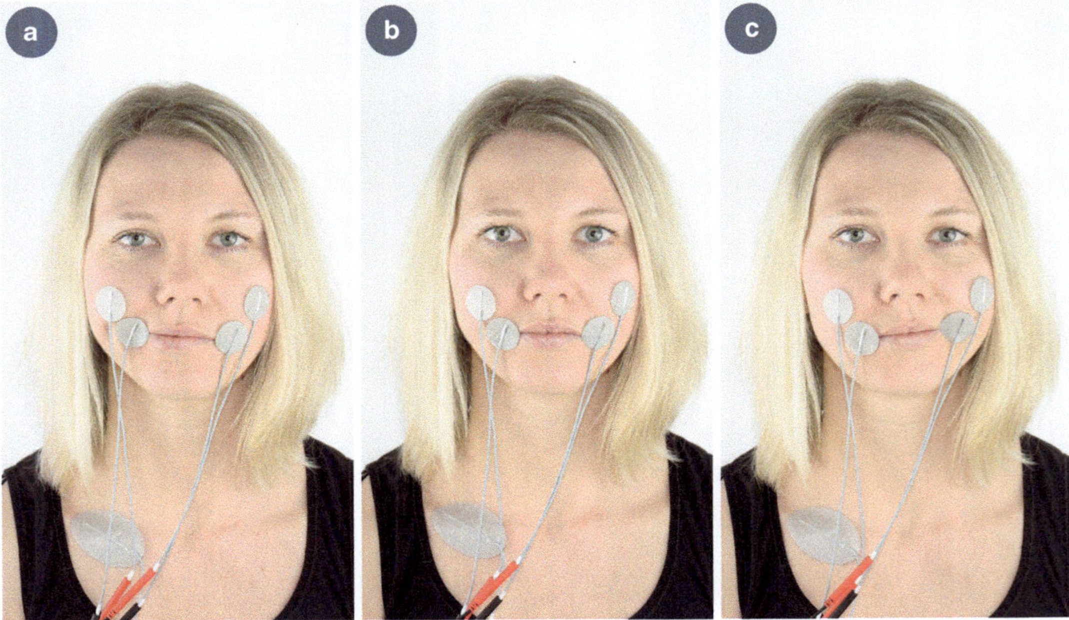

**Fig. 10.9** Coordination training of the Mm. zygomatici, alternating on both sides. (**a**) activation on the right side, (**b**) both sides in rest, (**c**) activation on the left side

## 10.13 FES at Completely Denervated FP

A completely denervated FP can occur, for example, in patients during a vestibular schwannoma surgery or a parotidectomy. In some cases, an injury of the facial nerve or complete severance can occur intraoperatively. In this case, the goal of postoperative FES would be to counteract atrophy of the facial muscles [14]. Regardless of the surgeon being able to preserve the nerve intraoperatively or surgical nerve reconstruction being performed, re-innervation of the muscles may take several months. Usually, a nerve regrows approximately 1 mm per day and every nerve suture requires approximately an additional 4 weeks for the axons to grow through. Without FES, atrophy of the mimic musculature would occur due to muscle inactivity. Therefore, FES is recommended to bridge the time till reinnervation to minimize denervation atrophy. So-called exponential or triangular currents with long pulse widths are used in FES as they immediately stimulate muscles rather than nerves. While a nerve can be stimulated with as little as 50 μs, a denervated muscle may need at least 10 ms (10,000 μs) pulse width to demonstrate a motor response. When selecting a suitable electrical stimulation device, ensure that the device offers the possibility of choosing between different current forms as well as long pulse widths to generate at least 250 ms [11]. Furthermore, a course FES may be deemed necessary before surgical intervention. This is because when target muscles stay preserved, a more complicated and invasive replacement surgery could be avoided and instead a reinnervation of the preserved original facial muscles could be achieved (Sect. 10.10). Thus, the significantly more complex free muscle transfer could be handed in. If the FP is completely denervated, long pulse times of up to 250 ms phase duration may be needed and sponge electrodes or large self-adhesive electrodes are typically used during stimulation. However, it should be noted that the electrical stimulation device must approve the use of such electrodes to do so (Table 10.4).

## 10.14 FES at Central FP

Personal experiences show that the application of FES must become viewed in a differentiated manner when treating central FP [14]. Treatment differentiates from peripheral FP due to the degree of impaired facial expression as well as the occurrence and duration of the disease. Of note, often a kind of pain may occur during early stages of stimulation. If a patient reports an uncomfortable stabbing sensation or pain during FES, stimulation should be discontinued. However, it is important to discriminate between pain experienced during stimulation and facial palsy trigeminal pain, which may occur simultaneously to FP. In some cases, FES may also have an analgesic effect on the patient. During the remission phase and when there are visible reinnervation potentials, biofeedback programs can be used in combination with emotionally supported facial expression movements.

## 10.15 FES After Operative Reanimated/Supplied FP

The term "surgically reanimated FP" describes reconstructive ways to improve symmetry and motor function of the paralyzed facial musculature. A distinction is made between three levels of function, which varies from the surgical options:

- The static plane.
- The dynamic-arbitrary level.
- The emotional level.

Azizzadeh [16] points out that after severe facial palsy with destruction of the nerve fibers and despite successful operation the original condition of the muscles cannot be fully restored. Regardless of spontaneous remission or surgical reconstruction, facial muscles will no longer be controlled as differentiated as before the onset of FP. In individual cases of nerve fiber loss, certain motor units and muscle fibers must be supplied by other axons. Incorrect or new innervations may be observed during the brain's motor learning process, for example,

**Table 10.4** Examples for the use of functional electrical stimulation (FES), including parameters and possible indications

| indication for FES in facial muscles | patient selection | parameters for FES in general | FES parameters practical examples |
|---|---|---|---|
| - FES as diagnostic tool<br>- verification of presence of stimulable and contractible muscle fibers | - Iatrogenic facial paralysis<br>- posttraumatic facial paralysis<br>- longstanding idipathic facial paralysis | - biphasic triangular impulses<br>- pulse phase width of 10 ms to 500 ms<br>- 1-3 Hz<br>- amplitudes of 1 mA to 30 mA<br><br>If facial muscle contractions can be triggered by FES, the presence of contractible muscle fibers is proven. The quantity of contraction correlates with the remaining muscle mass. Long pulse phase widths are typical for long time denervation. | - single pulses<br>- low frequency biphasic triangular impulses<br>- starting with a pulse phase width of 150 ms<br>- slowly increasing the amplitudes from 1mA till first contractions are visible<br><br>If no contractions can be detected, longer impulses of 250 ms or 500 ms should be tested. |
| - prevention or reduction of denervation atrophy<br>- facial reanimation | - Iatrogenic facial paralysis<br>- idiopathic facial paralysis with poor spontaneous remission<br>- facial nerve surgery (e.g., CFNTPL)<br>- muscle transplantation (e.g., M. gracilis) | - biphasic triangular impulses<br>- pulse phase width of 10 ms to 500 ms<br>- 1-10 Hz<br>- amplitudes of 1 mA to 30 mA<br>- optimum between muscles contractions and good tolerance by the patient should be found<br>- CFNTPL until the Tinel-Hoffman sign appears or at a minimum of 2 months until reinnervation signs are seen<br>- to avoid muscle fatigue due to overstimulation, stop the FES when the contractions vanish<br>- the amplitude of the electrical stimulation can be increased once to get back to stronger contractions<br>- if the contractions vanish a second time, FES should be paused for several hours | **1st week:**<br>- biphasic triangular impulses<br>- pulse phase width of 150 ms<br>- frequency as high as possible<br>- 2s on, 2s of time<br>- duration 20 minutes, or till the contractions vanish<br>- simultaneous to the FES-triggered muscle contractions, the patient should try to smile to activate the M. zygomaticus on both sides to keep the central representation active<br>- EMG-triggering from the non-paralytic side could be an option, to increase self-efficacy and central representation<br>- FES could be repeated twice a day with a minimum of 6-8h in between<br><br>**2nd week:**<br>- reduction of pulse phase width to 100 ms<br>- increase of stimulation frequency<br><br>**3rd week:**<br>- reduction of pulse phase width to 80 ms<br>- increase of stimulation frequency<br><br>…<br>Pulse phase width can be reduced in the next weeks because the training makes the denervated muscle more fatigue-resistance. |
| - EMG-biofeedback to improve control | - post paralytic synkinesis | - EMG-detection 1-2 channels without electrical stimulation | - EMG-biofeedback training to improve the relaxation<br>- 2 EMG-channel training for activation in one muscle while second muscle is relaxed<br>- 2 EMG-channel training for activation of both muscles of each side simultaneously to improve symmetry |

after cross-face nerve transplant (CFNTPL) or other neuromuscular surgeries. Therefore, FES may be a valuable contribution to motor learning, motor control, and ultimately improve the symmetry of the face (Figs. 10.5 and 10.6).

Muscle replacement surgeries, coupled with nerve surgeries, may also improve overall emotional muscle function. These include dynamic, arbitrary muscle substitute operations and nerve replacement operations. Examples of nerve replacement surgeries are hypoglossal facial nerve jump anastomosis, masseteric facial anastomosis, and accessory facial nerve anastomosis. The goal of a nerve transposition is for nerve fibers to sprout out to the facial muscles, discontinue muscular atrophy, and/or lower the increased muscle tone. As a result of surgery, patients should be able to activate movement potentials and trigger movement in the target muscles. One of the most frequently performed muscle replacement surgeries is the transplantation of the m. temporalis, the m. masseter, and the free gracilis graft. Especially after muscle and nerve replacement surgeries, postoperative therapy, including FES and biofeedback training, is recommended [14]. FES should be introduced 14 days post-surgery, as described in Sect. 10.10. During primary stimulation, it is recommended to use sponge pockets with rubber electrodes. Once complete sprouting of the nerve fibers in the target muscles has occurred and first action potentials in the target muscles appear, the use of biofeedback programs is recommended. At this time, the patient will learn to control individual muscles and increase perception of motor movements. From a speech and language therapy point of view, this approach is highly recommended as the patient increases awareness for the new structures and precision of motor movement. To generate emotionally coupled facial movements, a one- or two-stage surgery must be carried out. At the first stage, a so-called cross-face nerve graft is required. Therefore, the sural nerve, a sensitive nerve of the lower leg, is removed with the intend to relocate. The nerve graft is then connected to a nerve suture and attached to a strong branch of the n. facialis located at healthy side of the face. It is then connected to the paralyzed side through a subcutaneous tunnel extending underneath the upper lip. With the aim of reinnervation, the nerve graft is attached to the denervated mimic muscle, there

would be a low likelihood for successful reinnervation. In these cases, a free muscle graft may be connected during a follow-up surgery (approx. 9–12 months later). The m. gracilis from the thigh is often used for this procedure. FES can take on several functions in this complex two-stage surgery process [14]. A rarely used function is to use FES to locate denervated muscles.

If the treatment with exponential current demonstrates a contraction of the m. zygomaticus before the initial surgery, the patient should be informed, that if the original mimic musculature still will be reinnervated by FES and a free muscle transfer may be avoided. If gradual training over several weeks does not result in muscle contraction, it must be assumed that the musculature is too damaged to be used for reinnervation. In this case, e.g., a free muscle transfer is indicated. Until re-innervation occurs, exponential or triangular current treatment may minimize atrophy of the remaining facial muscles and the free muscle transplant. After successful reinnervation the EMG biofeedback programs may be used. This way, patients learn how to control the once immobile facial muscles and restore facial functions, such as the range of motion of mouth and cheek muscles and achieve a normal resting tone.

## 10.16 Patient Example

A 45-year-old patient presents in the specialized facial clinic 3 months after a surgical removal of a vestibular schwannoma. According to the surgical report, the n. facialis was stimulated throughout the surgical procedure. Postoperatively, the patient developed a complete unilateral FP and asks the SLP about his prognosis and therapy options. A needle electromyography was conducted but revealed no preserved arbitrary activity. However, excess pathological spontaneous activity could be observed, which may indicate severe axonal damage denervation of the facial muscles. A sonography of the paralyzed facial muscles revealed significantly smaller muscle mass as compared to muscles on the healthy side and no indications of voluntary movement. As a result of the absence of a spontaneous reinnervation, the option of surgical restoration using the hypoglossal nerve or the r. massetericus of the trigeminal nerve is discussed with the patient.

To counteract atrophy of the denervated mimic muscles up to the decision about the operation and the time after nerve reconstruction, electrical stimulation using long triangular pulses is recommended. A trial stimulation using a FES device is carried out during consultation. The stimulation using biphasic triangular pulses (150 ms, 5-7 mA) above the cheek and below the corner of the mouth (6x4 cm self-adhesive electrodes) triggers contraction of the m. orbicularis oculi and m. zygomaticus. Of note, proper electrode placement is adapted to the patient's individual needs and is photographically documented to serve as an instruction for the patient during home practice. Further, the patient is provided with detailed written instructions on how to properly place the electrodes and self-conduct electrical stimulation. Electrical stimulation should be carried out twice a day for 5 min each for the first week and at least 6 h apart (e.g., morning and evening). Further, stimulation should be conducted in front of a mirror to obtain immediate visual feedback. Triggering clearly visible contractions of the exercised muscles is crucial for minimizing the denervation atrophy of the affected facial muscles. Stretching of the trained muscles after each therapy unit as well as frequent breaks are recommended to prevent fatigue. From the second week onward, practice should increase to $2 \times 5$ min in the morning and $2 \times 5$ min in the evening with a 5-min break between sets. Finally, from the third week on, the patient should practice $3 \times 5$ min in the morning and evening with 5-min breaks between sets. A medical prescription is issued to the patient and a check-up appointment is scheduled for 3 months in the future. The patient is provided a telephone number in case any questions or problems with electrical stimulation occur during home practice. Further, the patient is educated that electrical stimulation may only minimize muscle atrophy, however, the chances of reinnervation do not increase through treatment. Surgical restoration is indicated even if the patient perceives the symptoms of FP as less severe following electrical stimulation.


**Summary**
Both, the literature and clinical practice recommend the use of FES in facial palsy therapy.



## References

1. Heckmann, Prof. Dr. Josef G. Therapie der idiopathischen Fazialisparese (Bell's Palsy). 3 31, 2017. Leitlinien für Diagnostik und Therapie in der Neurologie. https://dgn.org/wp-content/uploads/2013/01/030013_Therapie_der_idiopathischen_Fazialisparese.pdf.
2. Dobel C, et al. Emotionale Auswirkungen einer Fazialisparese (Emotional Impact of Facial Palsy). Laryngo-Rhino-Otol. 2013;92(01):9–23.
3. Ferner P. Anatomie des Nervensystems und der Sinnesorgane des Menschen. Ernst Reinhardt Verlag; 1967.
4. Mumenthaler M, Mattle H. Kurzlehrbuch Neurologie. 1. Auflage. Stuttgard: Georg Thieme Verlag; 2006.
5. Cheney M, Hadlock T. Facial surgery - plastic and reconstructive. 2014.
6. Facial Palsy UK. Physical Issues. Facial palsy UK; 2021. https://www.facialpalsy.org.uk/inform/what-is-facial-palsy/physical-issues/.
7. Willand MP, et al. Electrical stimulation to promote peripheral nerve regeneration. Neurorehabil Neural Repair. 2016;30(5):490–6.
8. Cararro U, et al. Persistent muscle fibre regeneration in long term denervation. Past, present, future. Muscle fibre regenration in longterm denervation. 2015, pp. 77–92.
9. Puls W, et al. Surface electrical stimulation for facial paralysis is not harmful. Muscle Nerve. 2020;61(3):347–53.
10. Fargher KA, Coulson S. Effectiveness of electrical stimulation for rehabilitation of facial nerve paralysis. Phys Therapy Rev. 2017;22(3-4):169–76.
11. Arnold D, et al. Selective surface electrostimulation of the denervated zygomaticus muscle. Diagnostics (Basel). 2021;11(2):188. https://doi.org/10.3390/diagnostics11020188.
12. Angelov DN, et al. Mechanical Stimulation of paralyzed vibrissal muscles following facial nerve injury in adult rat promotes full recovery od whisking. Neurobiol Dis. 2007;26(1):229–42.
13. Marotta N, et al. Neuromuscular electrical stimulation and shortwave diathermy in unrecovered Bell palsy - A randomized controlles study. Medicine. 2020;99(8)
14. Repitsch CA, Volk GF. Funktionelle Elektrostimulation bei Fazialisparesen. In: Schick T, editor. Funktionelle Elektrostimulation in der Neurorehabilitation. 2. Auflage. Deutschland: Springer Verlag GmbH; 2020. https://link.springer.com/chapter/10.1007%2F978-3-662-61705-2_10#DOI.
15. Volk GF, Finkensieper M, Guntinas-Lichius O. EMG Biofeedback Training zuhause zur Therapie der Defektheilung bei chronischer Fazialisparese. Laryngo-Rhino-Otol. 2014;93:15–24.
16. Azizzadeh B. Latest treatment options for facial paralysis. 062014. Latest treatment options for facial paralysis with Dr. Babak Azizzadeh; 2014. https://facialparalysisfound.wistia.com/medias/352hsepmqg

# Functional Electrical Stimulation in Dysphagia Treatment

**11**

Jan Faust and Carsten Kroker

## 11.1 Introduction

Neurogenic dysphagia is common after stroke and occurs in up to 80% of patients with acute stroke, although its prevalence varies depending on stroke severity, affected brain region, and diagnostic procedure employed [1, 2]. In addition, multiple complications are associated with dysphagia, including increased risk of aspiration pneumonia, malnutrition, and dehydration [3, 4]. Aspiration may occur in about half of acute stroke patients, with the risk of aspiration persisting in about a quarter of patients after 6 months [5], a condition that may continue even after 12 months [2]. Impaired food intake may be associated with significant impairment of quality of life [6] and may result in prolonged feeding via a gastric tube [3, 4]. High prevalence of dysphagia occurs in many neurological disorders, such as Parkinson's disease [1, 7], multiple sclerosis [8, 9], dementia [10, 11], or amyotrophic lateral sclerosis [12]. Therefore, dysphagia treatment is challenging due to the different underlying pathomechanism and patient-specific treatment options.

Conventional swallowing therapy includes oral-motor exercises, compensation through postural modification, and airway-protecting maneuvers to minimize risk of aspiration [13]. These methods can be accompanied by dietary interventions such as texture modification of foods and liquids [14]. However, evidence for conventional swallowing therapy is limited and the specific treatment effects often remain unclear [13, 15].

In recent years, the use of electrical stimulation in swallowing therapy has gained increasing attention including different application modalities such as functional electrical stimulation (FES), transcranial direct current stimulation (tDCS), repetitive transcranial magnetic stimulation (rTMS), or pharyngeal electrical stimulation (PES). In PES, the pharyngeal mucosa receives sensory stimulation via a catheter with a pair of bipolar ring electrodes at frequencies of 5–10 Hz. PES is expected to enhance functional reorganization of the swallowing cortex and increase sensory afferents, which may lead to improved swallowing function and early decannulation in severely dysphagic stroke patients with tracheostomy [16]. PES may be considered similar to surface FES, although it is not intended to induce contractions of the pharyngeal musculature [17]. In FES, the actual swallowing musculature is stimulated with

**Supplementary Information** The online version contains supplementary material available at [https://doi.org/10.1007/978-3-030-90123-3_11].

J. Faust (✉)
Helios Klinikum Krefeld, Department of Otolaryngology, Krefeld, Germany

C. Kroker
Praxis für Logopädie, Saarbrücken, Germany


T. Schick (ed.), *Functional Electrical Stimulation in Neurorehabilitation*,
https://doi.org/10.1007/978-3-030-90123-3_11

current on motor threshold, thus directly modulating the swallowing process. In addition, during stimulation with FES, motor actions take place that involve swallowing or functional exercises. FES is widely used in rehabilitation units for muscle strengthening and has consequently been applied to patients with acute or chronic dysphagia of various etiologies. FES usually requires the patient's cooperation as it involves assisted swallowing or motor exercises as well as behavioral approaches. However, if the patient is unable to cooperate, electrical stimulation might be performed to increase sensory afferents and consequently improve swallowing frequency and saliva management. In case of cognitive deficits, FES could be used more intuitively during swallowing attempts or at mealtime. Thus, the procedure is suitable even for severely dysphagic patients including those with tracheal cannula. From the authors' point of view, this is a decisive advantage over conventional dysphagia therapy, which is much more dependent on the patient's cooperation. Despite this, FES is often neglected in the treatment of dysphagia, which may be due to a lack of awareness or resources.

## 11.2 Dysphagia Assessment

### 11.2.1 Diagnostic Procedure

Before proceeding with electrical stimulation, a systematic evaluation of swallowing functions must be performed to determine the severity and type of dysphagia. Besides specific medical history and initial dysphagia screening, this involves a specialized clinical swallowing examination that includes cranial nerve assessment [14]. If further information on swallowing safety or underlying pathology is required, flexible endoscopic evaluation of swallowing (FEES) or videofluoroscopic swallowing study (VFSS) is recommended as the gold standard of dysphagia diagnostics [14]. FEES and VFSS provide objective information on swallowing pathology and are essential for the detection of silent aspiration [18].

### 11.2.2 Pathophysiology

Neurogenic dysphagia results from neurological disorders affecting the central or peripheral nervous system, neuromuscular transmission, or muscular structures [14]. Swallowing involves a variety of more than 30 muscles controlled by a complex neural network that includes the brainstem, basal ganglia, thalamus, limbic system, cerebellum, and motor and sensory cortex [19]. Safe and efficient swallowing depends on intact sensory afferents from the oral cavity, pharynx, and esophagus to the central nervous system (CNS), as well as motor coordination, both controlled by swallowing centers in the brainstem, cerebral cortex, and cerebellum [20]. Cortical lesions contribute to impairments of oral bolus control, lingual dyscoordination, contralateral facial weakness, and a delay in the initiation of volitionally induced swallowing [21, 22]. Whereas brainstem lesions are predominantly associated with paralysis of ipsilateral pharynx, larynx, or soft palate, as well as decreased upper esophageal sphincter (UES) opening and reflex triggering [19, 21, 23]. In infratentorial stroke, high incidence of dysphagia is reported in lesions of the lateral and medial medulla as well as the pons [24]. Brainstem infarcts occur less frequently than cortical strokes, but may result in more severe and prolonged dysphagia [21, 25]. A suggested pathophysiologic mechanism for severe dysphagia in brainstem infarcts could be a reverse pressure gradient due to dyscoordination of pharyngeal contraction and reduced cricopharyngeal relaxation [23]. Depending on the underlying structural and functional impairments, different pathophysiological mechanisms can be identified that may be related to several phenotypic dysphagia patterns [26].

### 11.2.3 Involved Cranial Nerves

There are mainly 5 cranial nerves involved in the swallowing process (V, VII, IX, X, XII) [27], almost all of which (except XII) have both motor and sensory function. Cranial nerve palsy may result in partial or complete loss of function of single or multiple cranial nerves, which can be observed in lesions resulting from tumors, trauma, head and neck surgery, infections, and stroke [28]. The pharyngeal plexus forms the major afferent and efferent fibers for swallowing, consisting of pharyngeal branches of the glossopharyngeus (IX) and vagus (X) nerves and sympathetic trunk branches that provide motor innervation to the pharyngeal constrictors and sensory innervation to the pharyngeal mucosa [29, 30]. After contributing to the pharyngeal plexus, the vagus nerve (X) forms branches to the superior laryngeal nerve (SLN) and the recurrent laryngeal nerve (RLN). The SLN is divided into the external motor branch and the internal sensory branch. The external branch of SLN innervates the cricothyroid muscle and may supply additional fibers to the pharyngeal plexus, while both the SLN and RLN are involved in innervation of the inferior pharyngeal constrictor and cricopharyngeal muscle [31–33]. The RLN innervates all other intrinsic muscles of the larynx and may also contain communicating branches between SLN and pharyngeal plexus [32]. Inadequate airway protection due to ipsilateral vocal cord paralysis may lead to possible aspiration after lesions of the nucleus ambiguous and lateral medulla [34, 35]. Cranial to the glottis, the larynx is supplied with sensory input by the inner branch of the SLN, which is essential for protective reflexes including glottic closure and coughing [36]. Thus, damage to the SLN, RLN, or pharyngeal plexus may result in decreased pharyngeal contraction, leading to hypopharyngeal residue and increased risk of aspiration [37]. Recovery from unilateral or bilateral cranial nerve palsy depends on the location and size of the lesion in the brain [28].

## 11.3 Evidence Base

Transcutaneous electrical stimulation has been the subject of numerous studies investigating its effectiveness in patients with dysphagia of various etiologies. However, conflicting results have been reported regarding functional effects on swallowing kinematics and outcome in dysphagic patients. This may result from the fact that stimulation protocols vary considerably in amplitude, frequency, duration, electrode placement, and especially the presence of simultaneous functional exercises. This makes it difficult to compare study results and determine their effectiveness in dysphagia treatment.

Most of the studies examine biphasic currents with 80 Hz and 700 µs square wave pulses that have been investigated for dysphagia of various etiologies. The method was first described in a study by Freed et al. using a slightly modified stimulation protocol of 80 Hz and 300 µs [38]. A general problem with most studies is the inconsistent nomenclature, with most studies using the term neuromuscular electrical stimulation (NMES). However, NMES is a passive stimulation without volitional activity of the patient, mainly used for muscle strengthening and atrophy prophylaxis in upper motor neuron lesions [39]. Whereas FES provides electrical stimulation to facilitate muscle contractions during a functional task in a timed coordinated manner. In this regard, electrical stimulation closely matched to a volitional muscle contraction may potentially activate more muscle fibers than without exercise [39]. Curiously, some authors refer to NMES as such, even though it is conducted according to the principles of FES. Therefore, some authors argue that NMES may be considered similar to FES in situations where a muscle contraction is facilitated simultaneously to a functional task [40]. However, many stimulation protocols do not include proper synchronization of current and fail to implement sufficient rest periods to prevent fatigue of the swallowing musculature.

There are various meta-analyses generally confirming the efficacy of transcutaneous electrical stimulation in the treatment of dysphagia [40–46], although varying in their conclusion. Restrictions must be made for the two initial reviews by Carnaby-Mann and Crary [40] and Tan et al. [46], including non-randomized studies and dysphagia of different etiologies. Controversially, in the review by Tan et al. [46], electrical stimulation was superior to conventional dysphagia treatment only in patients with dysphagia caused by non-stroke diseases, and in a later review by Chen et al. [45], superiority of electrical stimulation was found exclusively in stroke-associated dysphagia. For the latter, though, improvements were significant only when combining electrical stimulation with functional therapy [45]. However, a recent systematic review based exclusively on randomized controlled trials confirmed that in 10 of 11 analyzed studies electrical stimulation combined with conventional swallowing therapy resulted in significant improvements on swallowing function in patients with post-stroke dysphagia compared to control groups with conventional therapy only [47]. Another recent systematic review showed positive effects of electrical stimulation in the treatment of stroke-related dysphagia regarding improvement in quality of life, reduction of aspiration, restoration of oral intake, and socioeconomic integration. These effects were present with a sole application of electrical stimulation and could be increased further by combining it with functional exercises [48].

Accordingly, the National Institute for Health and Care Excellence (NICE) guidelines consider transcutaneous electrical stimulation to be safe for adults with post-stroke dysphagia, providing evidence for its potential benefit for this patient group. However, there was insufficient evidence supporting its clinical use in non-stroke patients [49].

## 11.4 Objectives and Implementation of FES in Dysphagia Treatment

FES generates muscle contractions due to depolarization of peripheral motor nerves under the electrodes. After CNS damage, when cortical control is disrupted, these electrically evoked contractions can be used to facilitate functional tasks and restore intentional movements [50]. At the same time, the afferent sensory response activates the involved motor networks and may induce reorganization of motor control [51]. The increased sensory feedback through central pathways leads to an activation of motor neurons,

similar to the recruitment of motor units during voluntary contractions [50]. Regeneration of swallowing function often depends not only on the functioning of the efferent motor pathways, but also on afferent sensory feedback. Here, the sensory problem is situated more at the level of the mucosal sensors and may affect swallowing control even in healthy individuals due to local anesthesia of the oropharyngeal mucosa [52]. Mucosal sensors as well as the laryngeal reflexes are dependent on the mechanical stimulus of inhalation and exhalation, which seems to be a major reason for high incidence of dysphagia in patients with a cuffed tracheostomy tube, including higher risk of silent aspiration when compared to cuff-deflated condition [53].

The specific objectives can be summarized as follows:

- Improvement of sensory input, bolus perception, and reflex triggering.
- Increase of hyolaryngeal excursion.
- Improvement of vocal cord closure.
- Reduction of penetration and aspiration.
- Improvement of upper esophageal sphincter opening.
- Increased pharyngeal muscle contraction and tongue base retraction.
- Increase in oral food intake and quality of life.

Since dysphagia is a disorder with a complex sequence of movements under exertion of time with different types of underlying pathomechanisms, FES parameters must be adapted to the individual patient's conditions. Accordingly, this results in different stimulation protocols, with different current forms, different application techniques, or amplitudes.

On the one hand, swallowing muscles are located in a confined space of the neck region, making them rather easy to access with electrodes. On the other hand, there is a large number of antagonists that must be considered, such as the laryngeal elevator and laryngeal depressor muscles or the glottal adductors and abductors [54]. It is essential to take these conditions into account when selecting the stimulation parameters. However, this requires special knowledge and experience of the healthcare professional, as even small changes in electrode placement or stimulation parameters can affect the functional outcome.

## 11.4.1 Preparation of the Stimulation Protocol

The use of FES in the neck area is subject to special regulatory approval criteria and is therefore not supported by all manufacturers. It is thus obligatory to use systems that have been approved for use in the head and neck region. Contraindications as specified by the medical device manufacturer must be considered, e.g. pregnancy, tumors, cardiac pacemakers, cranial stimulators, or metal implants in the head and neck area.

First of all, there is no standardized stimulation protocol, as currents may differ depending on the device used, electrode size, and pulse shape. Even when the same device is used, there are many variables that may cause muscles to respond differently. As described previously, a common stimulation protocol in dysphagia therapy uses a rather high stimulation frequency of 80 Hz, which may lead to fatigue of the swallowing muscles, especially when stimulation is applied continuously over a long duration and without sufficient rest periods [55]. In contrast, lower stimulation frequencies of 20 Hz were found to produce fatigue-resistant tetanic muscle contractions, whereas intensity and pulse width seem to be of minor concern [56]. Higher stimulation frequencies produce higher contractile force, but result in more rapid muscle fiber fatigue [39]. Electrical stimulation selectively recruits fast-twitch (type II) fibers before slow-twitch (type I) muscle fibers in a reverse recruitment order to regular contractions. Type II fibers may fatigue more quickly at higher stimulation frequencies than type I fibers, which are generally more resistant to fatigue [55]. However, unlike typical type I and type II fibers of the limb musculature, swallowing-related muscles may contain unique hybrid fibers to exhibit rapid contraction and fatigue resistance [57, 58]. There

is evidence to support this assumption for an optimal stimulation frequency of 30–60 Hz in dysphagia therapy, which includes synchronized functional tasks with sufficient rest periods to avoid fatigue [59–61]. Doeltgen et al. [62] showed that EMG-triggered 80 Hz current stimulation applied to submental muscles containing a 4-s stimulation phase synchronized to volitional swallows increased motor evoked potential (MEP) amplitudes at 30 and 60 min after stimulation. Changes in corticobulbar excitability induced by electrical stimulation were present only at higher frequencies of 80 Hz and when stimulation was synchronized with swallowing, whereas non-synchronized and continuous stimulation had no effect on MEP amplitudes [62]. These findings suggest that a short stimulation phase closely matched to volitional swallowing should be used to enhance corticobulbar excitability.

Regarding stimulation frequency, there is a need for further research on which frequencies are most appropriate for stimulating the swallowing musculature. On the one hand, higher frequencies of 80 Hz may increase swallow-associated CNS motor activity; on the other hand, muscle fatigue may occur more quickly than when using lower frequencies. In general, however, care should be taken with all frequencies that stimulation should be synchronized with swallowing and to implement sufficient rest periods in order to enhance motor learning and prevent muscle fatigue. This could be achieved by using electromyography (EMG)-triggered current, as demonstrated in a prospective study by Leelamanit et al., [59] in which 23 patients with chronic dysphagia of different etiologies were treated with a short phase of EMG-triggered 60 Hz stimulation current synchronized with swallowing. The results showed improvements in swallowing function in 20 of 23 patients, including increased laryngeal elevation during stimulation and reduced aspiration [59]. However, no control group was established. Since chronic dysphagic patients were recruited, these improvements after stimulation were unlikely to occur due to spontaneous recovery, though.

Pulse duration is another important parameter, while greater muscle force production is generated by increasing either pulse duration or stimulus amplitude [39]. In a study by Barikroo et al., a short pulse duration of 300 µs increased the maximum amplitude tolerance compared to a longer pulse duration of 700 µs [63]. Thus, a short pulse duration may lead to higher amplitude stimulation, which could facilitate stimulation of deeper swallowing muscles such as mylohyoid and geniohyoid, responsible for hyoid elevation [63, 64]. Another study by Humbert et al. found the hyolaryngeal complex to be pulled downward at rest and hyolaryngeal excursion to be reduced during swallowing when using the 80 Hz and 700 µs stimulation protocol in ten different electrode placements [65]. Ludlow et al. [66] confirmed this finding on hyoid depression at rest when using the identical stimulation parameters. Despite this adverse condition, there was a significant decrease in aspiration and pooling, albeit only when sensory stimulation was applied [66]. On the other hand, there is evidence that a short pulse duration of 300 µs may place the larynx in a more forward position prior to the onset of swallowing, reducing the range of anterior excursion by approximately 20% to its peak position during swallowing [64, 67]. This reduced hyoid range of motion may result in a shorter duration of hyoid excursion during swallowing when electrical stimulation is applied to the submental musculature. Hyoid elevation and tongue pressure generation can also be increased after surface electrical stimulation to the laryngeal region using a short pulse duration of 200 µs, as shown in a study by Takahashi et al. [68]. Therefore, it can be assumed that hyolaryngeal excursion may be facilitated by a short pulse duration rather than by electrode placement. To promote hyolaryngeal excursion, bipolar surface electrodes should be placed bilaterally on the anterior neck, either cranially or caudally to the hyoid bone or combined (see Fig. 11.1), using a rather short pulse duration to penetrate deeper tissue layers with higher amplitudes.

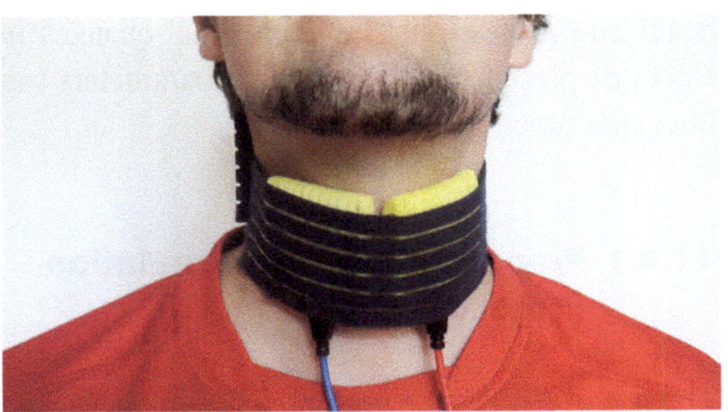

**Fig. 11.1** Bipolar: Two electrodes (anode, cathode) placed on each side of the thyroid cartilage, used for biphasic tetanizing currents

Although the use of sensory stimulation has demonstrated to increase swallowing safety in post-stroke patients [69–71], stimulation at motor level has been found to further improve swallowing kinematics and increase efficacy [72]. Moreover, sensory stimulation has been commonly used as a sham condition, which is questionable considering the residual effect on increasing afferent feedback.

**Summary**
- Bipolar surface electrodes should be used bilaterally on the anterior neck (either cranially or caudally to the hyoid bone or combined).
- Stimulation frequency should be applied at 30–80 Hz (while lower frequencies are less likely to cause fatigue).
- Pulsed current of 200–700 µs with square wave biphasic pulses should be used (while a shorter pulse duration may facilitate hyolaryngeal excursion).
- Stimulation current should be applied rather on motor than on sensory level.
- FES should be synchronized with a functional task (swallowing or motor exercise) and include sufficient rest periods.

*CAVE*: The use of tetanizing currents is only appropriate in case of damage to the upper motor neuron.

## 11.4.2 Kilohertz-Frequency Alternating Current (Medium-Frequency Current)

While low-frequency pulsed current (usually delivered in the range of 1–120 Hz) is associated with discomfort at higher amplitudes and thus limiting muscle force production, medium-frequency stimulation (MFS) at kilohertz frequencies may be more comfortable and is expected to penetrate deeper tissue layers [73, 74]. This may allow higher current amplitudes to be used, resulting in a greater stimulation effect. Consistent with this concept, a high-resolution manometry (HRM) study on 29 healthy participants found a significant increase in tongue base pressure after continuous MFS at 2.5 kHz with a burst modulation of 50 Hz (so-called "russian current"), but not after low-frequency stimulation at 100 Hz [75]. In a prospective study by Miller et al., [76] twelve patients were randomly assigned to either the stimulation group, which received conventional swallowing therapy combined with MFS (2-channel) at motor level or sham group receiving conventional swallowing therapy at sensory-level MFS. Each group showed significant improvements in dysphagia severity, but no significant differences were found between the study groups [76]. However, the small sample size, low interrater reliability, and differences in stroke onset may have limited the statistical power of this study. Another MFS protocol using interferential current (IFC) at sensory threshold was found to increase swallowing frequency in healthy subjects, at least during a 15-minute stimulation period [77]. A similar IFC stimulation protocol was used in a randomized controlled trial by Maeda et al. resulting in improved airway defense and nutrition in patients with dysphagia [78]. Since MFS seems to be unsuitable for stimulation of denervated musculature, its use is limited to upper motor neuron damage [74, 75, 79]. The potential benefit of medium-frequency current still needs to be confirmed by further clinical trials under real sham conditions.

**Summary**
- The use of kilohertz frequency current is a novel application form in dysphagia therapy.
- Kilohertz frequency currents can penetrate deeper tissue layers to potentially stimulate deeper swallowing muscles.
- Kilohertz frequency current may enhance pharyngeal swallowing phase by increasing tongue base pressure.
- MFS at sensory level may increase swallowing frequency and improve nutrition status.

## 11.4.3 Single Pulse Stimulation Current

Single pulse stimulation offers several advantages in the treatment of dysphagia compared to previously described currents that induce a tetanic contraction. Single pulses are commonly used to treat paralysis resulting from lower motor neuron damage, where the pulse duration can last up to 1000 ms. In this context, longer pulses of 500–1000 ms are used for the stimulation of severely damaged muscle-nerve units or after complete denervation. When the lower motor neuron is affected due to lesions of the peripheral nervous system, different degrees of denervation (neurapraxia, axonotmesis, or neurotmesis) may occur, resulting in paralysis of a single or multiple innervated muscles. If the peripheral nerve is disrupted, the muscle can no longer be made to contract with conventional tetanizing currents using pulses in the microsecond range [74]. Longer pulse widths are needed, while pulse duration increases with the degree of damage and higher intensities are needed to still produce a muscle contraction. A more precise evaluation of denervation is provided on the one hand by needle EMG or, alternatively, by accommodation measurement, which can be calculated with the help of modern electrical stimulation devices. As the paralyzed muscle fatigues faster than a healthy muscle, rapid successive stimulation may cause the contraction to become sluggish. Therefore, the refractory period must be considered and sufficient pauses must be provided in the course of stimulation. At the same time, regular stimulation of the muscle is necessary to protect it from atrophy. However, in case of damage to the upper motor neuron, denervation is not or hardly to be expected [51], so that the paralyzed muscles can be electrically stimulated even with shorter impulses of <1 ms in order to generate a fused contraction. Meanwhile, the aim of paralysis therapy is to reduce the long pulse widths to the point where they become small enough (<1 ms) to continue with tetanizing currents. Triangular pulses are commonly used to achieve selective muscle contraction of the impaired muscle unit and to reduce the influence of healthy antagonists. Another advantage of triangular pulses is the better tolerability due to the ramped rise compared to rectangular pulses. Due to accommodation, a stronger stimulus effect on damaged muscle units can be assumed, while healthy muscles and antagonists will contract with a delay. However, the shorter the pulse, the more the square and triangular characteristics converge, stimulating more healthy muscle units and antagonists, respectively.

In dysphagia therapy, though, shorter pulse widths are indicated, since the pulse should be executed synchronously with swallowing. Thus, a pulse width of 100–200 ms appears to be appropriate to produce a timed contraction of the glottal adductors and to support the initiation of swallowing. Moreover, FES in dysphagia treatment should include healthy muscles in order to activate as many motor units involved in swallowing as possible. This requires shorter pulses than in traditional paralysis therapy of lower motor neuron lesions. Therefore, the use of single pulses in dysphagia treatment must be distinguished from paralysis therapy in terms of pulse duration and amplitude. However, with very short pulses of <10 ms, much higher intensities are required to evoke a muscle contraction due to the very short stimulus duration.

In contrast to bipolar biphasic tetanizing currents, single pulses are usually offered monopolar and monophasic (direct current) in paralysis therapy, as this produces a stronger stimulation effect under the smaller electrode and paralyzed muscles can be addressed more specifically (see Fig. 11.2). In addition, lower amplitudes are usually required in the face and neck area compared to stimulation

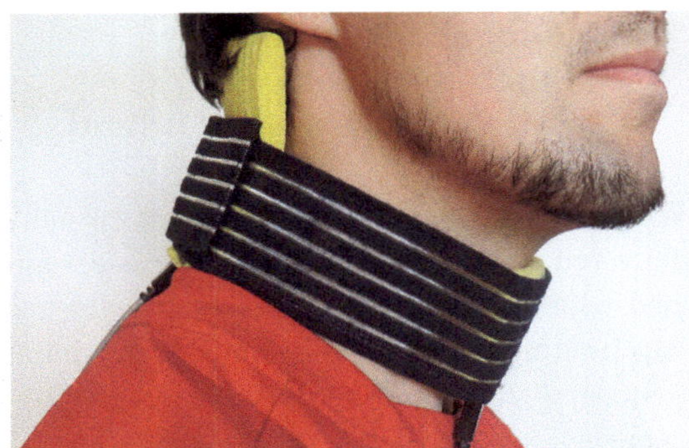

**Fig. 11.2** Monopolar: One passive electrode (anode) on the nape, one active electrode (cathode) placed centrally on thyroid cartilage (lateral view), used for single pulses

of the extremities. Since head and neck muscles are located closer under the skin than the extensive muscle courses on the arm and leg, damage to the skin is less likely. It is recommended to perform a galvanic or impulse galvanic (IG50/8 Hz) preparation phase in order to reduce skin resistance and increase motor nerve excitability (catelectrotonus) [74, 75, 79]. This creates favorable conditions for subsequent functional stimulation of the paralyzed muscle with single pulses. Stimulation with triangular single pulses in laryngeal electrode placement can induce endoscopically detectable contractions of the glottal adductor muscles [80], which may lead to an immediate swallowing response (Video 11.1). In addition, the laryngeal elevator muscles are likely to be activated with monophasic triangular pulses in the range of 200 ms (Video 11.2). Acoustic or visual feedback of the pulse generation ensures that the current has been applied properly. Electrically induced contractions of the vocal cords should be symmetrical under normal conditions but may be irregular due to accommodation in unilateral laryngeal paralysis.

If there is no denervation, significant vocal cord adduction may be observed using tetanizing current with a specific stimulation protocol including a short pulsed current of 200 µs and a biphasic pulse rate of 100 Hz with a cycle of 3 s on followed by 5 s off-phase, as shown by Seifpanahi et al. [81]. Another study by Humbert et al., which was based on a commonly used stimulation frequency of 80 Hz, failed to induce any or only minor contractions of the intrinsic laryngeal muscles with 10 different electrode placements [82]. Therefore, it seems that glottal closure may be achieved by modifying the current parameters rather than the electrode placement. However, in a study on 9 healthy subjects, a significantly shorter laryngeal vestibule closure reaction time was demonstrated after submandibular electrical stimulation with tetanizing current (30 Hz, 50–250 µs), which could lead to faster glottic closure in dysphagic patients and, accordingly, to a reduction in the risk of aspiration [83].

When using single pulses, it can be assumed that triangular pulses may result in greater laryngeal elevation by inhibiting the antagonistic lowering musculature. In addition to the rising shape of the curve, the intensity also plays a role in the activation of antagonists and must therefore be adjusted individually. Since intensity controls the number of activated fibers, higher amplitudes could potentially activate more antagonists despite a flat curve rise. Therefore, the amplitude should be adjusted individually up to the threshold of muscle contraction perceived by the patient or visible swallowing response. The functional effects of single pulse current can also be assessed endoscopically during FEES to determine the contractile threshold of the intrinsic laryngeal muscles, analogous to the evaluation of other therapeutic maneuvers. A contraction of the intrinsic laryngeal musculature triggered by single pulses can facilitate a reflective swallowing response, even if the patient is unable to initiate such voluntarily (Video 11.3). With the rising ramp of triangular pulses, a better reflex triggering can be expected compared to rectangular pulses. This could be due to the smoother rise to maximum amplitude, which in some ways resembles the dynamics of the physiological swallowing process. In this case, the peak of the rise ramp should be reached around the last third of the pulse, followed by a short drop (equivalent to sawtooth shape). Due to the reduced sensory function found in many dysphagic patients, such pulse-triggered swallowing responses may increase sensory input and consequently restore motor control. Therefore, when reflex triggering is impaired, single pulses should be administered only after the inspiratory phase to avoid nonphysiologic swallowing patterns. In order to synchronize swallowing activity with impulse delivery, EMG-systems are the first choice because

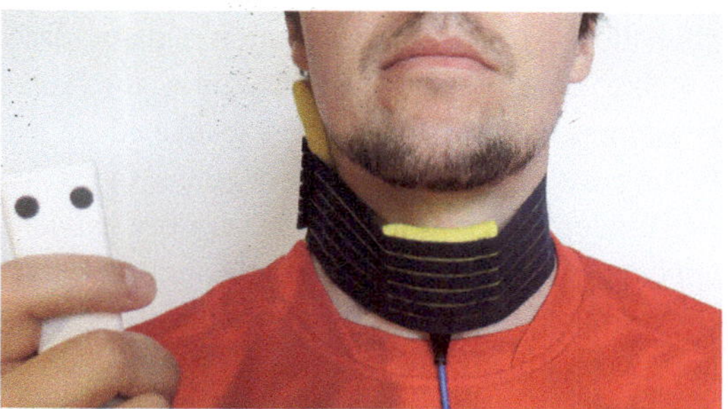

**Fig. 11.3** Monopolar: One passive electrode (anode) on the nape, one active electrode (cathode) placed centrally on thyroid cartilage (front view), for single pulses using a manual button

they detect swallowing activity by contraction of the submental muscles and immediately deliver an impulse of predefined length and amplitude when the threshold is exceeded. In practice, however, EMG-triggered systems are rare, and reliability may be limited by complete absence of the swallowing reflex or by inadvertently reaching the threshold in response to speech or chewing movements. Systems with a manual button, where the patient or alternatively the therapist triggers the pulses synchronously with the onset of swallowing, are more accessible (see Fig. 11.3). As the pulses have to be triggered manually at the right moment, this requires more coordination, but can usually be performed by the patient with some practice.

### 11.4.3.1 FES in Laryngeal Dysfunction

The use of single pulse current has been shown to be effective in the treatment of laryngeal palsy by inducing glottal closure, which is essential for swallowing safety. In a randomized controlled trial, FES with single triangular pulses was superior to conventional voice therapy resulting in a significant decrease of vocal fold irregularity measured by objective voice analysis in patients with unilateral RLN paralysis [84]. However, conventional voice therapy is considered a compensatory approach, whereas FES focuses more on restitution, making comparison difficult. The stimulation protocol introduced by Pahn and Pahn [54] involves a fixed scheme, consisting of a 7-min impulse galvanic (direct current) preparatory phase followed by individually adapted monophasic triangular pulses synchronized with phonation. Although galvanization is particularly suitable in traditional paralysis therapy, it can also be adapted to dysphagia therapy to take advantage of the positive effects for bridging the skin barrier. In a randomized controlled trial, sensory galvanic application to the bilateral masseter muscle in early stroke patients induced significantly greater improvements in dysphagia severity than the control group receiving conventional therapy [85]. Thus, galvanic treatment may have positive effects on swallowing safety by increasing sensory feedback. Vocal cord paralysis (VCP) may occur after peripheral damage to the vagus nerve or RLN, but may also be found after central lesions of the nucleus ambiguous and lateral medulla causing ipsilateral VCP [35, 86]. Meanwhile, several studies indicate a close relationship between laryngeal paralysis and concomitant dysphagia [37, 87, 88]. In this context, it has been shown that not only decreased glottic closure leads to an increased risk of aspiration, but also pharyngeal weakness and decreased UES relaxation can be found in patients with VCP [89, 90]. This can be explained by having both the RLN and the external branch of SLN involved in the innervation of the cricopharyngeal muscle, with the external branch of SLN providing additional fibers to the inferior pharyngeal constrictor [30, 33]. In contrast, however, VCP may also result in higher pharyngeal peak pressures as a result of compensation of the healthy contralateral pharyngeal muscles at chronic stage [91]. Additionally, dysphagic symptoms in patients with VCP may vary depending on etiology and may be more severe after central lesions and in acute onset [88, 92]. It can be assumed that reducing glottal incompetence through the use of FES will improve airway protection and lower the risk of aspiration. Under therapy-refractory conditions, this can also be achieved by surgical vocal cord medialization [14].

### 11.4.3.2 FES in Cricopharyngeal Dysfunction

In a HRM study by Heck et al. [93], when swallowing was synchronized with a short EMG-triggered 80 Hz stimulation phase, no immediate effect on UES dynamics was found in healthy adults.

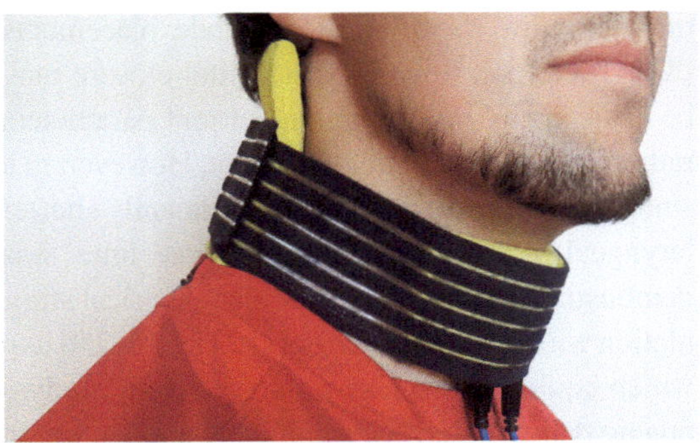

**Fig. 11.4** Monopolar: One neutral electrode (anode) on the nape, two smaller electrodes (cathodes) placed on each side of the thyroid cartilage, used for single pulses

However, a delayed effect of FES was measurable after 5- and 30-min intervals, consisting of an increased relaxation time of the UES and decreased hypopharyngeal pressure. Another HRM study in 26 healthy adults showed a significant prolongation of the relaxation time of the UES by 10% for short biphasic single pulses of 5 ms delivered synchronously with swallowing 5 ml of water compared to sham condition [94]. For this particular application, a monopolar electrode placement was selected, having two smaller electrodes (cathodes) on each side of the thyroid cartilage and one neutral electrode (anode) placed on the nape (see Fig. 11.4). This application may enhance UES opening due to bilateral application of short biphasic single pulses at the onset of swallowing.

Failed or reduced relaxation of the UES is associated with hypopharyngeal residue and may increase the risk of consecutive aspiration. FES with synchronized single pulses may reduce bolus residues in the piriform sinus by prolonging UES relaxation, resulting in lower risk of subsequent penetration or aspiration (Video 11.4). Consistently, Lee et al. found that decreased UES relaxation time was the primary risk factor for aspiration in post-acute stroke patients [95], making cricopharyngeal dysfunction (CPD) a major challenge in the treatment of oropharyngeal dysphagia. In chronic CPD with impaired UES opening, cricopharyngeal myotomy, dilation, or botulinum toxin injection may be considered [14]. Future clinical trials should investigate the effect of FES on UES opening dynamics in

**Summary**
- Single pulses can be used in paralysis therapy as well as in the treatment of dysphagia (but with different pulse widths and waveforms)
- Single pulses can be used for pathologies resulting from both upper and lower motor neuron lesions.
- Single pulses induce contraction of the intrinsic laryngeal muscles and may lead to airway protection.
- Single pulses are applied synchronously to swallowing using EMG-systems or a manual button at the onset of swallowing.
- Galvanic preparation phase should be administered in paralysis therapy and may be used as an adjunct in dysphagia therapy to improve sensory input.
  *CAVE:* Moist sponge pockets pulled over the electrodes protect the skin in case of longer pulse widths and galvanic current. Otherwise, the skin is at risk of cauterization! Direct current should be applied according to the principle of minimum dosage, as excessive exposure can lead to skin cauterization! This requires the amplitude to be adjusted to the size of the electrodes. The current density must not exceed $0.2 \text{ mA/cm}^2$ for the smallest reference electrode.

order to determine its impact on swallowing safety.

## 11.5 Combination of FES and Conventional Therapy

As already outlined before, there is evidence confirming that FES should be combined to swallowing exercises to achieve optimal results in dysphagia treatment. In this context, a combination of most functional exercises with FES is conceivable, as far as the electrode placement and cooperation of the patient is appropriate. In a randomized controlled trial on 61 subacute stroke patients, a combination of FES and effortful swallowing technique resulted in significantly greater improvements in hyolaryngeal excursion and swallowing function than without FES [96]. Regarding electrode placement when combining FES and effortful swallowing technique, Huh et al. found that a bipolar pair of electrodes placed horizontally on the suprahyoid and infrahyoid muscles may be the most appropriate position for this specific stimulation paradigm to improve swallowing function [97]. Byeon examined the combined effect of FES and Mendelsohn maneuver in subacute dysphagic patients after cerebral infarction, with the compound intervention group showing greater improvements in functional swallowing outcome and quality of life compared to the discrete treatment groups [98]. A compound intervention program was investigated in two studies, in which FES was conceptually combined with swallowing maneuvers and resistance exercises [60, 61]. A fatigue-resistant stimulation protocol was used with a frequency of 30 Hz and a short stimulation phase of 5 s followed by 15 s rest. Both studies demonstrated positive effects on swallowing safety and quality of life. Additionally, in the study by Sproson et al., a follow-up was performed at 1 month, at which time swallowing-related improvements were stable or even continued to improve [61].

These results show that FES can be combined with both functional exercises and swallowing maneuvers to enhance motor learning and swallowing safety. However, the parameters of the stimulation current should be adapted to the functional exercise in terms of duration, frequency, and electrode placement in order to facilitate the patient's movement and avoid fatigue. Depending on the exercise, both tetanizing and single pulses are suitable for this purpose, depending on the underlying pathomechanism. If reflex triggering or glottal closure is disturbed, single pulses may be considered as the first choice. For isometric exercises, tetanizing currents seem to be preferable to facilitate muscle contraction. For example, in dysphagic patients with insufficient glottic closure, both swallowing exercises and vocal cord adduction can be supported by FES using supraglottic swallowing technique. The choice of current parameters can be very specific to the individual and may be adapted to the best functional response and patients' preferences.

## 11.6 Discussion

The future potential of FES in dysphagia therapy is far from being exhausted. However, it seems that a combination of conventional therapy and FES offers the best prospects for improving swallowing function. Further research should be directed to determine which specific procedures can be linked to FES or even used conceptually. Standardized stimulation protocols that could guide and simplify application should reflect a more consistent and concrete nomenclature that allows clear inferences about the intervention. These shortcomings are certainly due to the still rather new use of electrical stimulation in dysphagiology. Technical advancements, such as EMG-triggering or alternating 2-channel technology for staggered stimulation, could make it possible to stimulate the swallowing musculature in a more targeted manner, up to and including the development of a neuroprosthesis. In addition, a combination of FES and central neurostimulation is conceivable, as shown in a study by Zhang et al. combining rTMS with FES. In this study, the combination of rTMS and FES was superior to FES alone, resulting in improved recovery of patients with post-stroke dysphagia [99]. The functional effects of FES should be further investigated in order to get a better understanding of its therapeutic impact and to further optimize the stimulation parameters. Apart from stroke-related dysphagia, the outcome of FES in other etiologies has been inconsistent or poorly studied. Thus, there is a need for robust evidence reflecting a more substantial rationale for which parameters to use in accordance with the principles of FES. It seems reasonable that different symptomatology may require different stimulation paradigms, especially in case of lower motor neuron lesions. However, this requires a well-

reflected handling of stimulus patterns, but also a better understanding of the variables and their individual adaptation to the corresponding task. Efforts should also be made to measure long-term effects and to develop the most appropriate regimen for treatment success.

Given the enormous challenges ahead in the field of dysphagia management, electrical stimulation can make an important contribution to improve patients' treatment options and quality of life. However, this requires expertise and well-trained users.

## References


1. Takizawa C, Gemmell E, Kenworthy J, Speyer R. A systematic review of the prevalence of oropharyngeal dysphagia in stroke, Parkinson's disease, Alzheimer's disease, head injury, and pneumonia. Dysphagia. 2016;31(3):434–41. https://doi.org/10.1007/s00455-016-9695-9.
2. Terré R, Mearin F. Resolution of tracheal aspiration after the acute phase of stroke-related oropharyngeal dysphagia. Am J Gastroenterol. 2009;104(4):923–32. https://doi.org/10.1038/ajg.2008.160.
3. Arnold M, Liesirova K, Broeg-Morvay A, Meisterernst J, Schlager M, Mono M-L, et al. Dysphagia in acute stroke: incidence, burden and impact on clinical outcome. PLoS One. 2016;11(2):e0148424. https://doi.org/10.1371/journal.pone.0148424.
4. Kumar S, Selim MH, Caplan LR. Medical complications after stroke. Lancet Neurol. 2010;9(1):105–18. https://doi.org/10.1016/S1474-4422(09)70266-2.
5. Mann G, Hankey GJ, Cameron D. Swallowing function after stroke: prognosis and prognostic factors at 6 months. Stroke. 1999;30(4):744–8. https://doi.org/10.1161/01.STR.30.4.744.
6. Ekberg O, Hamdy S, Woisard V, Wuttge-Hannig A, Ortega P. Social and psychological burden of dysphagia: its impact on diagnosis and treatment. Dysphagia. 2002;17(2):139–46. https://doi.org/10.1007/s00455-001-0113-5.
7. Kalf JG, de Swart BJM, Bloem BR, Munneke M. Prevalence of oropharyngeal dysphagia in Parkinson's disease: A meta-analysis. Parkinsonism Relat Disord. 2012;18(4):311–5. https://doi.org/10.1016/j.parkreldis.2011.11.006.
8. Barzegar M, Mirmosayeb O, Rezaei M, Bjørklund G, Nehzat N, Afshari-Safavi A, et al. Prevalence and risk factors of dysphagia in patients with multiple sclerosis. Dysphagia. 2021. http://link.springer.com/10.1007/s00455-021-10245-z. Accessed 5 Apr 2021
9. Solaro C, Cuccaro A, Gamberini G, Patti F, D'Amico E, Bergamaschi R, et al. Prevalence of dysphagia in a

consecutive cohort of subjects with MS using fibre-optic endoscopy. Neurol Sci. 2020;41(5):1075–9. https://doi.org/10.1007/s10072-019-04198-3.

10. Langmore SE, Olney RK, Lomen-Hoerth C, Miller BL. Dysphagia in patients with frontotemporal lobar dementia. Arch Neurol. 2007;64(1):58–62. https://doi.org/10.1001/archneur.64.1.58.

11. Suh MK, Kim H, Na DL. Dysphagia in patients with dementia: alzheimer versus vascular. Alzheimer Dis Assoc Disord. 2009;23(2):178–84. https://doi.org/10.1097/WAD.0b013e318192a539.

12. Kühnlein P, Gdynia H-J, Sperfeld A-D, Lindner-Pfleghar B, Ludolph AC, Prosiegel M, et al. Diagnosis and treatment of bulbar symptoms in amyotrophic lateral sclerosis. Nat Clin Pract Neurol. 2008;4(7):366–74. https://doi.org/10.1038/ncpneuro0853.

13. Bath PM, Lee HS, Everton LF. Swallowing therapy for dysphagia in acute and subacute stroke. Cochrane Stroke Group, editor. Cochrane Database Syst Rev. 2018. http://doi.wiley.com/10.1002/14651858. CD000323.pub3. Accessed 27 Feb 2021

14. Dziewas R, Allescher H-D, Aroyo I, Bartolome G, Beilenhoff U, Bohlender J, et al. Diagnosis and treatment of neurogenic dysphagia – S1 guideline of the German society of neurology. Neurol Res Pract. 2021;3(1):23. https://doi.org/10.1186/s42466-021-00122-3.

15. Speyer R, Baijens L, Heijnen M, Zwijnenberg I. Effects of therapy in oropharyngeal dysphagia by speech and language therapists: a systematic review. Dysphagia. 2010;25(1):40–65. https://doi.org/10.1007/s00455-009-9239-7.

16. Dziewas R, Stellato R, van der Tweel I, Walther E, Werner CJ, Braun T, et al. Pharyngeal electrical stimulation for early decannulation in tracheotomised patients with neurogenic dysphagia after stroke (PHAST-TRAC): a prospective, single-blinded, randomised trial. Lancet Neurol. 2018;17(10):849–59. https://doi.org/10.1016/S1474-4422(18)30255-2.

17. Hamdy S, Rothwell JC, Aziz Q, Singh KD, Thompson DG. Long-term reorganization of human motor cortex driven by short-term sensory stimulation. Nat Neurosci. 1998;1(1):64–8. https://doi.org/10.1038/264.

18. Lindner-Pfleghar B, Neugebauer H, Stösser S, Kassubek J, Ludolph A, Dziewas R, et al. Dysphagiemanagement beim akuten Schlaganfall: Eine prospektive Studie zur Überprüfung der gelten-den Empfehlungen. Nervenarzt. 2017;88(2):173–9. https://doi.org/10.1007/s00115-016-0271-1.

19. González-Fernández M, Ottenstein L, Atanelov L, Christian AB. Dysphagia after stroke: an overview. Curr Phys Med Rehabil Rep. 2013;1(3):187–96. https://doi.org/10.1007/s40141-013-0017-y.

20. Sasegbon A, Hamdy S. The role of the cerebellum in swallowing. Dysphagia. 2021. http://link.springer.com/10.1007/s00455-021-10271-x. Accessed 17 Apr 2021

21. Aydogdu I, Ertekin C, Tarlaci S, Turman B, Kiylioglu N, Secil Y. Dysphagia in lateral medullary infarction (Wallenberg's syndrome): an acute disconnection syndrome in premotor neurons related to swallowing activity? Stroke. 2001;32(9):2081–7. https://doi.org/10.1161/hs0901.094278.

22. Daniels SK, Brailey K, Foundas AL. Lingual discoordination and dysphagia following acute stroke: analyses of lesion localization. Dysphagia. 1999;14(2):85–92. https://doi.org/10.1007/PL00009592.

23. Kunieda K, Sugi T, Ohno T, Nomoto A, Shigematsu T, Kanazawa H, et al. Incoordination during the pharyngeal phase in severe dysphagia due to lateral medullary syndrome. Clin Case Rep. 2021;9(3):1728–31. https://doi.org/10.1002/ccr3.3890.

24. Flowers HL, Skoretz SA, Streiner DL, Silver FL, Martino R. MRI-based neuroanatomical predictors of dysphagia after acute ischemic stroke: a systematic review and meta-analysis. Cerebrovasc Dis. 2011;32(1):1–10. https://doi.org/10.1159/000324940.

25. Martino R, Foley N, Bhogal S, Diamant N, Speechley M, Teasell R. Dysphagia after stroke: incidence, diagnosis, and pulmonary complications. Stroke. 2005;36(12):2756–63. https://doi.org/10.1161/01.STR.0000190056.76543.eb.

26. Warnecke T, Labeit B, Schroeder J, Reckels A, Ahring S, Lapa S, et al. Neurogenic dysphagia: a systematic review and proposal of a classification system. Neurology. 2021;96(6):e876–89. https://doi.org/10.1212/WNL.0000000000011350.

27. Prosiegel M, Höling R, Heintze M, Wagner-Sonntag E, Wiseman K. The localization of central pattern generators for swallowing in humans – a clinical-anatomical study on patients with unilateral paresis of the vagal nerve, Avellis' syndrome, Wallenberg's syndrome, posterior fossa tumours and cerebellar hemorrhage. In: von Wild KRH, editor. Re-engineering of the damaged brain and spinal cord. Vienna: Springer; 2005. p. 85–8.

28. Florie MGMH, Pilz W, Dijkman RH, Kremer B, Wiersma A, Winkens B, et al. The effect of cranial nerve stimulation on swallowing: a systematic review. Dysphagia. 2021;36(2):216–30. https://doi.org/10.1007/s00455-020-10126-x.

29. Gutierrez S, Iwanaga J, Pekala P, Yilmaz E, Clifton WE, Dumont AS, et al. The pharyngeal plexus: an anatomical review for better understanding postoperative dysphagia. Neurosurg Rev. 2021;44(2):763–72. https://doi.org/10.1007/s10143-020-01303-5.

30. Mu L, Sanders I. Neuromuscular specializations within human pharyngeal constrictor muscles. Ann Otol Rhinol Laryngol. 2007;116(8):604–17. https://doi.org/10.1177/000348940711600809.

31. Sakamoto Y. Classification of pharyngeal muscles based on innervations from glossopharyngeal and vagus nerves in human. Surg Radiol Anat. 2009;31(10):755–61. https://doi.org/10.1007/s00276-009-0516-9.

32. Sakamoto Y. Interrelationships between the innervations from the laryngeal nerves and the pharyngeal plexus to the inferior pharyngeal constrictor. Surg Radiol Anat. 2013;35(8):721–8. https://doi.org/10.1007/s00276-013-1102-8.

33. Uludag M, Aygun N, Isgor A. Innervation of the human cricopharyngeal muscle by the recurrent laryngeal nerve and external branch of the superior laryngeal nerve. Langenbeck's Arch Surg. 2017;402(4):683–90. https://doi.org/10.1007/s00423-016-1376-5.

34. Rubin AD, Sataloff RT. Vocal fold paresis and paralysis. Otolaryngol Clin N Am. 2007;40(5):1109–31. https://doi.org/10.1016/j.otc.2007.05.012.

35. Venketasubramanian N, Seshadri R, Chee N. Vocal cord paresis in acute ischemic stroke. Cerebrovasc Dis. 1999;9(3):157–62. https://doi.org/10.1159/000015947.

36. Mu L, Sanders I. Sensory nerve supply of the human oro- and laryngopharynx: a preliminary study. Anat Rec. 2000;258(4):406–20. https://doi.org/10.1002/(SICI)1097-0185(20000401)258:4<406::AID-AR9>3.0.CO;2-5.

37. Stevens M, Schiedermayer B, Kendall KA, Ou Z, Presson AP, Barkmeier-Kraemer JM. Physiology of dysphagia in those with unilateral vocal fold immobility. Dysphagia. 2021. http://link.springer.com/10.1007/s00455-021-10286-4. Accessed 25 Apr 2021

38. Freed ML, Freed L, Chatburn RL, Christian M. Electrical stimulation for swallowing disorders caused by stroke. Respir Care. 2001;46(5):466–74.

39. Sheffler LR, Chae J. Neuromuscular electrical stimulation in neurorehabilitation. Muscle Nerve. 2007;35(5):562–90. https://doi.org/10.1002/mus.20758.

40. Carnaby-Mann GD, Crary MA. Examining the evidence on neuromuscular electrical stimulation for swallowing: a meta-analysis. Arch Otolaryngol Neck Surg. 2007;133(6):564. https://doi.org/10.1001/archotol.133.6.564.

41. Ding R, Ma F. Effectiveness of neuromuscular electrical stimulation on dysphagia treatment in patients with neurological impairments – a systematic review and meta-analysis. Ann Otolaryngol Rhinol. 2016;3(12):1151.

42. Speyer R, Sutt A-L, Bergström L, Hamdy S, Heijnen BJ, Remijn L, et al. Neurostimulation in people with oropharyngeal dysphagia: a systematic review and meta-analyses of randomised controlled trials—part i: pharyngeal and neuromuscular electrical stimulation. J Clin Med. 2022;11(3):776. https://doi.org/10.3390/jcm11030776.

43. Chiang C-F, Lin M-T, Hsiao M-Y, Yeh Y-C, Liang Y-C, Wang T-G. Comparative efficacy of noninvasive neurostimulation therapies for acute and subacute poststroke dysphagia: A systematic review and network meta-analysis. Arch Phys Med Rehabil. 2019;100(4):739–50.e4.

44. Wang T, Dong L, Cong X, Luo H, Li W, Meng P, et al. Comparative efficacy of non-invasive neurostimulation therapies for poststroke dysphagia: A systematic review and meta-analysis. Neurophysiol Clin. 2021;S0987705321000447. https://doi.org/10.1016/j.apmr.2018.09.117.

45. Chen Y-W, Chang K-H, Chen H-C, Liang W-M, Wang Y-H, Lin Y-N. The effects of surface neuromuscular electrical stimulation on post-stroke dysphagia: a systemic review and meta-analysis. Clin Rehabil. 2016;30(1):24–35. https://doi.org/10.1177/0269215515571681.

46. Tan C, Liu Y, Li W, Liu J, Chen L. Transcutaneous neuromuscular electrical stimulation can improve swallowing function in patients with dysphagia caused by non-stroke diseases: a meta-analysis. J Oral Rehabil. 2013;40(6):472–80. https://doi.org/10.1111/joor.12057.

47. Alamer A, Melese H, Nigussie F. Effectiveness of neuromuscular electrical stimulation on post-stroke dysphagia: a systematic review of randomized controlled trials. Clin Interv Aging. 2020;15:1521–31. https://doi.org/10.2147/CIA.S262596.

48. Diéguez-Pérez I, Leirós-Rodríguez R. Effectiveness of Different Application Parameters of Neuromuscular Electrical Stimulation for the Treatment of Dysphagia after a Stroke: A Systematic Review. J Clin Med. 2020;9(8):2618. https://doi.org/10.3390/jcm9082618.

49. National Institute for Health and Care Excellence Guidelines. Transcutaneous neuromuscular electrical stimulation for oropharyngeal dysphagia in adults; 2018. https://www.nice.org.uk/guidance/ipg634. Accessed 18 Jul 2021.

50. Bergquist AJ, Clair JM, Lagerquist O, Mang CS, Okuma Y, Collins DF. Neuromuscular electrical stimulation: implications of the electrically evoked sensory volley. Eur J Appl Physiol. 2011;111(10):2409–26. https://doi.org/10.1007/s00421-011-2087-9.

51. Hömberg V. Evidence based medicine in neurological rehabilitation - a critical review. In: von Wild KRH, editor. Re-engineering of the damaged brain and spinal cord. Vienna: Springer; 2005. p. 3–14.

52. Fraser C, Rothwell J, Power M, Hobson A, Thompson D, Hamdy S. Differential changes in human pharyngoesophageal motor excitability induced by swallowing, pharyngeal stimulation, and anesthesia. Am J Physiol Gastrointest Liver Physiol. 2003;285(1):G137–44. https://doi.org/10.1152/ajpgi.00399.2002.

53. Ding R, Logemann JA. Swallow physiology in patients with trach cuff inflated or deflated: a retrospective study. Head Neck. 2005;27(9):809–13. https://doi.org/10.1002/hed.20248.

54. Pahn J, Pahn E. Die Nasalierungsmethode: Übungsverfahren der Sprech- und Singstimme zur Therapie und Prophylaxe von Störungen und Erkrankungen; mit Verfahren der neuromuskulären elektrophonatorischen Stimulation (NMEPS) von Kehlkopfparesen. Roggentin/Rostock: Oehmke; 2000.

55. Vromans M, Faghri PD. Functional electrical stimulation-induced muscular fatigue: Effect of fiber composition and stimulation frequency on rate of fatigue development. J Electromyogr Kinesiol. 2018;38:67–72. https://doi.org/10.1016/j.jelekin.2017.11.006.

56. Behringer M, Grützner S, Montag J, McCourt M, Ring M, Mester J. Effects of stimulation frequency, ampli-

tude, and impulse width on muscle fatigue: stimulation parameters and fatigue. Muscle Nerve. 2016;53(4):608–16. https://doi.org/10.1002/mus.24893.

57. Burkhead LM, Sapienza CM, Rosenbek JC. Strength-training exercise in dysphagia rehabilitation: principles, procedures, and directions for future research. Dysphagia. 2007;22(3):251–65. https://doi.org/10.1007/s00455-006-9074-z.

58. Kent RD. The uniqueness of speech among motor systems. Clin Linguist Phon. 2004;18(6–8):495–505. https://doi.org/10.1080/02699200410001703600.

59. Leelamanit V, Limsakul C, Geater A. Synchronized Electrical Stimulation in Treating Pharyngeal Dysphagia. Laryngoscope. 2002;112(12):2204–10. https://doi.org/10.1097/00005537-200212000-00015.

60. Martindale N, Stephenson J, Pownall S. Neuromuscular electrical stimulation plus rehabilitative exercise as a treatment for dysphagia in stroke and non-stroke patients in an NHS setting: feasibility and outcomes. Geriatrics. 2019;4(4):53. https://doi.org/10.3390/geriatrics4040053.

61. Sproson L, Pownall S, Enderby P, Freeman J. Combined electrical stimulation and exercise for swallow rehabilitation post-stroke: a pilot randomized control trial. Int J Lang Commun Disord. 2018;53(2):405–17. https://doi.org/10.1111/1460-6984.12359.

62. Doeltgen SH, Dalrymple-Alford J, Ridding MC, Huckabee M-L. Differential effects of neuromuscular electrical stimulation parameters on submental motor-evoked potentials. Neurorehabil Neural Repair. 2010;24(6):519–27. https://doi.org/10.1177/1545968309360417.

63. Barikroo A, Carnaby G, Bolser D, Rozensky R, Crary M. Transcutaneous electrical stimulation on the anterior neck region: the impact of pulse duration and frequency on maximum amplitude tolerance and perceived discomfort. J Oral Rehabil. 2018;45(6):436–41. https://doi.org/10.1111/joor.12625.

64. Barikroo A, Clark AL. Effects of varying transcutaneous electrical stimulation pulse duration on swallowing kinematics in healthy adults. Dysphagia. 2021. http://link.springer.com/10.1007/s00455-021-10276-6. Accessed 23 May 2021

65. Humbert IA, Poletto CJ, Saxon KG, Kearney PR, Crujido L, Wright-Harp W, et al. The effect of surface electrical stimulation on hyolaryngeal movement in normal individuals at rest and during swallowing. J Appl Physiol. 2006;101(6):1657–63. https://doi.org/10.1152/japplphysiol.00348.2006.

66. Ludlow CL, Humbert I, Saxon K, Poletto C, Sonies B, Crujido L. Effects of surface electrical stimulation both at rest and during swallowing in chronic pharyngeal dysphagia. Dysphagia. 2007;22(1):1–10. https://doi.org/10.1007/s00455-006-9029-4.

67. Arslan SS, Azola A, Sunday K, Vose A, Plowman E, Tabor L, et al. Effects of submental surface electrical stimulation on swallowing kinematics in healthy adults: an error-based learning paradigm. Am J Speech Lang Pathol. 2018;27(4):1375–84. https://doi.org/10.1044/2018_AJSLP-17-0224.

68. Takahashi K, Hori K, Hayashi H, Fujiu-Kurachi M, Ono T, Tsujimura T, et al. Immediate effect of laryngeal surface electrical stimulation on swallowing performance. J Appl Physiol. 2018;124(1):10–5. https://doi.org/10.1152/japplphysiol.00512.2017.

69. Gallas S, Marie JP, Leroi AM, Verin E. Sensory transcutaneous electrical stimulation improves post-stroke dysphagic patients. Dysphagia. 2010;25(4):291–7. https://doi.org/10.1007/s00455-009-9259-3.

70. Hamada S, Yamaguchi H, Hara H. Does sensory transcutaneous electrical stimulation prevent pneumonia in the acute stage of stroke? A preliminary study. Int J Rehabil Res. 2017;40(1):94–6. https://doi.org/10.1097/MRR.0000000000000206.

71. Mituuti CT, Arone MM, Rosa RR, Berretin-Felix G. Effects of sensory neuromuscular electrical stimulation on swallowing in the elderly affected by stroke: a pilot study. Top Geriatr Rehabil. 2018;34(1):71–81. https://doi.org/10.1097/TGR.0000000000000176.

72. Rofes L, Arreola V, López I, Martin A, Sebastián M, Ciurana A, et al. Effect of surface sensory and motor electrical stimulation on chronic poststroke oropharyngeal dysfunction. Neurogastroenterol Motil. 2013;25(11):888–e701. https://doi.org/10.1111/nmo.12211.

73. Ward AR. Electrical stimulation using Kilohertz-frequency alternating current. Phys Ther. 2009;89(2):181–90. https://doi.org/10.2522/ptj.20080060.

74. Edel H, Güttler J-P, Schubert D. Fibel der elektrodiagnostik und elektrotherapie. 6th ed. Berlin: Verlag Gesundheit; 1991.

75. Jungheim M, Schubert C, Miller S, Ptok M. Swallowing function after continuous neuromuscular electrical stimulation of the submandibular region evaluated by high-resolution manometry. Dysphagia. 2017;32(4):501–8. https://doi.org/10.1007/s00455-017-9791-5.

76. Miller S, Diers D, Jungheim M, Schnittger C, Stürenburg HJ, Ptok M. Studying effects of neuromuscular electrostimulation therapy in patients with dysphagia: which pitfalls may occur? A translational phase I study. GMS Ger Med Sci. 2021. https://www.egms.de/en/journals/gms/2021-19/000294.shtml. Accessed 30 Jul 2021

77. Furuta T, Takemura M, Tsujita J, Oku Y. Interferential electric stimulation applied to the neck increases swallowing frequency. Dysphagia. 2012;27(1):94–100. https://doi.org/10.1007/s00455-011-9344-2.

78. Maeda K, Koga T, Akagi J. Interferential current sensory stimulation, through the neck skin, improves airway defense and oral nutrition intake in patients with dysphagia: a double-blind randomized controlled trial. Clin Interv Aging. 2017;12:1879–86. https://doi.org/10.2147/cia.s140746.

79. Wenk W, Ach F, Wolf U. Elektrotherapie: mit 25 Tabellen (Physiotherapie Basics). 2nd ed. Berlin, Heidelberg: Springer; 2011.

80. Kurz A, Leonhard M, Ho G, Kansy I, Schneider-Stickler B. Applicability of selective electrical surface stimulation in unilateral vocal fold paralysis. The Laryngoscope. 2021;131(9). https://doi.org/10.1002/lary.29538.

81. Seifpanahi S, Izadi F, Jamshidi A-A, Shirmohammadi N. Effects of transcutaneous electrical stimulation on vocal folds adduction. Eur Arch Otorhinolaryngol. 2017;274(9):3423–8. https://doi.org/10.1007/s00405-017-4619-3.

82. Humbert IA, Poletto CJ, Saxon KG, Kearney PR, Ludlow CL. The effect of surface electrical stimulation on vocal fold position. Laryngoscope. 2008;118(1):14–9. https://doi.org/10.1097/MLG.0b013e318155a47d.

83. Watts CR, Dumican MJ. The effect of transcutaneous neuromuscular electrical stimulation on laryngeal vestibule closure timing in swallowing. BMC Ear Nose Throat Disord. 2018;18(1):5. https://doi.org/10.1186/s12901-018-0054-3.

84. Ptok M, Strack D. Electrical stimulation-supported voice exercises are superior to voice exercise therapy alone in patients with unilateral recurrent laryngeal nerve paresis: results from a prospective, randomized clinical trial. Muscle Nerve. 2008;38(2):1005–11. https://doi.org/10.1002/mus.21063.

85. Umay E, Yaylaci A, Saylam G, Gundogdu I, Gurcay E, Akcapinar D, et al. The effect of sensory level electrical stimulation of the masseter muscle in early stroke patients with dysphagia: a randomized controlled study. Neurol India. 2017;65(4):734. https://doi.org/10.4103/neuroindia.NI_377_16.

86. Chen H-C, Jen Y-M, Wang C-H, Lee J-C, Lin Y-S. Etiology of vocal cord paralysis. ORL. 2007;69(3):167–71. https://doi.org/10.1159/000099226.

87. Leder SB, Suiter DM, Duffey D, Judson BL. Vocal fold immobility and aspiration status: a direct replication study. Dysphagia. 2012;27(2):265–70. https://doi.org/10.1007/s00455-011-9362-0.

88. Schiedermayer B, Kendall KA, Stevens M, Ou Z, Presson AP, Barkmeier-Kraemer JM. Prevalence, incidence, and characteristics of dysphagia in those with unilateral vocal fold paralysis. Laryngoscope. 2020;130(10):2397–404. https://doi.org/10.1002/lary.28401.

89. Domer AS, Leonard R, Belafsky PC. Pharyngeal weakness and upper esophageal sphincter opening in patients with unilateral vocal fold immobility. Laryngoscope. 2014;124(10):2371–4. https://doi.org/10.1002/lary.24779.

90. Jang YY, Lee SJ, Jeon JY, Lee SJ. Analysis of Video Fluoroscopic Swallowing Study in Patients with Vocal Cord Paralysis. Dysphagia. 2012;27(2):185–90. https://doi.org/10.1007/s00455-011-9351-3.

91. Erdur O, Gul O, Ozturk K. Evaluation of upper oesophageal sphincter in unilateral vocal fold paralysis. J Laryngol Otol. 2019;133(2):149–54. https://doi.org/10.1017/S0022215119000045.

92. Zhou D, Jafri M, Husain I. Identifying the Prevalence of Dysphagia among Patients Diagnosed with Unilateral Vocal Fold Immobility. Otolaryngol Neck Surg. 2019;160(6):955–64. https://doi.org/10.1177/0194599818815885.

93. Heck FM, Doeltgen SH, Huckabee M-L. Effects of Submental Neuromuscular Electrical Stimulation on Pharyngeal Pressure Generation. Arch Phys Med Rehabil. 2012;93(11):2000–7. https://doi.org/10.1016/j.apmr.2012.02.015.

94. Jungheim M, Janhsen AM, Miller S, Ptok M. Impact of Neuromuscular Electrical Stimulation on Upper Esophageal Sphincter Dynamics: A High-Resolution Manometry Study. Ann Otol Rhinol Laryngol. 2015;124(1):5–12. https://doi.org/10.1177/0003489414539132.

95. Lee T, Park JH, Sohn C, Yoon KJ, Lee Y-T, Park JH, et al. Failed Deglutitive Upper Esophageal Sphincter Relaxation Is a Risk Factor for Aspiration in Stroke Patients with Oropharyngeal Dysphagia. J Neurogastroenterol Motil. 2017;23(1):34–40. https://doi.org/10.5056/jnm16028.

96. Park J-S, Oh D-H, Hwang N-K, Lee J-H. Effects of neuromuscular electrical stimulation combined with effortful swallowing on post-stroke oropharyngeal dysphagia: a randomised controlled trial. J Oral Rehabil. 2016;43(6):426–34. https://doi.org/10.1111/joor.12390.

97. Huh J, Park E, Min Y, Kim A, Yang W, Oh H, et al. Optimal placement of electrodes for treatment of post-stroke dysphagia by neuromuscular electrical stimulation combined with effortful swallowing. Singap Med J. 2020;61(9):487–91. https://doi.org/10.11622/smedj.2019135.

98. Byeon H. Combined effects of NMES and Mendelsohn Maneuver on the swallowing function and swallowing–quality of life of patients with stroke-induced sub-acute swallowing disorders. Biomedicine. 2020;8(1):12. https://doi.org/10.3390/biomedicines8010012.

99. Zhang C, Zheng X, Lu R, Yun W, Yun H, Zhou X. Repetitive transcranial magnetic stimulation in combination with neuromuscular electrical stimulation for treatment of post-stroke dysphagia. J Int Med Res. 2019;47(2):662–72. https://doi.org/10.1177/0300060518807340.

Carsten Kroker and Jan Faust

## 12.1 Introduction

Dysarthria is the term used to describe acquired speech disorders following neurological disease. It is caused by a disorder of the speech motor system. Dysarthria is the most common acquired communication disorder. The incidence exceeds aphasia by about twice [1]. Dysarthria affects communication in everyday life (partnership and family) and in the outside world (work and contacts) [2]. Despite this relevance, there is relatively little research on this disorder. The German Society of Neurology [3] recommends in its guidelines only one exercise-based procedure, namely LSVT® (Lee Silverman Voice Treatment) [4], which was essentially developed for Parkinson's disease and is mainly designed to increase speech volume. However, most dysarthria results from non-progressive diseases of the brain (hemorrhage, insult, trauma), in which the focus of disturbance is articulation. The aim of this paper is to fill this gap and to show a viable alternative course of action. We describe the diagnosis and therapy of dysarthric movement disorders mainly of the lips, tongue, and mandible. We ask to see this as a very promising tool, which of course must be inserted into a treatment concept that also integrates other levels of the disorder, e.g., participation, according to the ICF. A complete concept can be found in Kroker et al. [5]. In this article, mainly the treatment on the level of body structure is described (treatment of lips, tongue, and jaw motor function). In a small group study [5] it was shown that no further transfer exercises are needed to improve body function (speech). Transfers to activity and participation, i.e., whether a patient benefits in everyday life were studied only to a limited extent. Additional research would be needed in this area.

## 12.2 General Preliminary Considerations for Stimulation in the Cervical Region

In general, electrotherapeutic treatment in the anterior neck region is viewed critically. However, this attitude is based only on individual expert opinions [6]. Theoretically, there are two sources of danger here: Electrical irritation of the vocal folds could lead to laryngospasm and thus respiratory distress. A second aspect is stimulation of the carotid sinus. This represents the beginning of the internal carotid artery behind the carotid

**Supplementary Information** The online version contains supplementary material available at [https://doi. org/10.1007/978-3-030-90123-3_12].

C. Kroker (✉)
Praxis für Logopädie, Saarbrücken, Germany

J. Faust
Helios Klinikum Krefeld, Department of
Otolaryngology, Krefeld, Germany

bifurcation. It is thus located approximately at the level of the thyroid—somewhat laterally, although the height can vary greatly from patient to patient. The vessel wall of this arterial segment contains baroreceptors, which are thought to cap blood pressure spikes in healthy individuals. When these receptors are stimulated, there is an increase in vagotone resulting in a decrease in heart rate (bradycardia) and blood pressure. Pathologically increased stimulation of these receptors is called carotid sinus syndrome. Here, even a slight pressure in the neck area, such as that produced by a tight shirt collar, can cause a patient to collapse. The therapy here is a pacemaker [7], which then intrinsically limits the use of other electrical stimulation. In practice, however, these two complications associated with electrical stimulation do not usually occur. Initial trials of electrical stimulation for dysphagia were conducted under intensive care conditions [8], but without corresponding complications.

Crary et al. [9] surveyed 5000 therapists who used cervical electrical stimulation for dysphagia. No serious complications occurred. This problem also did not occur with the use of medium frequency currents, which penetrate deeper into the tissue, at least in a small pilot study with stroke patients [10]. However, there have been some successful attempts to use carotid nerve stimulation therapeutically, e.g., in angina pectoris or essential hypertension. However, this was done with implanted electrodes [11]. Interestingly, similar stimulation parameters were used as are common in dysphagia treatment (20–80 Hz/0.35 ms). In the field of voice therapy, most authors do not refer to this problem at all, e.g. [12, 13], although here the electrodes are applied exclusively to the neck. It should be noted, however, that electrotherapy devices used in the anterior neck region must now be approved in most countries specifically for this area of application. The foregoing considerations are relevant to the treatment of dysarthria only when the voice is to be additionally treated; in articulation treatment, stimulation is not applied in the anterior neck region. However, the arguments should also be considered for dysphagia and laryngeal paresis.

- Articulation disorders in dysarthria can be treated with common approved stimulators.
- For FES in the anterior cervical region in voice and swallowing disorders, use devices that are approved for this application in most countries.

## 12.3 Symptomatology of Individual Forms of Dysarthria

Speech is an extraordinary fine-motor complex and fast process. Hardly any other organ of the human body performs such virtuoso movements [14]. Therefore, it is not sufficient to assess the articulators (tongue, lips, mandible, soft palate) only in their gross motor movements and muscle tone, but also to consider the complex interaction and neuromuscular prerequisites of these muscle groups.

The authors use articulation speed as the central test instrument for measuring articulatory skills in dysarthria [5]. Here, an attempt is made to reproduce the underlying movement disorder using defined consonant clusters and to draw conclusions about or classify certain phenotypes. To describe the speech exercises, we use the international phonetic alphabet. This is achieved by repeating syllables (/ʃla/, /bla/, /kla) representing different movement patterns under time pressure in a metronome beat.

The authors follow the commonly used classification [5, 14] for dysarthria according to the type of movement disorder:

- Spastic dysarthria results from damage to the upper motor neuron. On examination of non-speech tongue and lip movements, usually only mild facial paresis is detectable, but from our experience, this tends to have no real disease value with respect to articulation, as the lips produce complete closure when speaking bilabial sounds. The tongue, on the other hand, shows a gross motor normal mobility, mostly without deviation from the midline, because in case of unilateral brain damage the vagus nerve and hypoglossal nerve are supplied bilaterally, and central paralysis can be compensated to a certain degree [15]. The main pathology usually manifests itself in the fact that the tip of the tongue can no longer be raised quickly enough during speech. Thus, in our articulation test, the sound /l/ is omitted in the test syllable /ʃla/ if it is produced under time pressure. The voice may also be affected, but the dysphonia usually plays only a minor role.

- Flaccid dysarthria results from damage to the lower motor neuron, i.e., in the brain stem. Significant severe paresis of all articulators is quite possible and not uncommon. Often all test syllables (/ʃla/, /bla/, /kla/) are affected. Characteristic is the fatigue if a syllable is repeated over a longer period (>10s). This leads to weakness and thus to a deterioration of the articulation. This is called a myasthenic reaction [5]. Such a fatigue reaction is also a typical symptom of flaccid paresis in body motor function. Deviation of the tongue from the midline is quite possible; unilateral paresis of the genioglossus muscle causes the tongue to deviate toward the affected side. Articulatory significant restrictions in the mobility of the jaw, the lips, and the velum occur. The voice is often hissed to aphonic, and laryngoscopy may frequently reveal vocal fold paresis.

- Ataxic dysarthria usually results from damage to the cerebellum. Gross motor articulators usually show no deficits. The test syllables (/ʃla/, /bla/, /kla/) are not formed in a simplified way under time pressure. However, after a certain speed, the patient is no longer able to increase the tempo further and remains behind the given beat. One symptom of ataxic disturbed body motor function is intention tremor: this does not occur at rest, only during movement, and increases as the target is approached. In some patients, an intention tremor of the tongue can be observed during production of test syllables. The voice is often very loud and highly clenched, possibly due to a compensatory mechanism [14].

- Hypokinetic dysarthria occurs mostly in Parkinson's disease (PD). Since articulation is not the main symptom in most cases, but voice dysfunction is, this manifestation is not relevant for the present article. The gold standard here is LSVT® (Lee Silverman Voice Treatment), whose efficacy is now so well established by studies [4] that the authors do not wish to make any recommendations to the contrary here. Parkinson's patients often show fatigue when measured for articulation speed in the sense that they do not simplify the syllables but fall more and more behind the temporal target with increasing repetitions. This fatigue also occurs not infrequently in body motor skills, this is well observed in the writing pattern: This becomes progressively smaller over a line to the point of micrographia.

- Hyperkinetic dysarthria are rather rare in practice. They mostly occur in Huntington's disease or medication side effects. They manifest as exaggerated movements (dyskinesia) of the articulatory organs and voice. Due to the extreme rarity and the questionable treatability, the authors would like to exclude this form of dysarthria from our explanations as well.

## 12.4 Diagnostics of the Articulation Disorder

In this chapter, the authors would like to introduce the "Dys-SAAR-thrietherapie". The name is derived from "Saarland," the part of Germany where this form of therapy was developed.

The aim of diagnostics is to determine the type and extent of motor deficits on the part of the articulators. However, this does not allow a direct conclusion on the impairment of the ability to communicate, since articulation also depends on other contextual factors. For example, a slightly impaired articulatory motor function can be compensated by slow speech. In part, different dialects also specify different speech rates. Likewise, the phonation can be different. Thus, a (dental-alveolar) tongue-tip R (/r/) has a higher susceptibility to interference than a (uvular) tongue-back R (/R/). Similarly, different languages place different demands on articulatory motor skills due to different consonant clusters.

In sum, articulation speed does not necessarily represent speech clarity, but improving articulation speed will likely have the opposite effect on clarity. This was shown quite impressively in a pilot study with eight chronically dysarthric patients [5].

In the diagnostic procedure [5], the patient is given a metronome beat and instructed to repeat test syllables in this beat. The test syllables represent articulation movements that are important for speech:

- /bla/: Change from bilabial to alveolar phonation.
- /kla/: Change from velar to alveolar phonation.
- /ʃla/: Change within the alveolar zone.
- /amp/: Velum function.
- Each syllable is tested individually.

  If the patient can form the corresponding syllable at the given rate, the rate is increased. If motor errors occur, it is lowered. The articulation speed is the frequency in beats per minute (bpm) at which the syllable is just correctly formed. The normal velocity was over 208 bpm for the /ʃla/, /bla/, /kla/ clusters in a study of 10 patients with dysarthria. The normal articulation speed of the velar /amp/ was 180 [5]. In our experience, intermediate severities reach an articulation speed of 100 bpm. For this reason, it makes sense to start the measurement here. Severe disorders are below 50 bpm. Below this level, it becomes difficult for many patients to maintain such a slow beat. The speed of increasing the beat rate is up to the experience of the therapist. It is not a validated measurement. In addition to this quantitative value, the quality of the articulatory error must also be assessed. For this purpose, the affected articulator and the type of motor error are named:

- It should be noted that insufficient velum elevation has an influence on all clusters. If there is still a residual motor function, however, it can be assumed that there is a dependency on the frequency specification only for the syllable /amp/.

It is possible that in the case of very mild dysarthria, normal values are determined for the tested clusters. In this case, disturbed clusters must be taken from the spontaneous speech and threshold values must also be determined for them. Often it already represents an increase of the degree of difficulty, if the /a/ in the syllables is replaced by another vowel (e.g., /i/). This is because the formation of the /a/ requires contraction of the hyoglossus muscle and the /i/ requires activity of the genioglossus muscle, which seems to be more susceptible to interference. The most common simplifications result from elision of the /l/, which can be explained primarily by paresis of the intrinsic tongue muscles. Tip elevation and depression of the tongue is achieved primarily by the superior longitudinalis and inferior longitudinalis muscles, respectively (Table 12.1).

The elevation of the dorsum of the tongue (/k/) is mainly achieved by the extrinsic tongue muscles (styloglossus muscle, palatoglossus muscle).

The most complex sound is the /ʃ/, which is achieved by a complex interaction of intrinsic and extrinsic tongue muscles. Involved are: M. genioglossus, M. styloglossus, and M. longitudinalis inferior.

All intrinsic and extrinsic tongue muscles except the palatoglossus muscle are innervated by the hypoglossal nerve. Thus, electrical stimulation is performed at the floor of the mouth when hypoglossal motor function is impaired.

The most speech-relevant lip closure muscle is the orbicularis oris muscle. In the case of damage, this is not stimulated directly so as not to restrict the ability to move. The facialis main trunk is suitable here.

Jaw closure during articulation is essentially achieved by the pterygoid medius muscle but also by the masseter and temporal muscles. All are motorically innervated by the trigeminal nerve, on which stimulation is applied when indicated.

In addition, it is listed what kind of movement disorder can be identified:

- Spastic (simplification of the cluster without fatigue). The Video 12.1 shows a patient with spastic dysarthria speaking the cluster /ʃli/ at

**Table 12.1** Disturbed clusters and possible errors

| disturbed cluster | possible error | possible error |
|---|---|---|
| /bla/ | /b/<br>- incomplete lip closure | /l/<br>- incomplete tongue tip elevation<br>- lateralization |
| /kla/ | /k/<br>- incomplete tongue dorsum elevation | /l/<br>- incomplete tongue tip elevation<br>- lateralization |
| /ʃla/ | /ʃ/<br>- sagittal grooving is flattened<br>- lateralization<br>- insufficient jaw closure | /l/<br>- incomplete tongue tip elevation<br>- lateralization |
| /amp/ | /m/<br>- velopharyngeal closure<br>- incomplete lip closure | /p/<br>- incomplete lip closure<br>- incomplete velopharyngeal closure |

175 bpm correctly. At 179 bpm he simplifies the syllable to /ʃa/.

- Flaccid (simplification of the cluster with fatigue). The Video 12.2 shows a patient with flaccid dysarthria speaking the cluster /bla/ at 120 bpm. After a few seconds he simplifies the syllable to /ba/.
- Ataxic (deceleration without simplification and fatigue). The Video 12.3 shows a patient with ataxic dysarthria speaking the cluster /bla/ at 120 bpm correctly. At 125 bpm he can't follow the beat.

Movement disorder.

Additional videos with assessment examples of these disorders can be viewed at www.dysaarthrie.com. This form of diagnosis is the motor part of the Informal Dys-SAAR-thriediagnostik (DSD) [5]. The full implementation also includes a subtest that tests intelligibility on the telephone. However, for the everyday implementation of this therapy, this subtest is not necessary and can also be replaced by recordings of spontaneous speech at the beginning of therapy and as a follow-up, which is also a more comprehensible result for the patient. For scientific data collection, however, an intelligibility test can be useful. There are, of course, other alternatives, e.g., the German "Münchner Verständlichkeitsprofil (MVP)" [16].

- The first step in diagnostics is to determine how quickly the syllables /ʃla/, /bla/, /kla/ can be formed in the metronome beat. In addition, it should be documented which movement sequences are realized incorrectly and how.
- In a second step, the speech ability should be documented (e.g., by speech recording).

## 12.5 Therapy of the Articulation Disorder

An unconditional prerequisite for Dys-SAAR-thrietherapie (DST) [5] is the motor diagnosis described above. The aim of the therapy is to train the affected movement disorder under defined and influenceable conditions exactly at the limit of success.

For this purpose, the following assumptions are made:

1. Most dysarthric patients can perform almost all required articulation movements but slowed down. If they nevertheless adopt the usual speech tempo, this results in a fuzzy articulation, which, on closer analysis, consists of a simplification of the movement

sequences. Thus, there are two options for therapy: slowing down the speech tempo or helping the articulatory motor system to regain faster movement sequences. The authors would like to discuss the second option here. For the first option some approaches also exist [17, 18].

2. Dysarthria always consists of a sensory and motor component. Many affected persons lack direct feedback since they are in principle able to articulate clearly. Exceptions are only the most severe motor impairments. The normal speaker can easily compensate for certain impediments to articulation. This phenomenon is called the "pipe smoker effect". This is because a pipe smoker is perfectly capable of articulating clearly despite the obstruction located in the mouth [14]. The same applies to patients with peripheral hypoglossal palsy [5], who can compensate articulatory for the loss of unilateral tongue motor function via compensatory mechanisms. The therapeutic consequence of this is that a dysarthric patient usually cannot give himself correct feedback, and thus cannot optimally decide whether he is training at the correct difficulty level. Thus, the therapist is always responsible for the feedback as a crucial influencing factor.

3. The difficulty level is calibrated via the feedback. This is a form of shaping, which is crucial for successful neurological rehabilitation [19]. A time signature with metronome allows for over 100 bpm (if one starts at about 100 bpm for a moderately severe disorder with a goal of 208) different difficulty levels per trained consonant cluster. Absolute individual fine-tuning to the patient is thus possible. A forced-use effect is achieved through the feedback and the associated fixation of attention on the disordered movement [5].

4. The authors assume that electrical stimulation in the mouth and throat area can have a very positive influence on motor learning. At least in dysphagia, this has been quite well studied [20].

A high therapy frequency is an obligatory prerequisite for a successful neurorehabilitation—

this is true for the linguistic [21] as well as for the motor area [22]. Therapy with this approach should take place at least 3 weeks and optimally 5 weeks [5].

## 12.6 Practical Implementation

Choice of current parameters:

From the diagnostics, the first step is to determine the type of movement disorder. If it is a flaccid dysarthria, which has already existed for more than 4 weeks, it can be assumed with relative certainty that a muscle atrophy is present and that the affected musculature is probably no longer faradically excitable. Because faradic current cannot trigger a contraction in an atrophied muscle, much wider pulses are needed for this purpose. When selecting the current, it must be remembered here that the speech musculature works together in a complex manner. It can therefore be assumed, particularly in the case of hypoglossus-innervated muscles, that different muscles have different excitability thresholds. It is therefore recommended to use a current that stimulates the entire musculature if possible. Therefore, monophasic square-wave pulses with a pulse width of 100 ms are used. In the case of very severe atrophy, the pulse width can be extended up to 500 ms in the sense of classical paralysis treatment. The single pulses must be synchronized with the speech exercises by hand switch. The current is applied on motor threshold.

All other movement disorders (acute flaccid, ataxic, and spastic dysarthria) usually do not show an electrical degenerative response due to a lack of atrophy and can therefore be stimulated with normal biphasic faradic current (50 Hz/1 ms). This has the advantage that a tetanic contraction occurs, which does not have to be synchronized by hand switch. The stimulation is permanent throughout the exercise session. The current is applied on motor threshold.

▶ – In flaccid dysarthria, select rectangular current (monophasic) with 100 ms width and synchronize with speech exercises.

- In spastic and ataxic dysarthria, select a biphasic faradic current.
- Stimulate disturbed articulator during speech practice.

*Choice of stimulation site:*
Usually choose a monopolar electrode placement. The active electrode is placed on the disturbed articulator:

- Disturbed tongue movement: Hypoglossal nerve—floor of mouth (Figs. 12.1 and 12.2).
- Disturbed jaw closure: Trigeminal nerve—masseter muscles (Fig. 12.3).
- Disturbed lip closure: Facial nerve—facialis trunk (Fig. 12.4).

*Speech exercises:*
The speech exercises are performed over a treatment period of 30 min, during which the disturbed clusters identified with the help of diagnostics are repeated for 30s at a time under electrical stimulation at a metronome rate. If the patient articulates all clusters on one exhalation

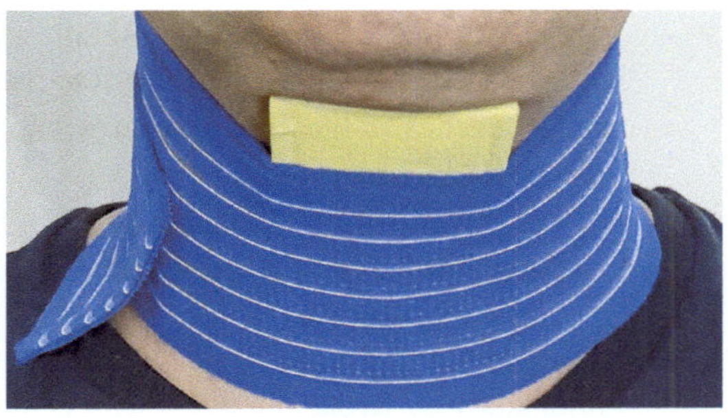

**Fig. 12.1** Hypoglossal nerve—monopolar stimulation

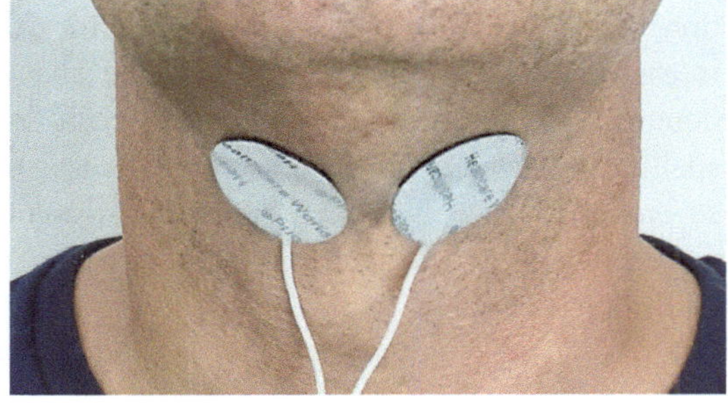

**Fig. 12.2** Hypoglossal nerve – bipolar stimulation

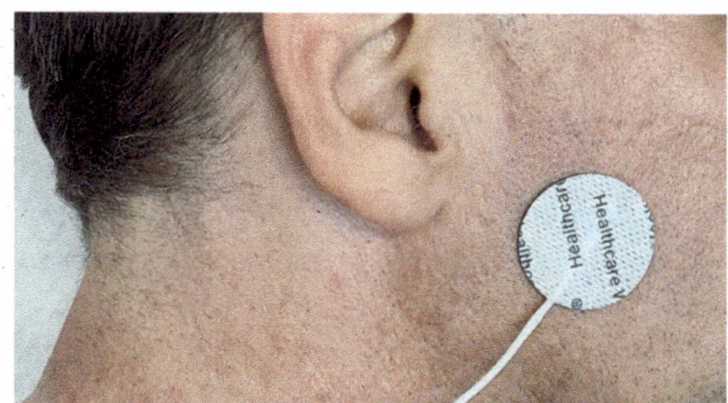

**Fig. 12.3** Masseter muscles—monopolar stimulation

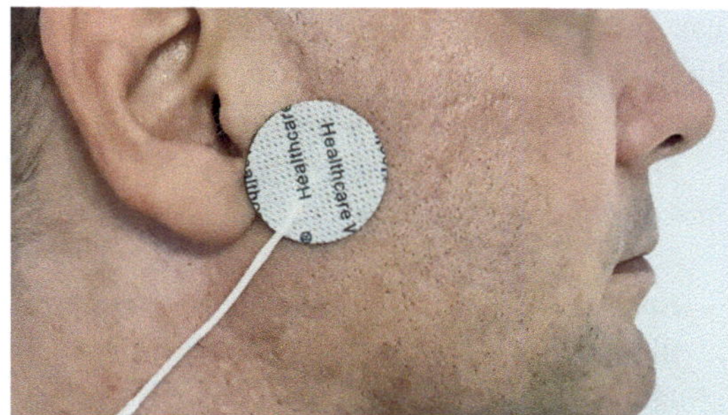

**Fig 12.4** Facial nerve monopolar stimulation

correctly and at the speed of the metronome, the metronome beat is increased by one bpm, if one cluster or more is simplified or if the patient does not follow the beat, the metronome frequency is reduced by one bpm. Thus, with each breath, the metronome frequency is adjusted. After 30s of speech practice, there is a 30s pause. During this pause, the patient is asked to watch for possible errors in articulation or speech tempo during the next pass. For example, if the syllable /la/ is reduced to /a/ at a certain frequency (e.g., 110 bpm), the patient is asked to pronounce the /l/ as clearly as possible without slowing down. With this concentration on the disturbed movement, the articulation speed can usually be increased by 2–3 bpm without loss of clarity (e.g., to 112 bpm). Thus, because of the therapist's feedback, there is a greater effort on the part of the patient, resulting in an increased articulatory rate. With practice, this type of attentional focus on the disordered movement is no longer necessary for the required rate. The perturbed movement can now be produced at a higher rate (112 bpm) without effort. If attention is now directed once again to the disordered movement, the articulation speed increases again (e.g., 114 bpm). In sum, it can be said that like CIMT therapy [22] a correct movement of the affected musculature is "forced."

For some disturbed movements, visual feedback via a mirror can also be beneficial, e.g., "Please try to close your lips completely on the /b/ of /bla/ in the metronome beat".

Some patients find it difficult to keep the beat. This is often the case when they have never had a connection to music. In this case, the therapist can guide the patient's hand in time, tapping along with the beat and speaking along with the first syllables.

*Goals of therapy according to the type of movement disorder:*

- Spastic dysarthria: Increase the speed of articulation for the affected syllable while maintaining distinctness. In this movement disorder, the syllable /ʃla/ is almost always exclusively affected. Usually this is reduced to /ʃa/ because the tip of the tongue cannot lift at a sufficient speed.
- Atactic dysarthria: Retention of articulation speed with increasing metronome beat. Simplifications do not usually occur. Usually, all three syllables need to be trained.
- Flaccid dysarthria: The problem here is that two goals must be pursued: increasing the speed of articulation on the affected syllable while maintaining distinctness, as in spastic dysarthria, and avoiding fatigue. To train myasthenic symptomatology, it is often useful to shorten the exercise/pause ratio of 30s/30s (e.g., exercise/pause = 7s/20s) and to approach the whole 30s:30s ratio in small steps. This could be done, for example, by increasing the exercise and pause interval by 1 s each new hour of therapy until the 30s/30s ratio is reached.

In flaccid dysarthria, it is not uncommon for all test syllables to be affected. Any articulator may be disrupted. Unfortunately, treatment of velum paresis is not possible with this procedure, at least not using plate electrodes. The velum can only be electrically stimulated by a point electrode on the soft palate, which makes additional speech exercises impossible. However, since there is relatively little experience with intraoral electrical stimulation, this procedure should be used with caution. Testing of the syllable /amp/ is nevertheless important, for consideration of other measures.

In a single case study of a chronic dysarthric patient [5], it was shown that training within the alveolar articulation zone also has generalization effects on untrained clusters of the same articulation zone. The three given training and testing clusters represent the most important articulation or coarticulation movements and are sufficient for training most dysarthria. In languages where the given clusters do not occur or practically do not occur (for example, there are far fewer clusters in Japanese than in German or English), the clusters must be replaced accordingly by similarly articulated forms (e.g., /ʃla/by/ʃta/) only the choice of articulation zone is crucial here.

► - 30s practice then 30s break over 30 min.
- Disturbed syllable should be spoken in the metronome beat at the limit of what is possible (regarding frequency).
- Always give feedback during breaks.
- Practice at least three times a week.

*Effectiveness:*

In a pilot study by Kroker et al. [5] with eight chronic dysarthric stroke patients (at least 12 months post onset), it was shown that training according to this principle improved communication skills in seven of eight patients after 20 intensive sessions. The test included the abandonment of compensatory strategies such as spelling or the use of gestures (in the case of severe forms) as well as intelligibility when communicating with strangers (directory assistance) on the telephone.

### 12.6.1 Procedure According to *Pahn and Pahn*

Pahn and Pahn [23] transferred their findings, which they had acquired in connection with the therapy of laryngeal paresis [13], to dysarthric disorders. In this approach, the accommodation of the tongue muscles was first measured. Based on the obtained accommodation quotient (alpha value), the pulse width of the stimulation pulse was chosen, which was applied to the floor of the mouth. Triangular pulses of 10 ms–1000 ms (depending on alpha value) were used. The pulses were synchronized with speech exercises by hand switch. Pahn and Pahn [23] suggests training with fricatives and plosives. These should be selected by the therapist. A standardized scheme is not provided for this. Case studies are not available for the approach.

## 12.7 Diagnosis and Therapy of Voice Disorders

Severe voice disorders occur mainly in ataxic and flaccid dysarthria. Since the ataxic voice disorder is probably a miscompensation of articulation [14], treatment of the same could also have a positive effect on the voice. Usually, the patient tries to produce a halfway intelligible articulation with a lot of pressing. From their own experience, the authors can confirm this hypothesis. Patients with ataxic dysarthria achieve a much higher articulation speed of all syllables when they form a strongly pressed voice. However, similar effects can be achieved in a more voice-sparing manner with an unpressed increase in speech volume [4].

The voice disorder of flaccid dysarthria corresponds to vocal fold paralysis. At least this symptom could be diagnosed and treated like one. To avoid redundancy, we would like to refer here to the chapter of Schneider-Stickler [24] in this book. However, all forms of dysarthria can also occur entirely without a voice disorder.

A particular vocal symptom of flaccid dysarthria is that in some cases voiceless phonemes are produced voiced. Ziegler et al. [14] attribute this to an additional existing velum paresis, thus there is a lack of counterpressure above the vocal folds, which could influence phonation. At the same time, it should be noted that both the velum and the laryngeal muscles are mainly innervated by the vagus nerve and this type of disorder usually occurs after damage to the lower motor neuron. Thus, severe velum palsy also makes impairment of laryngeal function likely. It was shown in a study from Venketasubramanian et al. [25], that vocal fold paralysis is strongly correlated with palatal weakness. Thus, one could hypothesize that in flaccid dysarthria, a change from voiced phonation to voiceless produced under time pressure could occur under electrical stimulation of the vocalis muscle. Patients with spastic dysarthria with mild voice disorder could also possibly benefit from this type of therapy by gaining fine motor control of the vocalis muscle. Unfortunately, there are neither normative values nor therapeutic experiences to support this consideration.

Voice dysfunction is the leading symptom of hypokinetic dysarthria, but since there is sufficient evidence base for LSVT© [4] we do not want to specify otherwise here.

## 12.8 Case Study

A 73-year-old female patient presented at the day clinic of our institution. She suffered a left middle infarction three years earlier and a right middle infarction two years earlier. The reason for admission was depression. She was born in Italy and moved to Germany at the age of 22. She stated that her voice was bad and that she had therefore problems being understood since the stroke. She said this was especially difficult in contact with strangers, but also in her own family. She had seen an ENT specialist and had a written report of a hyperfunctional voice disorder. In the outpatient therapy, voice-typical exercises were carried out (for breathing, as well as for reaching a low position of the larynx). However, there had not been a satisfactory result for her. In fact, the voice still sounded somewhat hoarse in the initial examination, but in our view, this was not to be attributed to such a high pathological value. However, communication was still somewhat difficult, and the examiner had to ask more than once. However, the speech did not sound typically dysarthric, rather strongly colored by an Italian accent. The measurement with the three test syllables showed a simplification of the syllable /ʃla/ to /ʃa/ at 85 bpm without fatigue response. The /bla/ and /kla/ clusters scanned near normal. The findings were in favor of spastic dysarthria, which would have been expected given the location of the brain damage. She herself stated that the syllable /ʃla/ was virtually rare in Italian and therefore it was slowed. Therefore, we tested other syllables of the same articulation zone (e.g., /ʃta/) and got similar results. We agreed to train this articulation zone for 20 sessions and to check whether there was an increase in distinctness. To do this, we had the patient call directory assistance ten times and ask for different names in different cities. She received the correct phone number within 1 min in only one of the 10 cases.

The therapy started over 20 sessions with a frequency of five times/week for 30 min each. Stimulation was at the floor of the mouth with biphasic faradic current (1 ms/50 Hz/5,8 mA). We started with three syllables from the alveolar-alveolar articulation zone (/ʃla/, /ʃli//ʃta/). The arithmetic mean was initially 82 bpm. After 20 sessions, she had increased 100% to 164 bpm.

After therapy, she stated that she could speak much more clearly, which was also confirmed by her relatives. In the telephone test, she was able to improve significantly to 9/10 successful attempts. She stated that she had significantly improved her quality of life.

This example shows that dysarthria cannot always be diagnosed with certainty. The problem was probably that the patient used the term "voice" incorrectly and doctors and therapists were misled by this. Often this diagnosis becomes difficult when several influencing factors coincide (e.g., poor dental status, foreign accent, additional aphasia). The test of articulation speed proved to be very valuable in this case. The outcome of the therapy is truly impressive for the duration of the condition. While the improvement in motor skills and clarity are most likely due to the therapy, the gain in quality of life is not necessarily due to the speech success alone, as the patient also received psychiatric treatment at the same time.

## 12.9 Discussion

The strength of Dys-SAAR-thrietherapie (DST) lies primarily in the treatment of articulatory fine motor skills. Dysarthria, as mentioned at the outset, is the most common communication disorder and articulatory dysfunction is the most common symptom of dysarthria. Thus, this type of therapy finds meaningful application in a broad patient population. Initial study results show a promising outcome in the intensive setting after only 20 sessions. Compared to LSVT ©, DST offers the following advantages: An increase in intelligibility is achieved in LSVT © essentially by increasing speech volume. However, this is close to normal in many non-progressive dysarthric patients, so that an increase in speech volume would not only appear very unnatural, but also have a questionable effect overall. DST does not require any change in speech volume. Furthermore, LSVT © is completed after 16 sessions and the result is then achieved. DST may also be useful in a second or third intensive interval. However, it should also be noted that DST makes high demands on a patient's motivation. Most patients perceive the 30 min therapy as very strenuous, but usually achieve success quickly. Experience shows that an audible improvement in speech occurs when the rate of articulation increases by 20%. This is usually achieved after about 5–7 sessions.

## References


1. Duffy JR. Motor speech disorders: substrates, differential diagnosis and management. St Louis, MO: Elsevier; 2005.
2. Kroker C, Chang C, Steiner J. Die Dys-SAAR-thrietherapie (DST) – Ein neuer Weg der Behandlung von akuten und chronischen neurogenen Sprechstörungen. Forum Logopädie. 2015;6:14–9.
3. DGN: Leitlinien für Diagnostik und Therapie in der Neurologie Neurogene Sprechstörungen (Dysarthrien); 2018. http://www.dgn.org. Accessed 01 Jul 2021.

4. LSVT Global. LSVT LOUD training and certification Workshop, Skript zum Workshop. Mainz: Selbstverlag; 2013.
5. Kroker C, Schock A, Steiner J. Dysarthrie als Störung im Zeittakt. 1st ed. Idstein: Schulz-Kirchner Verlag; 2018.
6. Bazin S, Kitchen S, Maskill D, Reed A, Skinner A, Walsh D, Watson T. Guidance for the clinical use of electrophysical agents 2006. In: Watson T, editor. Electrotherapy evidence-based practice. 12th ed. Philadelphia, PA: Elsevier; 2008. p. 361–86.
7. Brignole M, Moya A, de Lange F, Deharo JC, Elliot PM, Fanciulli A, Fedorowski A, Furlan R, Kenny AR, Martin A. 2018 ESC Guidelines for the diagnosis and management of syncope. Eur Heart J. 2018;39:1883–948. https://doi.org/10.1093/eurheart/ehy071.
8. Larson G. Conservative management for incomplete dysphagia paralytica. Arch Phys Med Rehabil. 1973;54(4):180–5.
9. Crary MA, Carnaby-Mann GD, Faunce A. Electrical stimulation therapy for dysphagia: descriptive results of two surveys. Dysphagia. 2007;22:165–73. https://doi.org/10.1007/s00455-006-9068-x.
10. Miller S, Diers D, Jungheim M, Schnittger C, Stürenberg HJ, Ptok M. Studying effects of neuromuscular electrostimulation therapy in patients with dysphagia: which pitfalls may occur? A translational phase I study. Ger Med Sci. 2021;19:30. https://doi.org/10.3205/000292.
11. Edel H. Fibel der Elektrodiagnostik und Elektrotherapie. Berlin: Verlag Volk und Gesundheit; 1983.
12. Bossert FP, Jenrich W, Vogedes K. Leitfaden Elektrotherapie. München: Elsevier Urban & Fischer; 2006.
13. Pahn J, Pahn E. Die Nasalierungsmethode. 1st ed. Rostock: Verlag Matthias Oehmke; 2000.
14. Ziegler W, Vogel M. Dysarthrie. 1st ed. Stuttgart: Thieme; 2010.
15. Poek K. Neurologie. 9th ed. Berlin: Springer; 1994.
16. Ziegler W, Zierdt A. Telediagnostic assessment of intelligibility in dysarthria: a pilot investigation of MVP-online. J Commun Disord. 2008;41:553–77. https://doi.org/10.1016/j.jcomdis.2008.05.001.
17. Yorkston K, Hammen V, Beukelman DR, Traynor CD. The effect of rate on the intelligibility and naturalness of dysarthric speech. J Speech Hear Disord. 1990;55:550–60. https://doi.org/10.1044/jshd.5503.550.
18. Hustard K, Sassano K. Effects of rate reduction on severe spastic dysarthria in central palsy. J Med Speech Lang Pathol. 2002;10:287–92.
19. Grötzbach H. Rehabilitation bei Sprach- und Sprechstörungen: Grundlagen und Management. In: Frommelt P, Lösslein H, editors. Neurorehabilitation. Berlin: Springer; 2010. p. 339–50.
20. Faust J, Kroker C. FES in dysphagia treatment. Functional electrical stimulation in neurorehabilitation. Schick T, in press, Springer Nature 2022.
21. Bhoghal SK, Teasell RW, Foley NC, Speechley MR. Rehabilitation of aphasia: more is better. Stroke. 2003;10(2):987–93. https://doi.org/10.1161/01.STR.000006234364383DO.
22. Taub E, Morris DM. Constrained induced movement therapy to enhace recovery after stroke. Curr Aterioscler Rep. 2001;3(4):279–86. https://doi.org/10.1007/s11883-001-0020-0.
23. Pahn J. Basis und Konzeption der Therapie von Aphasie, Dysphasie und Dysarthrie durch neuromuskuläre elektroartikulatorische Stimulation (NMEAS) einschließlich Dysphagie. In: Pahn J, Pahn E, Radü HJ, editors. Einführung in die Therapie mit vocaSTIM®. 1st ed. Schnaittach-Laipersdorf: Physiomed; 2001. p. 21–2.
24. Schneider-Stickler B. Applicability of selective electrical surface stimulation in unilateral vocal fold paralysis. This book. Schick T, editor. FES in neurorehabilitation in press 2022.
25. Venketasubramanian N, Seshadri R, Chee N. Vocal cord paresis in acute ischemic stroke. Cerebrovasc Disorders. 1999;9(3):157–62. https://doi.org/10.1159/000015947.

Berit Schneider-Stickler

## Abbreviations

| | |
|---|---|
| AMP | Amplitude |
| BoNT | Botulinum neurotoxin |
| BVFP | Bilateral vocal fold paralysis |
| FES | Functional electrical stimulation |
| LEMG | Laryngeal electromyography |
| PW | Pulse width |
| RLN | Recurrent laryngeal nerve |
| UVFP | Unilateral vocal fold paralysis |
| VF | Vocal fold |
| VQ | Voice quality |
| VT | Voice therapy |

## 13.1 Etiology and Clinical Evaluation of Unilateral Vocal Fold Paralysis

Proper and unimpaired bilateral vocal fold motion is mandatory for phonation, swallowing, breathing, and coughing. The prerequisite for this is an unrestricted functionality of the recurrent laryngeal nerves (RLN) on both sides.

Impairment of unilateral or bilateral RLN function causes either unilateral vocal fold paral-

ysis (**UVFP**) or bilateral vocal fold paralysis (**BVFP**) with resulting dysphonia, dyspnea, and/or dysphagia. Whereas UVFP affects more the voice function but less the respiratory function, BVFP usually results in acute shortness of breath with inspiratory stridor.

The etiology of RLN paralysis can be commonly divided into tumor/trauma-related, surgery-related (iatrogenic), and idiopathic. Mechanical injury to the RLN anywhere along its courses around the aortic arch (left side) and the subclavian artery (right side) due to organic reasons, tumor formation, or even surgery of the thyroid, neck, thorax, or heart can cause a nerve damage. The left RLN is more frequently involved, as undoubtedly the longer course around the aortic arch creates additional vulnerability.

During surgery, neural disruption can typically occur from thermal damage, crushing, stretching, cutting, compression, and vascular compromise.

Unilateral vocal fold paralysis (UVFP) is a common cause of so-called neurogenic dysphonia resulting in glottic closure insufficiency and irregular vocal fold vibrations. Important tools for voice assessment in UFVP are perception, acoustics, evaluation of vocal fold (**VF**) movement characteristics, aerodynamics, and self-rating questionnaires [1–3]. The most essential diagnostic tool for evaluation of VF motion is the laryngo(strobo-)

B. Schneider-Stickler (✉)
Division of Phoniatrics-Logopedics, Department of Otorhinolaryngology, Medical University of Vienna, Vienna, Austria
e-mail: berit.schneider-stickler@meduniwien.ac.at

scopy. Whereas the laryngoscopy is essential for evaluation of the respiratory vocal fold mobility, the stroboscopy is mandatory for evaluation of vocal fold vibration (glottal closure, amplitudes, mucosal waves, regularity/irregularity) during phonation. Due to motor denervation and resulting atrophy in UVFP, the paralyzed vocal fold tends to lose volume and tension. The position of the ailing vocal fold can be classified as median, paramedian, intermediate, or lateral (Fig. 13.1). The position of the paralyzed vocal fold does not allow any assumption about the type and location of the nerve lesion. Nevertheless, the position of the paralyzed vocal fold in UFVP has impact on voice quality. The larger the glottic gap, the breathier the voice sound is. In asymmetric tension of both vocal folds, roughness predominates the degree of hoarseness. Not only hoarseness due to roughness and/or breathiness may hamper patients' daily conversation, but also the limited phonation endurance with voice fatigue and laryngeal discomfort.

Clinical diagnostics of vocal fold motion impairment needs to consider routine laryngeal electromyography (**LEMG**), as only the LEMG can differentiate vocal fold paralyzes from other causes of vocal fold motion impairment (e.g., arytenoid fixation/ankylosis). Meanwhile, LEMG has been accepted as the most important tool for prognostic information about the nerve recovery or even synkinetic reinnervation. LEMG can be useful for not only confirming that the mobility disorder has a neurologic basis but also for establishing a management plan.

## 13.2 Course and Rationale of Therapy Options in Unilateral Vocal Fold Paralysis

It is well known that some patients can be vocally asymptomatic despite an immobile vocal fold as long as the ailing vocal fold is positioned in midline (median position). Median position of the VF can be preferably observed in synkinetic reinnervation.

In most cases of acute UVFP, the onset of nerve damage can be clearly determined because of typical clinical symptoms (hoarseness, roughness, breathiness, vocal fatigue).

Following the classification scheme for peripheral nerve injury by Sir Herbert Seddon, the RLN paralysis can be classified into nerve conduction blocks and axonal injuries [4, 5]. A nerve conduction block (neurapraxia) involves only a myelin injury with an intact axon. In such patients, neural function usually recovers within up to 8 weeks. However, when the axon is injured, which is known as axonotmesis, the recovery rate is poor. The severity of axonal injuries usually varies, as they may result in neuronal death or in re-innervation of the target muscles; this variation makes patients' recovery unpredictable. A spontaneous recovery of vocal fold mobility occurs usually within 6–12 months from the onset of UVFP and defines a temporary UVFP. After 12 months, a RLN recovery is unlikely and the UFVP is considered permanent. Even re-innervation processes don't necessarily have to lead to physiologic but also to synkinetic reinnervation [6, 7].

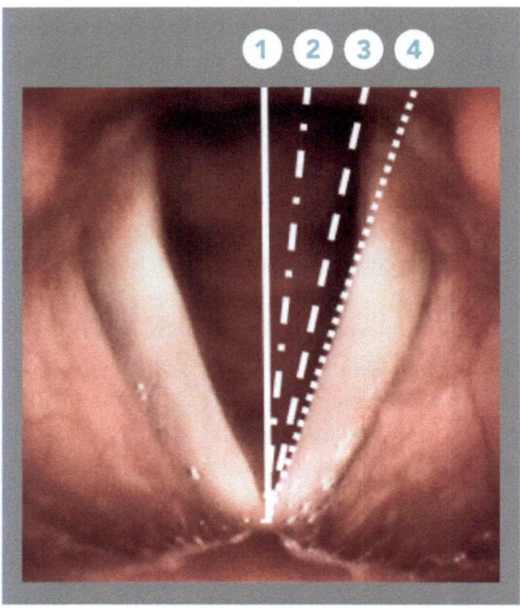


**Fig. 13.1** Possible position of the paralyzed vocal fold (1 = median, 2 = paramedian, 3 = intermediate, 4 = lateral)

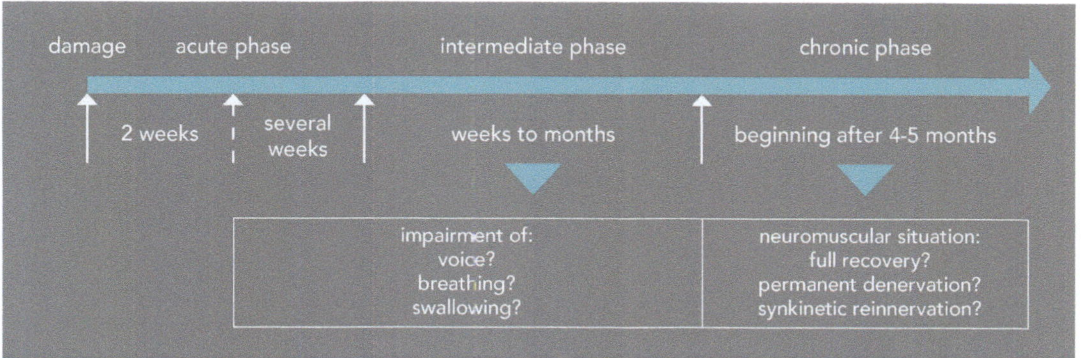



**Fig. 13.2** Course of vocal fold paralysis/paresis

Considering the timeline, the UFVP duration can be classified into acute, intermediate, and chronic phase (Fig. 13.2). The acute phase of UVFP comprises days to several weeks and the intermediate phase weeks to months. The acute and intermediate phases consider the remyelination of axon injuries by Schwann cells in potential neuropraxia with nerve restauration between 2 and 6 weeks after surgical damage. In more severe cases of RLN damage (e.g., axonotmesis und neurotmesis), an axonal re-growth of 1–1.5 mm per day can be seen resulting in reinnervation, either physiological or synkinetic.

An acute situation of RLN paralysis is given few weeks after onset of clinical symptoms, the intermediate phase considers weeks to several months and the chronic phase starts approximately 6 months after the onset of RLN symptoms. Any restitution of RLN function defines the previous phase of RL paralysis as temporary. The restitution of RLN can result in either physiologic or synkinetic reinnervation. In cases without RLN restitution the paralysis must be defined as permanent.

Clinicians can be guided during this time course by LEMG, voice assessment tools and laryngo(strobo)scopy to indicate optimum therapy for patients considering the time course of RLN paralysis, spontaneous recovery potential, chronic denervation or synkinetic reinnervation, and the patient's need for therapy.

Figure 13.2 clearly demonstrates the time course of RLN paralysis for both UFVP and BFVP.

## 13.3 Therapy Overview for Unilateral Vocal Fold Paralysis

▶ The consideration of the time course and assumed RLN is essential for further therapy considerations.

An overview of therapy alternatives considering the time course of RLN paralysis is outlined in Fig. 13.3.

▶ Whereas UVFP treatment approaches generally aim to improve glottal closure for better voice quality, treatment of BVFP needs to consider the respiratory situation more than the phonatory function and needs to find a balance between respiration and phonation.

In UVFP, the standard treatment is yet based on surgical intervention, voice therapy (**VT**), or a combination of the two [8–10]. Voice exercises aim to improve the voice quality (**VQ**); however, present studies lack objective evidence demonstrating the benefit of voice therapy [11]. Surgical approaches include different techniques of injection laryngoplasty [12], external VF medialization/thyroplasty type I [1, 13, 14], and reinnervation [15, 16].

In temporary UFVP, voice therapy and injection laryngoplasty with resorbable materials are still the preferred therapy options, whereas in permanent UFVP injection laryngoplasty with durable materials, nonselective reinnervation techniques, external vocal fold medialization

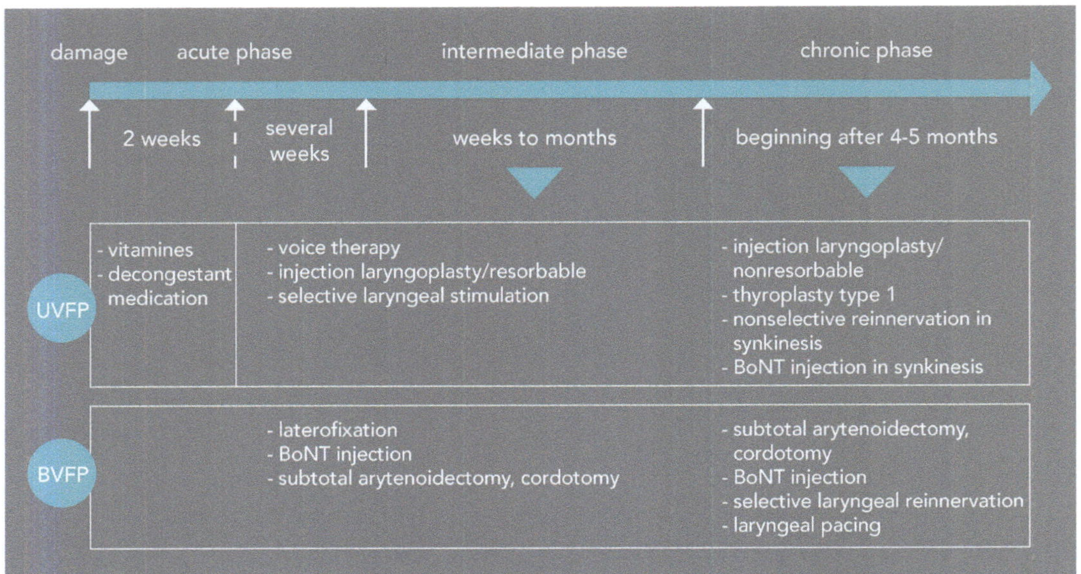


**Fig. 13.3** Therapy alternatives in UVFP and BVFP depending on the time course

(thyroplasty type I), and botulinum neurotoxin (BoNT) injections in cases with synkinetic reinnervation are indicated.

The implementation of functional electrical stimulation (FES) in UVFP therapy is still unconventional, although FES has been often used for the therapy of paralyzed muscles [17, 18].

Recently own studies could provide promising study results on the benefit of FES of the larynx in acute UVFP since similar vocal outcome and UVFP restitution rate could be achieved by FES in comparison to traditional voice therapy [19]. The systematic use of FES in UVFP is currently still limited, most likely due to the complexity of the laryngeal physiology, which makes it extremely difficult to determine a combination of parameters able to generate a therapeutic neuromuscular stimulation through superficial electrodes without causing undesirable side-effects.

## 13.4 Functional Electrical Stimulation in: Unilateral Vocal Fold Paralysis: Selective and Nonselective Effects

FES is an accepted therapeutic strategy for muscle strengthening, maintenance of muscle mass and strength during prolonged periods of immobilization, selective muscle retraining, and the control of tissue reaction as shown in other chapters of this textbook.

So far, FES in UFVP is not yet routinely considered as standard therapy, although FES has been successfully applied in the treatment of several other voice disorders like muscle tension disorders, benign vocal fold lesions, and presbyphonia [20, 21]. In an ovine model, the increase in volume of the thyroarytenoid muscle in elder animals could be shown after applying FES [22]. The selective effect of FES on human laryngeal muscles has been reported by Bidus et al. by endoscopic evaluation of adduction of the vocal folds under stimulation [20].

Up to now, only few papers reported on its effectiveness for the treatment of UVFP [11, 23, 24]. It is expected that FES helps preventing atrophy of denervated muscles and supports nerval regeneration process even in UVFP. In 2008, Ptok and Strack [11] reported on the results of 69/90 (after exclusion of 21 datasets for various reasons) UVFP patients (onset between 2 weeks and 6 months prior therapy) receiving 3 months traditional voice therapy alone or accompanied by FES. In the FES group, vocal fold irregularity decreased significantly more than in the voice therapy group, while maximum phonation time assessment failed to detect differences between the 2 groups. Garcia Perez et al. [24] published on the therapeutic effects of synchronous FES in chronic UVFP patients with paralysis onset between 10 and 24 months before therapy start. To this study, 20 patients (7 male and 13 female) were recruited, and 10 patients (3 male and 7 female) concluded the study. Several measures (maximum phonation time, jitter, shimmer, and harmonic-to-noise-ratio) showed a significant improvement after 10 FES sessions of 30 min performed once per week for 10 consecutive weeks. No significance was observed for the fundamental frequency. No safety issues were reported.

Recently, Kurz et al. [19] reported on FES in acute UVFP after thyroid surgery compared to standard voice therapy. It could be shown in 51/1519 patients with UFVP after thyroid surgery, that after up to 3 months of therapy, the UVFP restitution and the functional voice outcome following voice therapy or FES were comparable. The RLN recovery rate was statistically similar in both groups with 53.8% after voice therapy and 40.0% after FES. The glottic closure during phonation improved in both therapies. FES may allow a better closure in the anterior two-thirds of the glottis. With voice therapy, a better posterior closure seems to be achieved and the development of pathological compensations could occur less frequently. This result also seems logical since surface stimulation certainly does not reach the posterior laryngeal sections very well. As the vocal fold position of ailing vocal fold did not deteriorate under both therapy after up to 3 months, both voice therapy and FES maintain or even improve mass, tension, and volume of intrinsic laryngeal muscles.

The effect of FES of the larynx can be objectified by laryngo(strobe)scopy and perceptually. For individual assessment of FES applicability in UVFP, the adduction of the healthy and the ailing vocal fold with endoscopically visible vocal fold closure and/or auditively perceptual improvement of voice sound and frequency twitch during selective FES of the intrinsic laryngeal can be used. In a monocentric study, the first systematic data on the applicability of FES in UVFP therapy could be provided by Kurz et al. 2021 [25] very recently. The study has been designed to assess the most effective stimulation parameters for selective

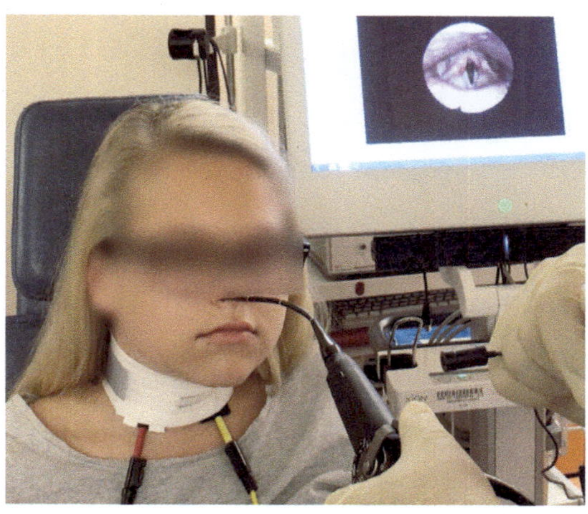

**Fig. 13.4** Clinical investigation situation of FES for individual assessment of stimulation parameters: FES application during flexible transnasal laryngoscopy

laryngeal stimulation in UVFP. Criteria were FES-induced bilateral adduction of the VFs in absence of, or in combination with limited side effects/unspecific laryngeal muscle activation and discomfort. The effects of FES have been assessed by flexible laryngoscopy in terms of vocal fold adduction at both respiration/rest endoscopically and phonation. An example of clinical investigation situation is given in Fig. 13.4.

The position of the electrodes should consider laryngeal anatomy and dimensions. The thyroid cartilage is located on top of the cricoid cartilage and protects the vocal folds in the endolaryngeal space (Fig. 13.5). Thus, the surface electrodes should be placed in front of both sides of the thyroid cartilage.

The chosen electrodes have a surface sufficiently large to deliver the stimulation without causing damages to the tissue, but sufficiently small to reduce the occurrence of unspecific activation of other laryngeal muscles besides the adductor muscles (Fig. 13.6).

The electrodes need to be accurately placed to promote the selective activation of the adductor muscles. The applied pulse widths (PW) and amplitudes (AMP) combination have to be precisely assessed to avoid discomfort or unspecific stimulation of the laryngeal muscles, while inducing synchronous adduction of both VFs.

Sensitivity, and discomfort thresholds and any undesirable nonselective side-effects (swallow-

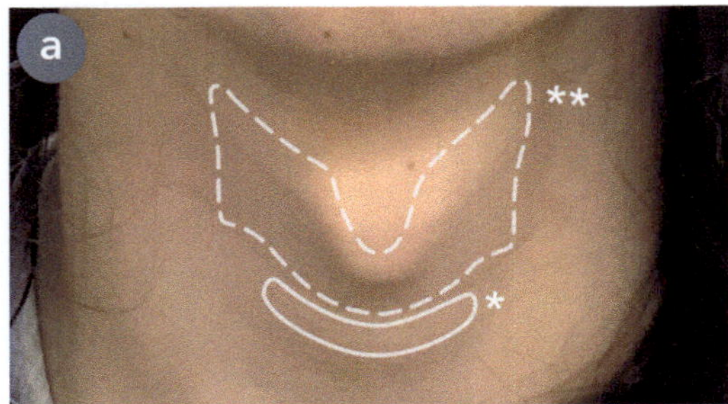

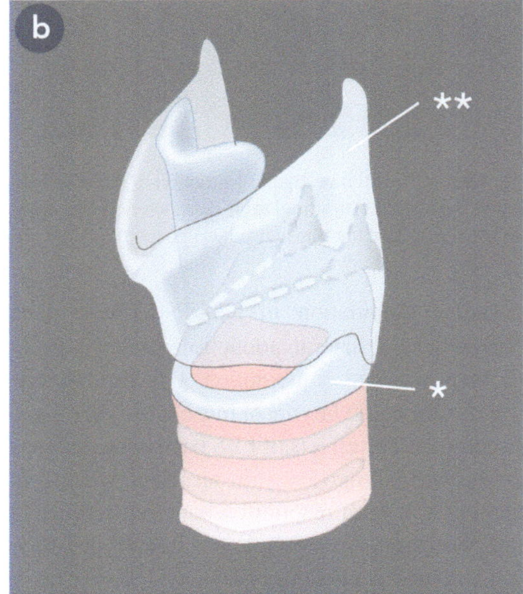

**Fig. 13.5** Schematic anatomy of the larynx (* cricoid, ** thyroid) with vocal folds located in the endolarynx. (**a**) Clinical evaluation of laryngeal anatomy: landmarks for inspection and palpation (* cricoid, ** thyroid). (**b**) Vocal folds with their origin from the inside of the thyroid leading to the arytenoid cartilages

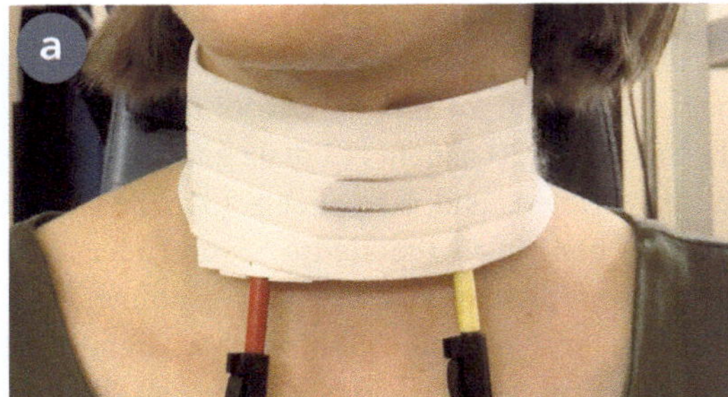

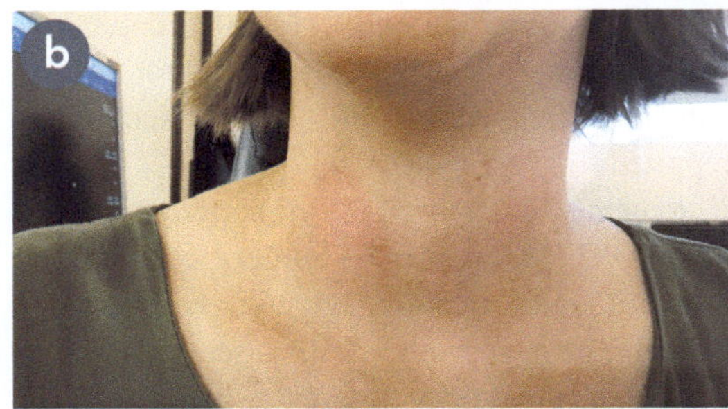

**Fig. 13.6** Clinical situation during FES. (**a**) Placement of the surface electrodes in front of the thyroid cartilage fixated by a neck band. (**b**) Mild local prelaryngeal erythema of the skin after FES because of hyperemia

ing, coughing, unspecific strap muscle/platysma response) have to be documented (Table 13.1) for the different combinations of amplitude (AMP) and pulse width (PW) during individual assessment of FES, before defining any stimulation parameters for selective functional electrical stimulation of the larynx.

A monocentric study on 32 adult patients with UFVP was performed by Kurz et al. [25] to provide systematic data on the applicability of SES in UVFP therapy. Symmetric triangular-shape, charge-balanced PW of 1, 10, 25, 50, 100, 250, and 500 ms were tested with increasing AMPs between 1 mA and 20 mA. The investigation started with administering a PW of 100 ms, and

went down to 1 ms and up to 250 and 500 ms. Generally, the administration of PWs lower than 25 ms was a rare event since, if an unspecific strap muscle/platysma response, coughing and/or swallowing reflexes could be seen, or the patient reported discomfort already at 25 ms; here no shorter PWs were administered to reduce the burden for the patient. The stimulation was delivered as a train of 5 pulses using 2 wet surface square electrodes of 40x28 mm (anode and cathode, respectively) placed on the region corresponding to each thyroarytenoid muscle by means of neck palpation, fixed in place with a neck-brace, and connected to the external stimulator (see also Fig. 13.4). Initially, the sensitivity and the discomfort thresholds should be detected (Table 13.1). The sensitivity threshold describes for each administered PW the lowest amplitude at which the patient feels the stimulation. It can be exclusively assessed by means of patient's feedback. The stimulation parameters causing undesirable side-effects need to be registered, such as those triggering the unspecific strap muscle/platysma response (grade 1 = mild superficial muscle contraction of the neck skin; grade 2 = moderate muscle response with involvement

**Table 13.1** Documentation of parameters for individual FES in UVFP

| sensibility threshold | discomfort threshold | undesirable side effects | selective laryngeal effect |
|---|---|---|---|
| the minimal AMP at which the patient perceives the stimulation | the AMP at which the stimulation does trigger discomfort/pain | the AMP at which the stimulation does trigger strap muscles (platysma response, coughing or swallowing | the AMP at which the stimulation does trigger bilateral vocal fold adduction and/or perceptible frequency change/voice sound improvement during phonation |

of the mouth floor/chin; grade 3 = strong response of the extrinsic laryngeal strap muscles causing involuntary head nodding or contractions in the clavicular region), coughing and/or swallowing reflexes.

FES in UVFP can be considered successful when it elicits bilateral VF adduction sufficient to cause their adduction at rest and/or during phonation or when a voice sound change is perceptible during phonation (improved voice quality, frequency change).

Kurz et al. [25] reported that the median sensitivity threshold was below 5 mA, and the median discomfort threshold was below 17 mA, independently from the applied PW. In this study, FES triggered a swallow reflex in 41% and 44% of the assessed patients when a PW of 250 or 500 ms, respectively was used. Swallow reflex was triggered by SES in 22% of the patients at a PW of 50 ms, and in ≤6% of the patients tested with a PW of 100 ms or ≤ 25 ms. Almost a third of the patients tested with a PW of 100 ms experienced a SES-elicited coughing reflex within an AMP range of 5–19 mA. Mild platysma response occurred in 34% of the patients assessed with a PW of 500 ms; in 44% with a PW of 250 ms; in 66% with a PW of 100 ms; and in a percentage above 70% in patients assessed with shorter PWs. In general, the use of shorter PWs was accompanied by an increased percentage of unspecific strap/platysma muscle responses. Moderate platysma response occurred in 19% of the patients assessed with a PW of 500 ms; in 25% with a PW of 250 ms; in 50% with a PW of 100 ms; and in a

percentage above 59% in patients assessed with shorter PWs. The use of shorter PWs was accompanied by an increased percentage of unspecific strap/platysma muscle responses. Severe platysma response occurred in 6% of the patients assessed with a PW of 500 ms; in 13% with a PW of 250 ms; in 34% with a PW of 100 ms; and in a percentage above 38% in patients assessed with shorter PWs. The use of shorter PWs was accompanied by an increased percentage of unspecific strap/platysma muscle responses. A selective laryngeal response during SES could be observed in 28/32 (87.5%) of the patients. Of the responsive patients, 71% responded with a PW of 50 ms and 75% with a PW of 100 ms within a median AMP range of 6–7 mA. The response rate strongly decreased with shorter PWs (26% with 25 ms, 4% with 1 ms, and 14% with 10 ms) and moderately decreased with longer PWs (64% with 250 ms and 46% with 500 ms).

▶ In agreement with the findings of previous studies [11, 23, 24], Kurz et al. [25] could demonstrate that the use of a PW of 50 or 100 ms in combination with a median AMP comprised between 5 and 10 mA delivers the best results in terms of bilateral adduction of the VFs, while ensuring the lowest rate of side effects and/or discomfort (Fig. 13.7).

Kurz et al. could point out that the administration of FES with a PW of 50 ms is capable to effectively induce a bilateral adduction of the VFs at respiration/rest or during phonation in 71% and

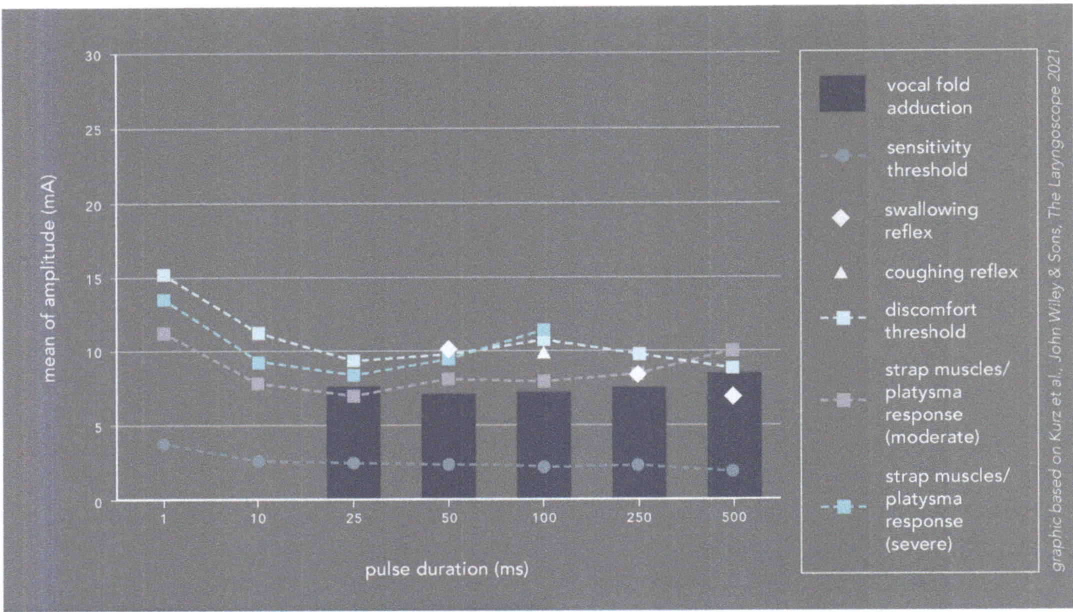


**Fig. 13.7** Selective bilateral adduction of the vocal folds (VFs) while ensuring the lowest rate of side effects and/or discomfort (in [25])

77% of the responsive patients UVFP, respectively. However, this property is lost by stimulations delivered at lower PWs. For instance, for PWs $\leq$ 25 ms, mild platysma response occurred between 64 and 91%, moderate platysma response between 59 and 72%, and severe platysma response between 38 and 53% of the assessed patients. For stimulations delivered within a PW range between 50 and 250, the median sensitivity threshold was found between 1.0 and 2.0 mA, while relevant unspecific laryngeal muscle response is observed with a median AMP between 8 and 11.5. With stimulations delivered within this PW range, the most effective bilateral adduction of the VFs either at respiration/rest or during phonation can be elicited with a median AMP between 6 and 7.5 mA effectiveness point of view. This finding strongly suggests that it is possible to use SES to induce VF adduction within an AMP range below the discomfort threshold of most of the patients suffering from UVFP.

The success of FES-induced bilateral adduction of the VFs at respiration/rest or during phonation in absence or in presence of limited

**Summary**
It can be summarized that the use of PWs shorter than 50 ms is mostly ineffective and accompanied by undesirable side-effects. The use of 500 ms too is expected to have a low efficacy and be consistently accompanied by increased swallowing reflex. On the contrary, the use of a PW comprised between 50 and 250 ms has shown the highest effectiveness accompanied with the lowest rate of side effects for the patients. The choice of the PW within this range should be taken considering the characteristics of the single patients and the presence of comorbidities for which, for instance, the induction of a swallowing reflex may be of use.

unspecific reactions is strictly related to applied PW and AMP, it also depends on the size and type of surface electrodes, as well as their correct placement in front of the larynx.

Taken these study results into consideration, FES should be more often considered as therapy option in acute UVFP, especially if patients prefer to be independent from medical institutions and therapists. A major benefit of FES of the larynx in UFVP is the flexible home training after personalized fitting.

Since the Covid-19 pandemic with social distancing and lockdowns, FES is gaining even more importance in the therapy of UVFP.

## References


1. Benninger MS, Crumley RL, Ford CN, et al. Evaluation and treatment of the unilateral paralyzed vocal fold. Otolaryngol Head Neck Surg. 1994;111(4):497–508.
2. Ryu C, Kwon T, Kim H, et al. Guidelines for the management of unilateral vocal fold paralysis from the Korean society of laryngology, phoniatrics and logopedics. Clin Exp Otorhinolaryngol. 2020 Nov;13(4):340–60.
3. Mattei A, Desuter G, Roux M, Lee JB, Louges MA, Osipenko E, Sadoughi B, Schneider-Stickler B, Fanous A, Giovanni A. International consensus (ICON) on basic voice assessment for unilateral vocal fold paralysis. Eur Ann Otorhinolaryngol Head Neck Dis. 2018;135(1S):S11–5.
4. Seddon HJ, Medawar PB, Smith H. Rate of regeneration of peripheral nerves in man. J Physiol. 1943;102(2):191–215.
5. Kaya Y, Sarikcioglu L. Sir Herbert Seddon (1903–1977) and his classification scheme for peripheral nerve injury. Childs Nerv Syst. 2015;31:177–80.
6. Crumley RL. Laryngeal synkinesis revisited. Ann Otol Rhino Laryngol. 2000;109(4):365–71.
7. Crumley RL. Laryngeal synkinesis: its significance to the laryngologist. Ann Oto Rhino Laryngol. 1989;98(2):87–92.
8. Miller S. Voice therapy for vocal fold paralysis. Otolaryngol Clin North America. 2004;37(1):105–19.
9. Busto-Crespo O, Uzcanga-Lacabe M, Abad-Marco A, et al. Longitudinal voice outcomes after voice therapy in unilateral vocal fold paralysis. J Voice. 2016;30(6):767.e9–767.e715.
10. Walton C, Carding P, Flanagan K. Perspectives on voice treatment for unilateral vocal fold paralysis. Curr Opinion Otolaryngol Head Neck Surg. 2018;26(3):157–61.
11. Ptok M, Strack D. Electrical stimulation-supported voice exercises are superior to voice exercise therapy alone in patients with unilateral recurrent laryngeal nerve paresis: results from a prospective, randomized clinical trial. Muscle Nerve. 2008;38(2):1005–11.
12. Prendes BL, Yung KC, Likhterov I, Schneider SL, Al-Jurf SA, Courey MS. Long-term effects of injection laryngoplasty with a temporary agent on voice quality and vocal fold position. Laryngoscope. 2012;122(10):2227–33.
13. Schneider B, Bigenzahn W, End A, Denk DM, Klepetko W. External vocal fold medialization in patients with recurrent nerve paralysis following cardiothoracic surgery. Eur J Cardiothorac Surg. 2003;23(4):477–83.
14. Daniero JJ, Garrett CG, Francis DO. Framework surgery for treatment of unilateral vocal fold paralysis. Curr Otorhinolaryngol Rep. 2014;2(2):119–30.
15. Marie JP, Dehesdin D, Ducastelle T, Senant J. Selective reinnervation of the abductor and adductor muscles of the canine larynx after recurrent nerve paralysis. Ann Otol Rhino Laryngol. 1989;98(7 Pt 1):530–6.
16. Paniello RC, Edgar JD, Kallogjeri D, Piccirillo JF. Medialization versus reinnervation for unilateral vocal fold paralysis: a multicenter randomized clinical trial. Laryngoscope. 2011;121(10):2172–9.
17. Martin F, Witt TN. Elektrodiagnostische und histometrische Untersuchungen über den Einfluss von Reizstrom auf die Atrophie der denervierten Kehlkopfmuskulatur im Tierexperiment. Laryngol Rhinol Otol. 1983;62(12):590–6.
18. Lake DA. Neuromuscular electrical stimulation. An overview and its application in the treatment of sports injuries. Sports Med. 1992;13(5):320–36.
19. Kurz A, Leonhard M, Denk-Linnert DM, Mayr W, Kansy I, Schneider-Stickler B. Comparison of voice therapy and selective electrical stimulation of the larynx in early unilateral vocal fold paralysis after thyroid surgery: a retrospective data analysis. Clin Otolaryngol. 2021;46:530–7.
20. Bidus KA, Thomas GR, Ludlow CL. Effects of adductor muscle stimulation on speech in abductor spasmodic dysphonia. Laryngoscope. 2000;110(11):1943–9.
21. Gilman M, Gilman SL. Electrotherapy and the human voice: a literature review of the historical origins and contemporary applications. J Voice. 2008;22(2):219–27.
22. Gugatschka M, Jarvis JC, Perkins JD, et al. Functional electrical stimulation leads to increased volume of the aged thyroarytenoid muscle. Laryngoscope. 2018;128(12):2852–7.

23. Ptok M, Strack D. Voice exercise therapy versus electrostimulation therapy in patients with unilateral vocal fold paralysis. HNO. 2005;53(12):1092–7.
24. Garcia Perez A, Hernandez Lopez X, Valadez Jimenez VM, Minor Martinez A, Ysunza PA. Synchronous electrical stimulation of laryngeal muscles: an alternative for enhancing recovery of unilateral recurrent laryngeal nerve paralysis. J Voice. 2014;28(4):524.e521–7.
25. Kurz A, Leonhard M, Denk-Linnert DM, Mayr W, Kansy I, Schneider-Stickler B. Comparison of voice therapy and selective electrical stimulation of the larynx in early unilateral vocal fold paralysis after thyroid surgery: a retrospective data analysis. Clin Otolaryngol. 2021;46:530–7..

Thomas Schick, Christian Dohle,
and Klemens Fheodoroff

## 14.1 Introduction

Functional electrical stimulation (FES) is used for a wide variety of applications in neurorehabilitation, as described in detail in the previous chapters. The variety of neurological symptom manifestations, which show up in clinical routine, often require the modification of the different therapeutic approaches. From this requirement, the combination of FES with other successful therapies emerged.

The combination of FES with other therapeutic approaches, such as mirror therapy or botulinum neurotoxin therapy (BoNT-A), has proven to be effective in rehabilitation. Both mirror therapy and BoNT-A are recognized and established treatment methods in neurorehabilitation. The combination of these therapies with FES has proven to enhance the therapeutic effects and, in some cases, to produce lasting improvements (Sect. 14.2).

Several studies showed that the combination of FES and mirror therapy in neurorehabilitation of stroke patients [1–3] brought benefits in motor recovery. A systematic review and meta-analysis [4] in 2020 highlight the synergistic effects of mirror therapy combined with EMG-triggered FES. Section 14.2 provides a detailed overview of this combination modality.

▶ The combination of functional electrical stimulation (FES) and mirror therapy is well suited for the treatment of motor deficits in stroke patients in neurorehabilitation.

FES, applied in addition to BoNT-A therapy, can have a beneficial effect on spastic movement disorders.

The use of mirror therapy in stroke rehabilitation is excellently suited for the treatment of stroke patients with severe motor deficits [5]. This also explains why the combination of FES and mirror therapy is preferred here. Furthermore, it was shown that the usually available treatment time of 30 min does not inhibit the successful implementation of these combined therapy procedures [1].

The combination of BoNT-A therapy with immediately following (F)ES is clinically useful in spastic movement disorders. It is described in a systematic review [6] and discussed in Sect. 14.3.

T. Schick (✉)
MED-EL, Department Neurorehabilitation
STIWELL, Innsbruck, Austria
e-mail: schick@neuro-reha.info

C. Dohle
P.A.N. Center for Post-Acute Neurorehabilitation,
Fürst-Donnersmarck-Stiftung, Berlin and
Center for Stroke Research, Charité—University
Medicine Berlin, Berlin, Germany
e-mail: Dohle.fdh@fdst.de

K. Fheodoroff
Gailtal Klinik Hermagor, Hermagor, Austria
e-mail: klemens.fheodoroff@kabeg.at

This chapter is intended to provide a basis from which consistent stimulation protocols, supported by further studies, can be developed in the future. Furthermore, it should be understood as a basis for discussion in order to use both therapy methods combined in a standardized way for the treatment of spastic movement disorders.

## 14.2 Combination of Functional Electrical Stimulation and Mirror Therapy

Christian Dohle

### 14.2.1 Introduction

The effect of electrical stimulation on recovery after stroke is based on different mechanisms. On the one hand, electrical stimulation elicits movements that should resemble those that were performed prior to the stroke, promoting motor learning. On the other hand, electrical stimulation causes direct afferent stimulation that might contribute to recovery as well. However, both effects (proprioception, sensory electrical stimulation) are mediated by peripheral sensory afferent pathways that might be affected by the stroke as well.

Thus, especially for severe arm paresis, therapies with direct (central) stimulation of motor representation are recommended, such as movement observation, mental imagery, or mirror therapy. During mirror therapy, a mirror is placed in a patient's mid-sagittal plane in such a way that the mirror image of the non-affected limb appears as if it were the affected one. Imaging studies demonstrated that the effect of the mirror illusion on brain activity can also be recorded neurophysiologically: When presenting a moving limb via a mirror, there is additional brain activity in the hemisphere contralateral to the visual image, i.e., the affected hemisphere in patients. The number of studies providing evidence for the effect of mirror therapy after stroke has virtually exploded over the last years. In their search in August 2018 for a Cochrane review, Thieme and co-workers (2019) identified 62 randomized controlled studies with a total number of 1982 participants, employing mirror therapy either isolated or in combination with other therapies [7]. As mirror therapy does not require any motor capabilities at all, it is a very suitable candidate for combination with electrical stimulation.

### 14.2.2 Evidence

The Cochrane review (2019) already found seven studies on the combination of mirror therapy with electrical stimulation. A hand search in February 2020 identified two additional studies in which these therapy regimes were combined. These studies should help to answer two different questions:

1. Can the effect of mirror therapy be enhanced by electrical stimulation?
2. Can the effect of electrical stimulation be enhanced by application of a mirror?

For both questions, three randomized controlled studies could be identified. Additionally, three studies with a three-arm design were found, comparing electrical stimulation and mirror therapy isolated with its combination. However, for electrical stimulation, different protocols were applied. In the following, the results of the studies are summarized.

### 14.2.3 Improvement of the Effect of Electrical Stimulation by Mirror Therapy

In the study of Kim and co-workers 2014 [8], 23 subacute stroke patients received functional electrical stimulation in addition to their regular therapy program. Patients could switch on stimulation of the musculi extensor digitorum, musculi carpi radialis longus and brevis by performing a similar movement with their non-affected side. During the procedure, patients were instructed to move both hands simultaneously. In the experimental group, the image of the non-affected side was presented via a mirror. When comparing the relative improvement of the three Fugl Meyer subscores, patients receiving the combination therapy showed stronger improvement in the distal scores (finger and hand), but not in the proximal ones. In the Box and Block test, there was no significant difference between the two groups.

Schick and co-workers [9] applied bilateral EMG-triggered multichannel electrical stimulation of the Musculi extensor carpi radialis longus and Musculi flexor digitorum superficialis on both sides in 33 subacute stroke patients (Fig. 14.1). In this design, stimulation was elicited by the EMG signal of the non-affected side. In this study as well, therapy procedure of both groups only differed in the additional placement of a mirror between both sides. After the intervention, there was no difference between both groups as a whole. However, in a subgroup analysis, a significant difference in the proximal Fugl Meyer score in patients with very severe paresis (total Fugl Meyer score < 17 points) was found.

In the study of Lee and Lee 2019 [10], a total number of 30 chronic, ambulatory stroke patients received afferent stimulation with a "mesh sock." In the intervention group (15 patients), this therapy was combined with mirror therapy during dorsiflexion of the foot. Here, significant differences between both groups in muscular strength and balance (Berg Balance Scale) as well as in specific gait parameters (gait velocity, step length, stride length) were recorded.

## 14.2.4 Improvement of the Effect of Mirror Therapy by Electrical Stimulation

Unfortunately, studies for the reverse question are sparse. Only one study by Lin and co-workers 2014 [11] compared the effect of the application of a "mesh glove" in addition to mirror therapy of the upper extremity. In this small study with $2 \times 8$ patients, the additional stimulation appeared to result in significant improvements in the Action Research Arm Test (ARAT) and the Box and Block test, but not spasticity.

Two other studies focused on the lower extremity: Ji and co-workers 2014 [12] treated three groups with 10 chronic stroke patients each. Two groups trained with a mirror. In one of these groups, this was combined with electrical stimulation, eliciting a foot dorsiflexion of the affected side by a dorsiflexion switch on the non-affected side. A third patient group received a sham therapy with neither mirror therapy nor electrical stimulation. Outcome variables were different parameters of a gait measurement system. In this study, both mirror groups showed improvement in gait velocity when compared to the sham group. Step length and stride length only improved in the combination therapy.

A further study with a similar design, but higher number of participants, was presented by Xu and co-workers 2017 [13]. In this study with

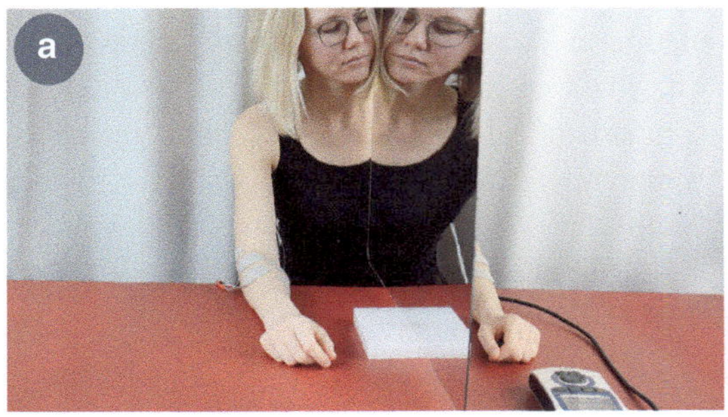
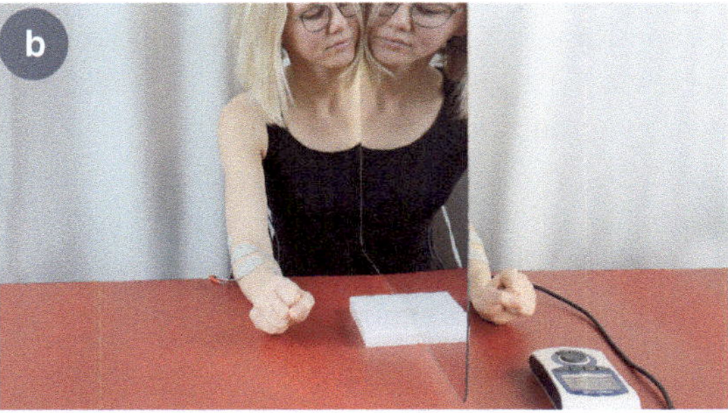

**Fig. 14.1** Combination of bilateral functional EMG-triggered multichannel electrical stimulation with mirror therapy. (**a**) mirror therapy before pulse triggering by EMG-triggered multichannel electrical stimulation, (**b**) mirror therapy with EMG-triggerered multichannel electrical stimulation. (from Schick and Co-workers, 2017 [9])

3 × 23 subacute stroke patients, there was greater improvement in the primary outcome variable (10 m gait test) in the combination therapy when compared to mirror therapy group and control therapy group (without additional therapy). The Brunnström stages of motor recovery of the lower limb showed greater improvement in both therapy groups receiving mirror therapy when compared to the control group. However, in this variable, there was no additional effect of the electrical stimulation. The same picture appeared in the passive range of motion. For spasticity (Ashworth scale), the combination therapy was found to be superior to isolated mirror therapy and the control group.

## 14.2.5 Combination Studies

In the three-arm study of Yun and co-workers 2001 [3] 20 subacute stroke patients in each group received either cyclical electrical stimulation of the Musculi extensor digitorum communis and extensor pollicis brevis, mirror therapy, or a combination of both. This study showed no difference between both isolated therapy regimes. However, the combination of both regimes showed to be superior in all subtests of the upper extremity Fugl Meyer score and hand extension force.

In another three-arm study, Nagapattinam and co-workers 2015 [14] compared the effect of electrical stimulation, mirror therapy, and its combination in three groups of 20 subacute stroke patients each. In all conditions, patients had to grasp for a bottle cyclically (task-specific training). In the primary outcome variable, the Action Research Arm Test (ARAT) with its four subtests, no significant difference between the therapy groups could be established, even as visual inspection of the data suggested a slight advantage for the combination therapy.

The third study of Mathieson and co-workers 2018 [15] applied a similar design and compared the two isolated therapies with its combination. A total of 50 subacute stroke patients participated. Here as well, functional electrical stimulation was cyclical with stimulation of the Musculi extensors digitorum and extensor pollicis brevis. In this study, the per-protocol analysis showed no difference between the three therapy regimes in any of the outcome variables (Fugl Meyer scores, ARAT, ADL scales), but with slightly different baseline values. An additional ANCOVA of the ARAT, considering these differences, provided a superior effect of functional electrical stimulation compared to mirror therapy and the combination.

## 14.2.6 Summary

Taking all evidence together, most of the studies detailed above suggest that the effect of functional electrical stimulation in subacute stroke patients can be enhanced by means of a mirror. The data of Nagapattinam and co-workers hint, however, that this effect is more prominent on the ICF functional level (e.g., Fugl Meyer score) when compared to ICF activity level (e.g., Action Research Arm Test).

For the reverse question (can mirror therapy be enhanced by electrical stimulation?) there are fewer studies. Two out of three studies described treatment of the lower extremity, where the rationale of employing mirror therapy is less clear. These few data suggest that mirror therapy might be enhanced by electrical stimulation.

Thus, taking all evidence together, there are clear hints that mirror therapy and electrical stimulation are complementary therapy approaches. The studies available so far do not allow a direct comparison of the effect of both therapies. Apparently, however, the combination provides additive effects. Data are more robust for enhancing electrical stimulation by means of a mirror than vice versa.

## 14.3 Botulinum Toxin A and (Functional) Electrical Stimulation

Klemens Fheodoroff

**Abstract**

This section presents the impact of spastic movement disorder (SMD) on movement control and the ability to act as well as treatment approaches. Injections with botulinum toxin A have become the gold standard of medical treatment for SMD, opening a "therapeutic window" in which the affected individuals can exercise under therapeutic guidance how to deal with SMD (stretching, positioning) and how to practice residual control of voluntary movements (strengthening, repetitive exercise) which may be disguised by muscle tone increase or synkinesis.

Electrical stimulation has been increasingly established as an ideal supplement. Through neuromuscular electrical stimulation (NMES), muscle tone in spastic agonists can be reduced and the effect of botulinum neurotoxin type A (BoNT-A) injections can be enhanced. By means of functional electrical stimulation (*FES*), action-related movement patterns can be reinforced and trained with frequent repetitions.

The foundations, the practical implementation, and goals for a combined treatment are discussed in detail.

**Keywords**

Spastic movement disorder; Botulinum toxin A; Neuromuscular and functional electrical stimulation; Treatment goals

### 14.3.1 Spastic Movement Disorder

Spastic movement disorder (SMD) [16] is one of the most frequent consequences of a central nervous system impairment (brain/spinal cord). Nowadays, only the plus phenomena of the pyramidal tract syndrome (upper motor neuron syndrome, UMNS) are subsumed under the term SMD. Prominent features of SMD are: enhanced proprioceptive muscle reflexes, a velocity-dependent increase in muscle tone during passive stretching, and the appearance of involuntary movement reactions (synkinesis, spastic dystonia). The minus phenomena—impaired muscle strength, impaired control of voluntary movements, and reduced muscle endurance—must be distinguished from SMD. Furthermore, muscle tissue changes developing over time with muscle shortening and restricted segmental joint mobility up to the development of contractures is considered as a consequence of SMD/UMNS [17–19].

---

**b760 Control of Voluntary Movement Functions** [20]

Functions associated with control and coordination of voluntary movements.
*Including*: Functions of control of simple and complex voluntary movements, coordination of voluntary movements, supportive functions of arm or leg, right left motor coordination, eye-hand coordination, eye-foot coordination; impairments such as control and coordination problems, e.g., dysdiadochokinesia.
*Excluding*: muscle power functions (b730); involuntary movement functions (b765); gait pattern functions (b770).

---

The Fugl-Meyer test has become standard for assessing control of voluntary movement with or without synkinesis. 30 instructions with increasing level of difficulty are used for assessing arm function (max. 60 points); 11 instructions with increasing difficulty are used for assessing leg function (max. 22 points). Reflexes, coordination, sensitivity, and balance tasks are evaluated separately [21–23].

▶ The systematic evaluation of control of voluntary movements functions should be an integral component of initial and final disability assessment for each intervention.

According to the International Classification of Functioning, Disability and Health (ICF), all of the above-mentioned parameters belong to the body functions components. As described in Chap. 5, body function impairments constitute internal barriers for the performance of various actions and tasks and constitute a need for external facilitators (aids/assistance) to partially compensate these internal barriers.

To categorize individual capacity in walking (d450), the *Functional Ambulation Categories*—a 6-point scale (from "*cannot walk/assistance of 2 persons*" to "*can walk everywhere independently, including stairs*") has been well-established.

**Table 14.1** Arm-hand activity scale [27]

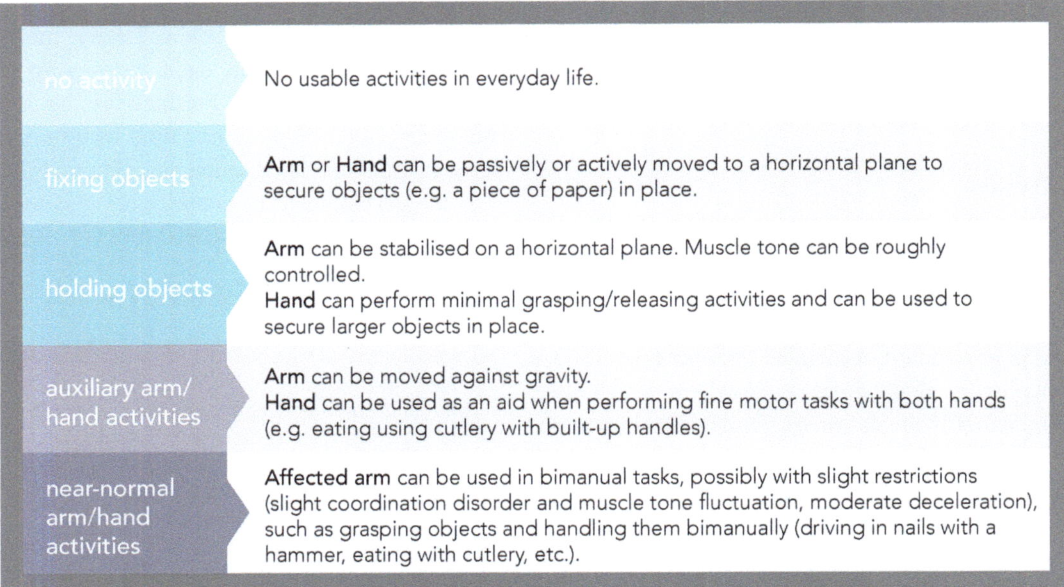



[24–26]. Regarding arm-hand activities, a similar 5-point scale has been developed recently, facilitating the choice of appropriate treatment strategies according to the current level of arm-hand activities [27] (Table 14.1).

In recent years, reliable clinical parameters have been published allowing to predict recovery of mobility within first 6 months after stroke already 48/72 h after onset of symptoms.

If the affected person can sit stable and without assistance 72 h after onset of stroke symptoms and can move hip/knee/ankle joint of the affected leg voluntarily to a small extent, there is a high (98%) probability that he/she will be able to walk independently and without aids 6 months after the stroke. Conversely, individuals who cannot sit unassisted for at least 30 s only have a 27% probability of being able to walk independently [28]. Here it is worth noticing that changes in gait pattern persist for a long time and are characterized by an abnormal muscle tone, gait asymmetry, and flexion synkinesis of the affected arm. Affected persons use up 50–70% more energy when walking compared to healthy individuals walking at the same gait speed [29, 30].

Similar parameters were determined for recovery of arm and hand activities. If the affected person is able to voluntarily abduct shoulder and stretch fingers of the paretic arm within 48 h after stroke, there is a high probability (98%) for near-normal arm/hand activities 6 months after the stroke. On the contrary, individuals without control of voluntary movements only have a 25% chance to regain arm/hand activities usable in daily routine. If shoulder abduction/finger extension still cannot be actively performed on day five and nine, this probability is reduced to less than 15%; on the contrary, there is a 13-fold increased risk for developing a SMD in the next months [31, 32].

Motor recovery after stroke has been described in six stages by Brunnström [33]. Yet it must be emphasized that, depending on the extent of the CNS damage, motor recovery can stop at any of these stages (Table 14.2).

In the early stages after brain lesions, a (flaccid) paresis usually is present. Depending on size and localization of brain lesion, the grade of the paresis, and the presence of pain and sensory and proprioceptive functions, an increase in muscle tone develops within the first 4 weeks after stroke in 4–27% of affected persons; in another 19–27% of affected persons, SMD develops within the first 3 months. 17–42% of stroke patients suffer from a chronic SMD [34]. With persisting SMD, muscle tissue changes in the paretic muscles

**Table 14.2** Stages of motor recovery (Brunnström 1966)

| level | denomination | characteristics |
| --- | --- | --- |
| 1 | muscle hypotonus | no voluntary movements |
| 2 | developing spasticity | basal flexor/extensor synergies |
| 3 | marked spasticity | components of flexor/extensor synergies can be initiated voluntarily |
| 4 | decrease in spasticity | voluntary movements deviating from basal flexor/extensor synergies can be initiated |
| 5 | disappearance of spasticity | voluntary movements can be initiated independent from basal flexor/extensor synergies |
| 6 | minimal spasticity | near-normal movements/coordination |

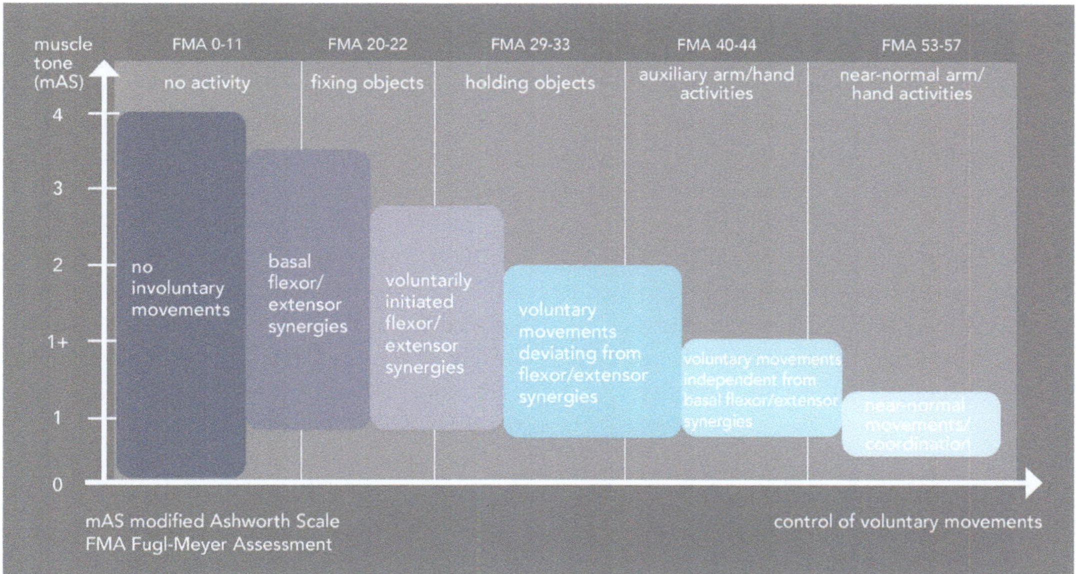


**Fig. 14.2** Impact of muscle tone on control of voluntary movements

(loss of elastic fibers, increase of connective and fatty tissue, ion channel proteins alterations) appear frequently [35]. These changes lead to further reduction of passive range of motion (pROM) in the spastic segment. Therefore, an early treatment of SMD appears reasonable [36].

However, further research is required if secondary changes can be prevented by early BoNT-A treatment (Fig. 14.2).

Given the development of SMD over time, different treatment goals should be considered. In the first 6–12 months, the focus is on reducing spasticity-associated muscle pain, maintaining the (passive) range of motion in the spastic segment, and reducing muscle tone to promote control of voluntary movements for arm/hand activities such as securing objects in place, grasping and releasing objects as well as standing up/sitting down and walking (barefoot). In the chronic phase of SMD, however, the focus should be on goals such as reducing involuntary movements/synkinesis and enabling (self) stretching exercises in the spastic movement segments to facilitate self-care activities (such as washing oneself/caring for body parts/dressing) [37–39] (Table 14.3).

Here it is important to emphasize that neither the paresis nor the muscle tone itself can be directly influenced by the affected individuals themselves, but by medication (BoNT-A injections), by (electrical-) stimulation, and by soft tissue surgery. However, during neurorehabilitation, affected persons should learn to deal with these impairments as efficiently as possible by being taught interventions related to a (guided) self-management. This also helps patients to optimize their self-determination by learning to counteract SMD through regular stretching and positioning as well as moving segments repetitively within their residual control of voluntary movements, including synkinetic movement patterns, to carry out tasks and actions (e.g., to secure objects in place; to carry objects in a bag with a flexed elbow)—if necessary, supported by dynamic splints and electrical stimulation.

For treatment of moderate/severe SMD, BoNT-A injections have proven effective.

## 14.3.2 Botulinum Toxin: Pharmacology, Mode of Action, and Use

### 14.3.2.1 Botulinum Toxin—Pharmacology

Botulinum neurotoxins (BoNT) are produced by anaerobic, spore-forming bacteria of the species *Clostridium botulinum*. These naturally occurring complex protein molecules are characterized by high neurotoxicity. All BoNTs bind to peripheral cholinergic nerve endings in both, smooth and striated muscle and to glands with cholinergic transmission inhibiting the release of the neurotransmitter acetylcholine (ACh) at the presynaptic membrane. Thus, they cause a reversible slack paralysis of the skeletal muscles or a secretion inhibition of the treated glands.

### 14.3.2.2 Mode of Action (Onset of Action—Maximum Effect—Duration of Action)

Of the seven known serotypes (A-G), almost exclusively serotype A (BoNT-A) is used for clinical purpose at the moment. BoNT-A consists of a heavy (100 kDa) and a light (50 kDa) chain connected by a disulfide bond. The heavy chain is responsible for binding BoNT-A to the presynaptic nerve terminals as part of ACh vesicle recycling process and for translocating from the ACh vesicles into the cytosol of the neuron. BoNT-A uptake into the terminal nerve ending is thus dependent on ACh release. Only when ACh vesicles fuse with the presynaptic nerve cell membrane, the specific binding receptor for the heavy BoNT-A chain is displayed (Fig. 14.3). The more ACh released after the injection, the more BoNT-A is incorporated into the presynaptic nerve endings. Thus, inactivity after BoNT-A treatment (e.g., bed rest) should be avoided.

The light chain causes the biological response by destroying proteins responsible for fusing ACh vesicles with the presynaptic membrane. Depending on the BoNT type and the destroyed fusion proteins, ACh release into the synaptic cleft is suppressed for a type-specific time period (between 2 and 24 weeks) [40, 41].

Due to this biological transformation, BoNT-A does not take effect right after the injection but three to five days later. The maximum effect of BoNT-A-induced chemodenervation can be expected after seven to ten days and lasts for 8–12 weeks. As ACh release is reduced at both, the extrafusal and the intrafusal (muscle spindle) endplates, the neuromuscular afferents (as part of the spastic reflex arc) are also blocked.

The neurotoxin is subsequently degraded by proteases in the preterminal axon; no further fusion proteins are destroyed. The fusion

**Table 14.3**  Common patterns in spastic movement disorders, muscles involved, and goals for treatment

| pattern | involved muscles | treatment goals |
|---|---|---|
| shoulder adduction,<br>- internal rotation,<br>- retraction | - pectoralis major<br>- latissimus dorsi<br>- teres major/minor<br>- subscapularis<br>- rhomboideus major/minor | - sitting/standing/walking with mild arm flexion synkineses<br>- cleaning armpit<br>- dressing upper body<br>- resting arm on table<br>- reaching for objects |
| elbow flexion | - biceps brachii, brachialis<br>- brachioradialis<br>- pronator teres | |
| pronated forearm | - pronator teres<br>- pronator quadratus | - resting arm on table<br>- reaching for objects |
| wrist and finger flexion (clenched fist) | - flexor carpi ulnaris/radialis<br>- flexor digitorum superficialis/profundus<br>- flexor pollicis longus | - washing/caring for hand<br>- stretching fingers against low resistance<br>- securing objects in place/grasping/releasing |
| thumb flexion, "lumbrical hand" (MCP joint flexion) | - flexor pollicis brevis<br>- oppones/adductpr pollicis<br>- interossei volares | |
| hip adduction | - adductor longus, brevis, (magnus)<br>- pectineus | - performing intimate hygiene/urinary catheterisation against mild resistance<br>- putting on trousers<br>- walking without crossed legs (scissor gait) |
| hip and knee flexion | - psoas major/iliacus<br>- gracilis/semimembranosus/semitendinosus | - putting on trousers<br>- standing up/standing with leg extended |
| knee extension | - rectus femoris<br>- quadriceps group | - sitting in (wheel) chair without thigh spasms/cramps<br>- walking with knee flexion in leg swing phase |
| spastic plantarflexion (pes equinovarus) | - soleus, gastrocnemius<br>- tibialis posterior/(anterior)<br>- flexor digitorum longus | - standing up/standing/walking with heel/sole/forefoot contact<br>- walking without splint/barefoot |
| toe claws | - flexor digitorum/hallucis longus<br>- flexor digitorum/hallucis brevis | - putting on shoes<br>- walking without splint/barefoot<br>- walking without foot cramps |
| tonic hallux extension (striatal toe) | - extensor hallucis longus | - putting on shoes<br>- walking with shoes without foot cramps |

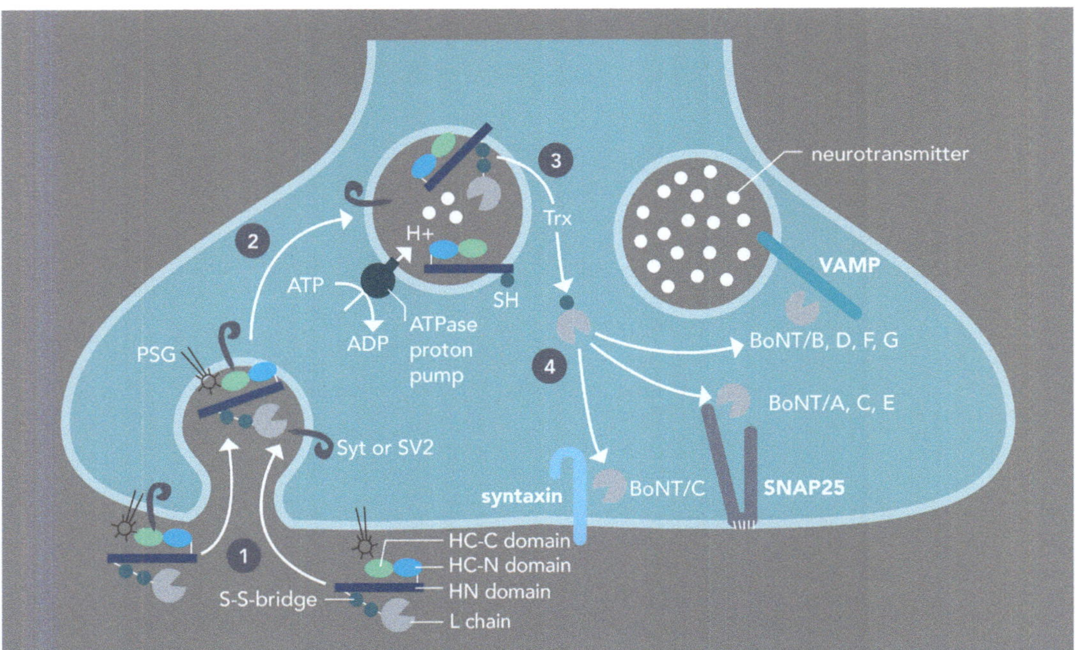


**Fig. 14.3** Mode of action of botulinum neurotoxins. The heavy BoNT chain with its carboxy-terminal end ("HC-C domain") specifically binds to a polysialoganglioside receptor ("PSG") of the presynaptic membrane and to one of two protein receptors (syntagmin—"Syt" or "SV2") located in the ACh vesicle membrane. It is then taken up into the terminal nerve end as part of ACh vesicle recycling process (1). The vesicle content is enriched with protons ("H⁺") via ATPase proton pump to reabsorb excess ACh into the vesicle. In this acidic environment, a structural change of the BoNT molecule occurs. The N-terminal end of the heavy chain ("HN domain") forms a kind of pore in the vesicle membrane through which the light BoNT chain ("L chain") is discharged from the ves- icle (2). The enzyme thioredoxin reductase ("Trx") cleaves the light chain at the disulfide bond ("S-S bridge"/"SH"). Now the light chain can develop its proteolytic activity in the cytosol (3). The protein complex for fusing the ACh vesicles with the presynaptic membrane and for ACh release into the synaptic cleft consists of three proteins that twist helically around each other: Syntaxin, SNAP-25 (Synaptosomal-Associated Protein), and VAMP (Vesicle-Associated Membrane Protein). BoNT types B, D, F, and G cleave VAMP, BoNT types A, C, and E cleave SNAP-25 (at different sites), and BoNT type C cleaves syntaxin (4), all of which result in neurotransmitter release inhibition and neuroparalysis (4). *ATP* adenosintriphosphate, *ADP* adenosindiphosphate

complexes necessary for exocytosis are newly formed so that the synapse can resume its function 8–12 weeks after treatment with BoNT-A. Particularly in the treatment of spastic movement disorder, this period of blocked neuromuscular transmission is also labeled as the "therapeutic window", which can be used to work out new movement patterns. Thus, the clinical duration of action can be extended.

The various commercially available BoNT-A products differ in protein content and excipients and thus also in potency. Therefore, the products are only comparable to a limited extent. So far, direct comparative studies of the different prod- ucts regarding duration and strength of action as well as safety and effectiveness in different indications are lacking. Therefore, the choice for one of the registered BoNT-A products heavily depends on the regional availability of the product and the clinical experience of the treating physician [41].

### 14.3.2.3 Licensed Indications—Off-Label Use

BoNT-A injections are medically indicated for diseases associated with increased striated or smooth muscle tone and spasms and for diseases with increased glandular secretion (saliva, sweat).

**Table 14.4** Licensed BoNT-A treatments and off-label use

| licensed indications[1] | related indications[2] |
| --- | --- |
| blepharospasm, hemifacial spasm | meige syndrome (blepharospasms plus oromandibular dystonia) |
| cervical dystonia (torticollis spasmodicus) | oromandibular dystonia; lingual and laryngeal dystonia, spasmodic dysphonia; focal dystonia of the arms/legs (writer's cramp); head and hand tremor |
| arm and hand spasticity after stroke | trunk and shoulder muscle spasms after stroke or severe traumatic brain injury |
| spasticity of the lower leg/ankle after stroke or severe traumatic brain injury | hip and thigh muscles after stroke/severe stroke/ severe traumatic brain injury |
| dynamic toe walking in children with cerebral palsy from age 2 onwards | hip and thigh musculature in children with cerebral palsy from age 2 onwards |
| axillary hyperhidrosis | palmoplantar hyperhidrosis |
| excessive saliva production with involuntary loss of saliva from the oral cavity (sialorrhoea) | |
| symptomatic treatment for chronic migraine | |
| overactive bladder with urinary incontinence | |

[1] for details: see country-specific licensing and summary of product characteristics
[2] Standardised information leaflets for obtaining written informed consent are available.

Up to now, a number of diseases have been officially registered for treatment using BoNT-A. However, BoNT-A is also used for off-label treatment in similar conditions (Table 14.4).

### 14.3.2.4 Treatment Techniques

Due to the size of the molecules, BoNTs can neither cross the skin barrier nor the blood-brain barrier. The protein must therefore be injected into the target structures. Consequently, knowledge of functional anatomy and spastic movement patterns to appropriately select overactive muscles as well as a precise injection technique are essential for treatment success. In addition to anatomical landmarks, ultrasound (US), electromyography (EMG), and electrical stimulation (ES) are used for localization control. A review by Grigoriu et al. demonstrated that the use of US or ES for injection control leads to better treatment results in both, arm and leg spasticity, than using anatomical landmarks or EMG-guided injections. [42]. Depending on severity of SMD, the spastic movement pattern, and the treatment goals, an average of five muscles in arm spasticity and four muscles in leg spasticity are treated with BoNT-A (see Table 14.3. Common patterns in spastic movement disorders).

### 14.3.2.5 Adverse Effects

Apart from pain and haematomas at injection sites, excessive local weakness and generalized weakness may occur in individual cases. Especially at higher dosages, dry mouth and eyes, double vision, dysphagia, flu-like symptoms, gallbladder motility disorders, and bladder emptying disorders have been observed. The adverse effects are reversible similar to the desired effects. Thorough information of patients and relatives on the expected effects and goals for treatment, possible local and systemic adverse effects should therefore be discussed and documented in a standardized way and written informed and signed consent should be obtained before injections.

### 14.3.2.6 Follow-up Examinations

As treatment effects vary individually and are dose-dependent, follow-up examinations on a regular basis are of importance. If not determined otherwise, the need for concomitant treatment should be assessed and determined after seven to fourteen days. After 4–6 weeks, it should be assessed whether or to what extent the treatment goals have been achieved, if the concomitant therapies have been carried out as planned, and if any adverse effects have occurred. At the same time, treatment plan modifications for the next injection (need for treatment of additional muscles, dosage adjustment) can be determined. After 12–20 weeks, the pharmacological effect of the treatment has subsided. By now at the latest, the need for further treatment cycles should be evaluated and further treatments should be planned/carried out [43].

### 14.3.3 Combined Treatment BoNT-A and Electrical Stimulation

Treatment of SMD with BoNT-A opens a "therapeutic window" which allows for applying non-pharmacological treatments aiming to develop new movement patterns and to expand the ability to act. By now, sound data for a number of combined treatments are available [6, 44].

As BoNT-A uptake depends on motor endplate activity, it is reasonable to force muscle contraction of the treated muscles by means of cyclic neuromuscular electrical stimulation (NMES). In fact, best clinical evidence for enhancing the effect of BoNT-A injections currently exists for NMES of the injected muscles immediately and in the first few days after treatment [45–47]. Duration of stimulation per NMES

session should be 30 min. The level of intensity should be chosen so that visible muscle contractions are elicited without provoking unwanted movements of non-involved muscle groups. Depending on the size of the affected muscle groups, the current intensities are usually between 15 and 90 mA. Direct current rectangular pulses with a duration of 200 μs are most frequently used in existing studies. Biphasic rectangular pulses with pulse widths of 200 μs to 400 μs, as delivered by some mobile electrical stimulation devices, are also suitable for therapy. The frequencies range from 3 to 8 Hz (to reduce muscle tone in the agonists) and 20 to 35 Hz (to increase muscle tone in the antagonists or activate the antagonists).

Only two high-quality studies have been conducted and published so far on functional electrical stimulation (*FES*) after BoNT-A treatment. The study by Weber and colleagues [48] examined combined treatment of BoNT-A injections in the forearm flexors and *FES*, compared to task-oriented training in chronic patients. The agonists as well as the antagonists of the group that received *FES* treatment were stimulated with a prefabricated myoelectric orthosis for 60 min per day for a total of 12 weeks from day seven onward after BoNT-A injections to induce grasping movements. Each stimulation cycle consisted of stimulating the forearm extensors (opening/closing fingers) for five seconds, followed by stimulating the finger flexors (5 s) and a break of 2 s. The reaching movement (moving the arm towards an object) was used as *FES* trigger. The control group completed a task-oriented training (stacking objects, wiping surfaces, sorting coins) with a similar level of intensity. The results, however, did not confirm any significant improvements in the group which received FES compared to the control group (activities were measures using the Motor Activity Log and the Action Research Arm Test).

In their study, Johnson and colleagues [49] combined BoNT-A treatment of the calf muscles with *FES* (biphasic electrical pulses with a frequency of 40 Hz, a pulse width of 30–350 ms, and currents up to 100 mA of the peroneal and the anterior tibial muscle for ankle joint extension and eversion in the leg swing phase, caused by a heel switch) and compared this course of treatment to conventional physiotherapy (two to three times per week for 45 min) without BoNT-A therapy. All patients were in their first year after stroke and were experiencing problems with heel contact at initial stance phase due to premature calf muscle activation during walking (measured through surface EMG). Although the study was only conducted in a small number of patients, a significant reduction in calf muscle tone, an increase in gait speed, and a decrease in effort (measured with the Physiological Cost Index) were evidenced.

At present, there are still insufficient data to make definitive recommendations on indications, stimulation parameters, programs, and outcome parameters for *FES*. Future studies on combined treatment of BoNT-A and *FES* should also consider and include standardized comparisons of different stimulation parameters (reduction of muscle tone in spastic agonists/increase of muscle tone in atrophic paretic antagonists, frequency and duration of ES) while trying to achieve the most homogeneous grouping possible (in terms of chronicity, control of voluntary movements and ability to act).

## 14.3.4 Case Example and Recommendations

The case described in Chap. 5 is presented here in detail.

61-year-old farmer suffering from the consequences of a hypertensive right basal ganglia hemorrhage. Three months after onset, he exhibited spastic plegia of the left arm and hand. Passive elbow and wrist extension as well as finger extension were painful against a moderate resistance (mAS 2°); stretching fingers was painful at the end of passive range of motion. Moderate spastic flexor synkinesis of left elbow and hand. Minimal control of voluntary elbow flexion was present; distally no selective movement control retrievable. Due to finger and wrist flexor spasticity, performing daily hygiene of the

left hand was painful and possible only to a very limited extent.

A combined treatment consisting of BoNT-A injections and *(F)ES* was used to treat left arm flexor spasticity.

### 14.3.4.1 Treatment Goals

Stretch fingers against low resistance without pain—within 4 weeks (d210). Wash and towel off left hand independently—within 6 weeks (d520). Secure objects in place on a table using the paretic hand—within 6 weeks (d440).

The following muscles in the left arm were treated:

| | | |
|---|---|---|
| m. brachialis | 0.5 vials | (2 sites) |
| m. pronator teres | 0.3 vials | (1 site) |
| m. flexor carpi radialis | 0.3 vials | (1 site) |
| m. flexor carpi ulnaris | 0.3 vials | (1 site) |
| m. flexor pollicis longus | 0.3 vials | (1 site) |
| m. flexor digitorum profundus | 0.3 vials | (2 sites) |
| m. flexor digitorum superficialis | 1.0 vial | (2 sites) |
| In total: | 3.0 vials | (6.0 ml) |

Chemodenervation was performed in a sonography-targeted manner and was well-tolerated.

Immediately afterward and during the following three days, the injected upper and forearm flexors were stimulated for 30 min using neuromuscular electrical stimulation (NMES) with biphasic rectangular pulses at a frequency of 3 Hz and a pulse width of 200 μs. Subsequently, also the antagonistic elbow and forearm extensors were stimulated using NMES with biphasic rectangular pulses for over 30 min once per day. Additionally, a positioning and stretching program for the left arm was compiled.

After ten days, the muscle tone in the elbow and wrist had reduced considerably (however still against moderate resistance—mAS 2°); stretching fingers against low resistance (mAS 1+) was possible free of pain. For the first time, minimal voluntary elbow extension and voluntary finger flexion within flexion synkinesis could be noticed; no selective finger extension retrievable. Only low-degree spastic flexion synkinesis in the left elbow and hand.

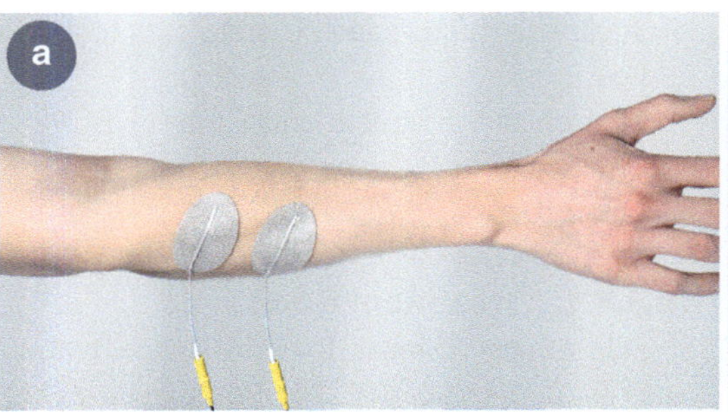
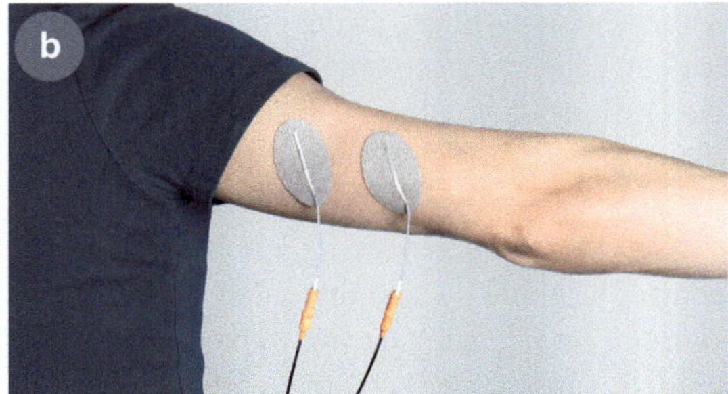

**Fig. 14.4** Electrode placement for *FES*

In the following weeks, an EMG-triggered *FES* of the antagonistically acting wrist, finger, and elbow extensors was performed daily (see Fig. 14.4. Electrode placement for *FES*). Again, biphasic rectangular pulses with a frequency of 30 Hz and a pulse width of 200 μs were used for FES. Predefined plateau and pause times were included in the timed sequence of stimulation channels. M. triceps brachii served as trigger muscle for EMG function. This allowed for initial extensor activity that was enhanced by means of additional electrical stimulation. The stimulation of the second channel for the hand and finger extensors was performed with a time lag of 2 s. To avoid a stimulation-induced increase in flexor muscle tone via stretch reflex, an adequately long current rise time of 3 s and a corresponding fall time of 2 s were chosen. The current intensity was selected individually and on a daily basis in order to allow the target muscles to contract as clearly visibly as possible, but to avoid a simultaneous spill over on the arm flexors. In parallel, an occupational training (washing, dressing, fixing objects) was established.

Four weeks after start of treatment, the muscle tone in the elbow, wrist, and fingers was significantly lower (mAS 1+); stretching the fingers continued to be pain-free and against low resistance (mAS1+). Repetitive voluntary elbow extension and finger flexion was possible deviating from basal flexion synkinesis. Selective finger extension was retrievable to some extent but rapidly exhausted. Mild spastic flexion synkinesis in the left elbow and the hand were occurring only in phases of simultaneous tension of several muscle groups, e.g., when standing up or walk-

ing. After a little stretching preparation, the hand could be placed on the table with the fingers extended.

### 14.3.4.2 Goal Evaluation

Stretch fingers against low resistance free of pain—within 4 weeks (d210)—achieved. Wash and dry the left hand independently—within 6 weeks (d520)—partially achieved. Secure objects in place on a table using the paretic hand—within 6 weeks (d440)—partially achieved.

The family members were trained to continue the *FES* therapy program at home. A check-up appointment for further BoNT-A treatment (if needed) and for modification of *FES* (if necessary) was set and agreed on 12–16 weeks after the first treatment.

### 14.3.5 Summary

Treatment of SMD using BoNT-A injections has become a standard intervention in neurorehabilitation. Various goals, depending on the duration and severity of SMD, can be pursued. There are now sufficient data on combined treatment using NMES after BoNT-A injections available supporting the use of ES for the therapy of SMD in routine clinical practice.

Both, muscle tone reduction in spastic muscles and voluntarily triggered electrical stimulation of paretic-atrophic antagonists by a proximal muscle in the context of rudimentary actions (e.g., reaching for something) should be offered for treatment. When using *FES*, control of voluntary movements, endurance, and ability to act should be carefully recorded in addition to changes in SMD.

## References


1. Schick T, Schlake H-P, Kallusky J, Hohlfeld G, Steinmetz M, Tripp F, Krakow K, Pinter M, Dohle C. Synergy effects of combined multichannel EMG-triggered electrical stimulation and mirror therapy in subacute stroke patients with severe or very severe arm/hand paresis. Restor Neurol Neurosci. 2017;3:319–32.
2. Kim H, Lee G, Song C. Effect of functional electrical stimulation with mirror therapy on upper extremity motor function in poststroke patients. J Stroke Cerebrovasc Dis. 2014;23(4):655–61.
3. Yun G, Chun M, Park J, Kim B. The synergic effects of mirror therapy and neuromuscular electrical stimulation for hand function in stroke patients. Ann Rehabil Med. 2011;35(3):316–21.
4. Luo Z, Zhou Y, He H, Lin S, Zhu R, Liu Z, Liu J, Liu X, Chen S, Zou J, Zeng Q. Synergistic effect of combined mirror therapy on upper extremity in patients with stroke: a systematic review and meta-analysis. Front Neurol. 2020;11:155. https://doi.org/10.3389/fneur.2020.00155.
5. Dohle C, Püllen J, Nakaten A, Küst J, Rietz C, Karbe H. Mirror therapy promotes recovery from severe hemiparesis: a randomized controlled trial. Neurorehabil Neural Repair. 2009;23(3):209–17.
6. Intiso D, Santamato A, Di Rienzo F. Effect of electrical stimulation as an adjunct to botulinum toxin type A in the treatment of adult spasticity: a systematic review. Disabil Rehabil. 2017;39(21):2123–33.
7. Thieme H, Morkisch N, Mehrholz J, Pohl M, Behrens J, Borgetto B, Mirror therapy for improving motor function after stroke. Cochrane Stroke Group, Herausgeber. Cochrane Database Syst Rev 11. 2018 [zitiert 21. August 2018]; available: http://doi.wiley.com/10.1002/14651858.CD008449.pub3
8. Kim H, Lee G, Song C. Effect of functional electrical stimulation with mirror therapy on upper extremity motor function in poststroke patients. J Stroke Cerebrovasc Dis Off J Natl Stroke Assoc. 2014;23(4):655–61.
9. Schick T, Schlake H-P, Kallusky J, Hohlfeld G, Steinmetz M, Tripp F. Synergy effects of combined multichannel EMG-triggered electrical stimulation and mirror therapy in subacute stroke patients with severe or very severe arm/hand paresis. Restor Neurol Neurosci. 2017;35(3):319–32.
10. Lee D, Lee G. Effect of afferent electrical stimulation with mirror therapy on motor function, balance, and gait in chronic stroke survivors: a randomized controlled trial. Eur J Phys Rehabil Med 2019;55(4). [zitiert 18. Februar 2020]; Available: https://www.minervamedica.it/index2.php?show=R33Y2019N04A0442
11. Lin K, Huang P, Chen Y, Wu C, Huang W. Combining afferent stimulation and mirror therapy for rehabilitating motor function, motor control, ambulation, and daily functions after stroke. Neurorehabil Neural Repair. 2014;28(2):153–62.
12. Ji S-G, Cha H-G, Kim M-K, Lee C-R. The effect of mirror therapy integrating functional electrical stimulation on the gait of stroke patients. J Phys Ther Sci. 2014;26(4):497–9.
13. Xu Q, Guo F, Salem HMA, Chen H, Huang X. Effects of mirror therapy combined with neuromuscular electrical stimulation on motor recovery of lower limbs and walking ability of patients with stroke: a randomized controlled study. Clin Rehabil. 2017;31(12):1583–91.
14. Nagapattinam S, Vinod Babu K, Sai Kumar N, Ayyappan VR. Effect of task specific mirror therapy withf unctional electrical stimulation on upper limb function for subacute Hemiplegia. Int J Physiother 2015;2(5). [cited 15. Oktober 2018] available: http://ijphy.org/view_issue.php?title=EFFECT-OF-TASK-SPECIFIC-MIRROR-THERAPY-WITH-FUNCTIONAL-ELECTRICAL-STIMULATION-ON-UPPER-LIMB-FUNCTION-FOR-SUBACUTE-HEMIPLEGIA.
15. Mathieson S, Parsons J, Kaplan M, Parsons M. Combining functional electrical stimulation and mirror therapy for upper limb motor recovery following stroke: a randomised trial. Eur J Physiother. 2018;20(4):244–9.
16. Dressler D, Bhidayasiri R, Bohlega S, Chana P, Chien HF, Chung TM, et al. Defining spasticity: a new approach considering current movement disorders terminology and botulinum toxin therapy. J Neurol. 2018;265(4):856–62.
17. Platz T. Therapie des spastischen syndroms, S2k-Leitlinie [S2k-Leitlinie]. online: Deutsche Gesellschaft für Neurologie; 2018 [updated 26.06.2019]. www.dgn.org/leitlinien.
18. Gracies J. Pathophysiology of spastic paresis. I: Paresis and soft tissue changes. Muscle Nerve. 2005;31(5):535–51.
19. Gracies J. Pathophysiology of spastic paresis. II: emergence of muscle overactivity. Muscle Nerve. 2005;31(5):552–71.
20. WHO. International classification of functioning, disability and health: ICF. Organization WH, editor. Geneva: World Health Organization; 2001.
21. Crow JL, Kwakkel G, Bussmann JB, Goos JA, Harmeling-van der Wel BC. Are the hierarchical properties of the Fugl-Meyer assessment scale the same in acute stroke and chronic stroke? Phys Ther. 2014;94(7):977–86.
22. Woodbury ML, Velozo CA, Richards LG, Duncan PW. Rasch analysis staging methodology to classify upper extremity movement impairment after stroke. Arch Phys Med Rehabil. 2013;94(8):1527–33.

23. Fugl-Meyer AR, Jaasko L, Leyman I, Olsson S, Steglind S. The post-stroke hemiplegic patient. 1. A method for evaluation of physical performance. Scand J Rehabil Med. 1975;7(1):13–31.

24. Mehrholz J, Wagner K, Rutte K, Meissner D, Pohl M. Predictive validity and responsiveness of the functional ambulation category in hemiparetic patients after stroke. Arch Phys Med Rehabil. 2007;88(10):1314–9.

25. Holden MK, Gill KM, Magliozzi MR. Gait assessment for neurologically impaired patients. Standards for outcome assessment. Phys Ther. 1986;66(10):1530–9.

26. Holden MK, Gill KM, Magliozzi MR, Nathan J, Piehl-Baker L. Clinical gait assessment in the neurologically impaired. Reliability and meaningfulness. Phys Ther. 1984;64(1):35–40.

27. Berger M, Freimueller M, Fheodoroff K. Evaluating the comprehensibility of the Arm-Hand-Activity-Scale (AHAS-German version) as part of establishing psychometric quality criteria. In: Dettmers C, Schönle P, Weiller C, editors. 5th European Congress of Neurorehabilitation (ECNR). Budapest. Bad Honnef: Neurologie & Rehabilitation; 2019. p. S50.

28. Veerbeek JM, Van Wegen EE, Harmeling-Van der Wel BC, Kwakkel G. Is accurate prediction of gait in non-ambulatory stroke patients possible within 72 hours poststroke? The EPOS study. Neurorehabil Neural Repair. 2011;25(3):268–74.

29. Awad LN, Reisman DS, Pohlig RT, Binder-Macleod SA. Reducing The cost of transport and increasing walking distance after stroke: a randomized controlled trial on fast locomotor training combined with functional electrical stimulation. Neurorehabil Neural Repair. 2016;30(7):661–70.

30. Pereira S, Mehta S, McIntyre A, Lobo L, Teasell RW. Functional electrical stimulation for improving gait in persons with chronic stroke. Top Stroke Rehabil. 2012;19(6):491–8.

31. de Jong LD, Hoonhorst MH, Stuive I, Dijkstra PU. Arm motor control as predictor for hypertonia after stroke: a prospective cohort study. Arch Phys Med Rehabil. 2011;92(9):1411–7.

32. Nijland RH, van Wegen EE, Harmeling-van der Wel BC, Kwakkel G. Presence of finger extension and shoulder abduction within 72 hours after stroke predicts functional recovery: early prediction of functional outcome after stroke: the EPOS cohort study. Stroke. 2010;41(4):745–50.

33. Brunnstrom S. Motor testing procedures in hemiplegia: based on sequential recovery stages. Phys Ther. 1966;46(4):357–75.

34. Wissel J, Manack A, Brainin M. Toward an epidemiology of poststroke spasticity. Neurology. 2013;80(3 Suppl 2):S13–9.

35. McKenzie MJ, Yu S, Macko RF, McLenithan JC, Hafer-Macko CE. Human genome comparison of paretic and nonparetic vastus lateralis muscle in patients with hemiparetic stroke. J Rehabil Res Dev. 2008;45(2):273–81.

36. Rosales RL, Efendy F, Teleg ES, Delos Santos MM, Rosales MC, Ostrea M, et al. Botulinum toxin as early intervention for spasticity after stroke or non-progressive brain lesion: A meta-analysis. J Neurol Sci. 2016;371:6–14.

37. Fheodoroff K, Ashford S, Jacinto J, Maisonobe P, Balcaitiene J, Turner-Stokes L. Factors influencing goal attainment in patients with post-stroke upper limb spasticity following treatment with botulinum toxin A in real-life clinical practice: sub-analyses from the upper limb international spasticity (ULIS)-II study. Toxins (Basel). 2015;7(4):1192–205.

38. Fheodoroff K, Scheschonka A, Ramusch S, Wissel J. Mapping of 1,633 goals from the tower study reveals a higher proportion of activity and participation-related goals in spasticity patients. International Congress of Parkinson's Disease and Movement Disorders; September 22–26, 2019; Nice, France2019. p. 1.

39. Wissel J, Fheodoroff K, Hoonhorst M, Mungersdorf M, Gallien P, Meier N, et al. Effectiveness of abobotulinumtoxinA in post-stroke upper limb spasticity in relation to timing of treatment. Front Neurol. 2020;11(104):104.

40. Rossetto O, Pirazzini M, Montecucco C. Botulinum neurotoxins: genetic, structural and mechanistic insights. Nat Rev Microbiol. 2014;12(8):535–49.

41. Field M, Splevins A, Picaut P, van der Schans M, Langenberg J, Noort D, et al. AbobotulinumtoxinA (Dysport((R))), OnabotulinumtoxinA (Botox((R))), and IncobotulinumtoxinA (Xeomin((R))) Neurotoxin Content and Potential Implications for Duration of Response in Patients. Toxins (Basel). 2018;10(12):535.

42. Grigoriu AI, Dinomais M, Remy-Neris O, Brochard S. Impact of injection-guiding techniques on the effectiveness of botulinum toxin for the treatment of focal spasticity and dystonia: a systematic review. Arch Phys Med Rehabil. 2015;96(11):2067–78. e1

43. Ashford S, Turner-Stokes LF, Allison R, Duke L, Moore P, Bavikatte G, et al. Spasticity in adults: management using botulinum toxin. National guidelines. 2nd ed. London: Royal College of Physicians; 2018.

44. Mills PB, Finlayson H, Sudol M, O'Connor R. Systematic review of adjunct therapies to improve outcomes following botulinum toxin injection for treatment of limb spasticity. Clin Rehabil. 2016;30(6):537–48.

45. Frasson E, Priori A, Ruzzante B, Didone G, Bertolasi L. Nerve stimulation boosts botulinum toxin action in spasticity. Mov Disord. 2005;20(5):624–9.

46. Hesse S, Jahnke MT, Luecke D, Mauritz KH. Short-term electrical stimulation enhances the effectiveness of Botulinum toxin in the treatment of lower limb spasticity in hemiparetic patients. Neurosci Lett. 1995;201(1):37–40.

47. Hesse S, Reiter F, Konrad M, Jahnke MT. Botulinum toxin type A and short-term electrical stimulation in the treatment of upper limb flexor spasticity

after stroke: a randomized, double-blind, placebo-controlled trial. Clin Rehabil. 1998;12(5):381–8.

48. Weber DJ, Skidmore ER, Niyonkuru C, Chang CL, Huber LM, Munin MC. Cyclic functional electrical stimulation does not enhance gains in hand grasp function when used as an adjunct to onabotulinumtoxinA and task practice therapy: a single-blind, randomized controlled pilot study. Arch Phys Med Rehabil. 2010;91(5):679–86.

49. Johnson CA, Burridge JH, Strike PW, Wood DE, Swain ID. The effect of combined use of botulinum toxin type A and functional electric stimulation in the treatment of spastic drop foot after stroke: a preliminary investigation. Arch Phys Med Rehabil. 2004;85(6):902–9.

Jürgen Pannek and Jens Wöllner

Main tasks of the lower urinary tract (LUT) are to store and voluntarily evacuate the urine. To fulfil these tasks, complex regulation mechanisms at different levels of the nervous system are involved. Any neurologic disorder may lead to a neurogenic lower urinary tract dysfunction (NLUTD). Clinical symptoms do not correlate with the type and severity of the dysfunction. Therefore, an exact diagnosis of NLUTD by video-urodynamic examination is important. Depending on the type of NLUTD, an adequate therapy is essential to preserve renal function and to sustain the best possible quality of life (QoL).

By video-urodynamic examination, risk factors for the upper urinary tract can be evaluated. If risk factors are present, treatment should be based on these objective parameters to protect renal function. If no risk factors are present, bladder management can be based on symptoms, e.g. urgency, frequency, incontinence, difficulty to void, or urinary tract infections.

Neuromodulation for the treatment of neurogenic lower urinary tract dysfunction (NLUTD) in patients with SCI is under rapid development.

Functional electrical stimulation (FES) of the LUT can be applied via peripheral nerves (vaginal/rectal/genital), tibial nerve stimulation, by intra-vesical stimulation, and by magnetic or electrical stimulation of the spinal cord. Although especially the spinal cord stimulations are at an experimental stage, they carry the potential to become treatment options in the future. In addition, neuromodulation may even be suited to prevent NLUTD instead of just treating it, which will significantly improve the quality of life of the affected persons.

## 15.1 Physiology and Pathophysiology of the Lower Urinary Tract

Main tasks of the lower urinary tract (LUT) are to store and voluntarily evacuate the urine. To fulfil these tasks, complex regulation mechanisms at different levels of the nervous system are involved. Supraspinal centres such as the frontal cortex, the pontine micturition centre and the insula are responsible for the voluntary control of micturition [1, 2]. The spinal cord is essential for the transmission of information originating from the LUT to the supraspinal neural networks. Together with descending efferent fibres from the cortical micturition centres to the lowest sacral segments, they form a closed-loop system to control urine storage and voiding. The integrity of the connections between cortical, supraspinal centres and spinal neurons is essential and must therefore be preserved. As a consequence, any neurologic disorder may lead to a neurogenic lower urinary tract dysfunction (NLUTD).

J. Pannek (✉) · J. Wöllner
Swiss Paraplegic Center, Department Neuro-Urology,
Nottwil, Switzerland
e-mail: juergen.pannek@paraplegie.ch;
jens.woellner@paraplegie.ch

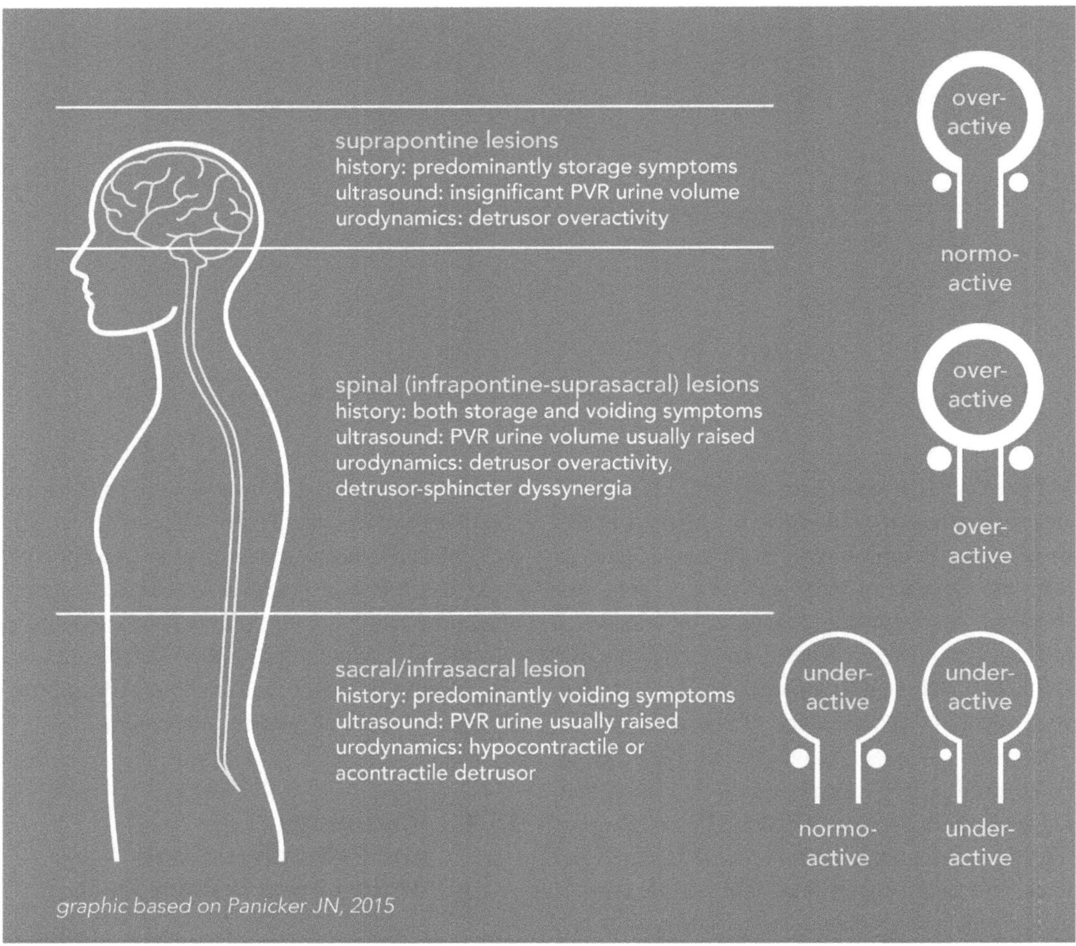


**Fig. 15.1** Neurogenic lower urinary tract dysfunction (NLUTD) based on the level of lesion

Treatment of NLUTD is not mainly based on the type of neurogenic disorder, but on the resulting type of lower urinary tract dysfunction in the storage and voiding phase. Depending on the level and completeness of the neurogenic lesion, different clinical manifestations of NLUTD can occur [3]. Basically, cortical or subcortical lesions above the pontine micturition centre (e.g. stroke, traumatic brain injury) leads to a loss of inhibition of detrusor activity. As a consequence, neurogenic detrusor overactivity (NDO), an unvoluntary contraction of the detrusor, is frequent in these patients, leading to elevated pressure in the bladder during the storage phase and may result in urgency and/or urinary incontinence. An infrapontine, suprasacral spinal lesion carries the highest risk for renal function. In these types of lesion, often the coordination between the detrusor muscle and the urethral sphincter is affected. Thus, simultaneous contractions of the bladder and the sphincter occur, leading to elevated intravesical pressure due to functional obstruction during bladder contraction. This phenomenon, referred to as detrusor-sphincter dyssynergia (DSD), can have detrimental consequences for renal function by either reflux or obstruction of the upper urinary tract. In addition, it can lead to incomplete voiding and elevated post-void residual urine, often leading to recurrent urinary tract infections (UTI) [4]. Subsacral spinal lesions or peripheral nerve lesions typically result in an acontractile bladder with insufficient or incomplete drainage. In addition, a flaccid urethral sphincter can cause stress urinary incontinence.

Unfortunately, clinical symptoms do not correlate with the type and severity of dysfunction. Up to 70% of patients with spinal cord injury (SCI) representing the group with a worsening of the pattern of the NLUTD and would require treatment, do not show additional symptoms [5]. It is of utmost importance to know that in one-third of the affected patients, the type of NLUTD is different from the prediction based on the level of lesion [3] (Fig. 15.1). Therefore, an accurate diagnosis of NLUTD by video-urodynamic examination is essential.

Depending on the type of NLUTD, an adequate therapy is essential to preserve renal function and to sustain the best possible quality of life (QoL). In the management of NLUTD, the general status, motor impairments, patient compliance, cognition, and social circumstances must be taken into account. Basically, as the type of NLUTD can change over time, a life-long follow-up is mandatory in these patients.

**Summary**
Neurological disorders can affect the integrity of the lower urinary tract. Depending on the underlying disease, extent of the lesion and the location of the lesion (central, peripheral), various dysfunctions of the storage and voiding phase can occur. NLUTD can affect the function of the upper urinary tract and can impair renal function. Furthermore, symptoms like urinary incontinence and voiding difficulties can have a negative impact on patients' quality of life.

## 15.2 Examination

The most important instrument to evaluate the function of the lower urinary tract is the (video)-urodynamic examination/study ([V]UDS). During this examination, the storage and voiding phase of the urinary bladder are evaluated. This is established by the insertion of a small transurethral double-lumened catheter. Via one channel of the catheter, the bladder is filled with sterile body-warm fluid at a defined filling speed. In urodynamic studies, saline is used. For video-urodynamic

studies, a mixture of contrast media and saline is instilled. The second channel of the catheter is used for a permanent recording of the intravesical pressure. This allows to permanently record intravesical pressure and volume. The sphincter EMG is measured with surface electrodes. In video-urodynamics, measurement is combined with fluoroscopy. By filling the bladder with contrast media, structural alterations of the lower urinary tract and potential risk factors for renal function (e.g. vesico-ureteral-renal reflux) can be detected. In persons with SCI, the examination is most frequently performed in the sitting or lying position.

By video-urodynamic examination, risk factors for the upper urinary tract, e.g. detrusor overactivity during the storage phase exceeding $40\,cm$ , $H_2O$, DSD, vesico-renal reflux, or loss of elasticity (low compliance) can be evaluated. If risk factors are present, treatment should be based on these objective parameters to protect renal function. If no risk factors are present, bladder management can be based on symptoms. The most common symptoms are:

– Urgency.
– Frequency.
– Incontinence.
– Difficulty to void/feeling of incomplete voiding.
– Recurrent urinary tract infections (UTI).

## 15.3 FES Techniques in NLUTD

As neuromodulation is regulated via afferent nerves, an at least partially preserved sacral reflex arch is a prerequisite for any neuromodulatory technique, including peripheral electrical stimulation [6]. Therefore, electrical stimulation does not seem to be indicated in persons with complete spinal cord injury but for cortical lesions like multiple sclerosis, stroke and traumatic brain injury.

### 15.3.1 Intravesical Stimulation

Intravesical electrical stimulation (IVES), first introduced by Katona [7], aims at activating detrusor contractions to improve voiding in patients with neurogenic non-obstructive urine retention. Usually, a monopolar active electrode is inserted in the bladder via a catheter using monophasic rectangular impulses with a frequency between 10 and 20 Hz. To either manifest or prove the failure of this treatment, 3 weeks of daily 1-h IVES sessions seem to be sufficient. The largest single-centre study in patients with chronic retention requiring intermittent catheterization demonstrated a minimum reduction of 50% both in the number of daily catheterizations and residual urine in 38 of these 102 patients (37.2%). After 8–15 months, these parameters returned to baseline, but a second IVES cycle led to similar improvements as the first ones [8]. Due to the low success rate and the short duration of the effect, IVES seems to be merely useful for a limited, well-selected group of patients.

### 15.3.2 Nervus Pudendus Stimulation

Temporary peripheral electrical stimulation.

This therapeutic approach offers a non-invasive alternative to medical therapy for detrusor overactivity in patients with neurogenic disorders. Due to the non-invasive approach and the easy handling, it can be used as home therapy, which increases patients' acceptance and compliance.

#### 15.3.2.1 Vaginal/Rectal Electrical Stimulation

Detrusor overactivity can be suppressed by afferent stimulation of the pudendal nerve and suppression of pelvic nerve activity by activation of central inhibition. Frequencies between 5 and 10 Hz were most successful in animal experiments and clinical studies [9, 10].

#### Electrical Stimulation

Transcutaneous electrical nerve stimulation can be applied by various routes. Whereas stimulation in non-neurogenic patients is frequently performed via rectal or vaginal electrodes (Fig. 15.2), hardly any data regarding this method can be found in persons with SCI. There are few studies

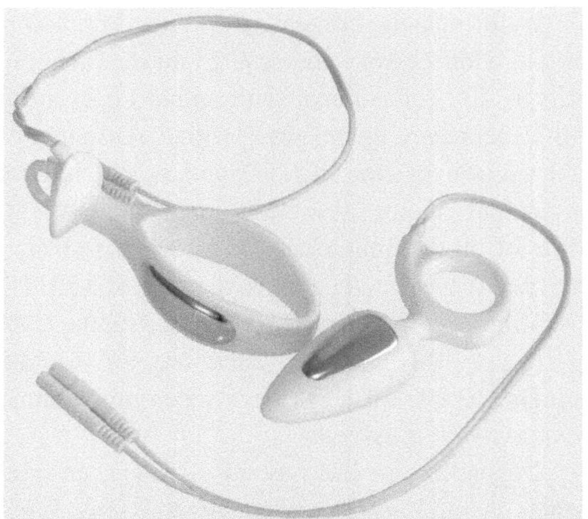

**Fig. 15.2** Rectal or vaginal electrodes

examining persons with neurogenic OAB due to various neurologic disorders, predominantly multiple sclerosis, pointing out that this stimulation may improve detrusor overactivity by daily stimulation at home. Whereas one study found a long-term effect [11], other studies described an effect duration of about 2 months in patients with MS [12]. In the study of Pannek et al., stimulation was applied twice a day for 20 min, using vaginal probes for women and rectal probes for men, with a frequency of 8 Hz and a pulse width of 400 μs over a period of 3 months. On the contrary, Primus et al. performed 15 20-min sessions over 3 weeks, with a pulse width of 1 ms and a frequency of 20 Hz. In both studies, the maximum tolerable stimulus was chosen by slowly increasing the intensity. The significant differences in both, stimulation frequency and stimulation parameters, may at least partially explain the different results.

#### 15.3.2.2 Genital Electrical Stimulation

The pudendal nerve originates in the nerve roots of S2–S4. It innervates the pelvic floor and external sphincter. The dorsal penile and clitoral nerves are the most superficial and exclusively afferent branches of the pudendal nerve. These branches have frequently been used for electrical stimulation, as they are inhibitory to the micturition reflex. In animal and human studies, spontaneous bladder contractions could be inhibited with stimulation of pudendal nerves. In persons with SCI, genital (penile/clitoral) stimulation is used more frequently than electrical stimulation with vaginal or rectal probes. Most frequently, 200 microsecond width square waves at a frequency of 25 Hz and a mean stimulus amplitude of 26 mA are applied. Both, acute continuous or conditional stimulation, lead to an increase in bladder capacity [13] and to an improvement of urodynamic parameters [14]. Data on chronic genital electrical stimulation in persons with SCI, however, is rather scarce. Lee et al. demonstrated an improvement in bladder capacity and detrusor overactivity in five out of six participants 2–4 weeks after a stimulation period of 14–28 days [15]. In the most recent study, five participants with chronic SCI used penile stimulation for seven days, which led to an improvement in continence, bladder capacity, and detrusor overactivity [16]. A retained sensation seems to be a prerequisite for treatment success. Genital stimulation is either used constantly or conditionally (event-driven). Both techniques can result in an inhibition of detrusor contractions and lead to an increase in functional bladder capacity [17], but both techniques require constantly wearing genital electrodes. This belongs to the apparent drawbacks of this type of stimulation.

### 15.3.2.3 Sacral Stimulation

Sacral neuromodulation by implantable electrodes is an established therapy for the treatment of overactive bladder and non-obstructive urinary retention and constipation. Non-invasive procedures, such as transcutaneous stimulation, are an option for patients who do not want to undergo surgery, even if it is minimally invasive. With surface electrodes placed above the sacral foramina S2 and S3, symptoms of overactive bladder can resolve. Different stimulation parameters are reported in the literature, applying a frequency of 10 to 50 Hz and pulse duration of 100 to 500 µs. Also, the stimulation duration (twice daily to 12 h for 3 months) is not clearly defined. As some studies and case series show a therapeutic effect of percutaneous sacral stimulation, this technique

might be an alternative option in patients who reject invasive sacral neuromodulation [18].

## 15.4 Tibial Nerve Stimulation (TNS)

Electrical stimulation of the tibial nerve, which proximally enters the sciatic nerve and the L4/5-S3 roots, is believed to modulate spinal cord and/or brain reflexes to exert its clinical effect on detrusor overactivity in persons with SCI (Fig. 15.3) [19]. Electrical percutaneous neuromodulation therapy (PTN) has been delivered transcutaneously, percutaneously, and via implanted electrodes. As the latter is a minimally invasive procedure, this paragraph will focus on the former techniques.

Percutaneous tibial nerve stimulation (PTNS) involves the placement of a needle electrode and usually requires weekly visits to the clinic for at least 12 weeks for stimulation, followed by monthly visits to maintain the effect [20]. In a study using PTNS utilizing the schedule mentioned above, including a monthly maintenance stimulation, the authors demonstrated a significant improvement in patients with neurogenic as in idiopathic detrusor overactivity for a period of 4 years [20]. The majority of studies is related to tibial nerve stimulation and neurogenic bladder dysfunction has been performed in persons with multiple sclerosis. In this group of patients, several researchers reported clinical as well as urodynamic improvements in detrusor overactivity/overactive bladder [21, 22].

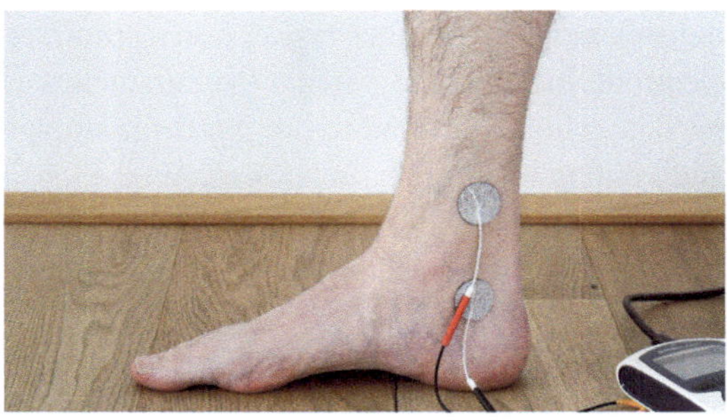

**Fig. 15.3** Tibial nerve electrode placement for detrusor overactivity

Transcutaneous tibial nerve stimulation (TTNS) is applied through skin electrodes and can be performed by the individuals themselves continuously or on demand [19]. Thus, TTNS is easier to perform and can be used by the patients themselves at home. Results, however, are conflicting. In a randomized study, TTNS was not effective in treating idiopathic or neurogenic detrusor overactivity [23]. In the study using TTNS specifically in persons with SCI, the authors applied this technique in the acute phase, and found deterioration in neurogenic bladder dysfunction in those without TTNS, but not in the TTNS group. Thus, they concluded that the method may be useful for preventing neurogenic bladder dysfunction in SCI [24]. This study, however, comprised of 19 patients only. To further explore this subject, a multicentred, prospective, randomized, sham-controlled study for TTNs in persons with acute SCI has started recently [25].

## 15.5 Spinal Cord Stimulation (SCS)

Case reports described mixed results of lumbosacral spinal cord epidural electrical stimulation (SCEES) on bladder function after SCI. SCEES was performed via an epidural spinal cord stimulator and a 16-electrode array that was surgically placed at the spinal segments L1-S1, 3.3 years after traumatic SCI. The individual may turn the stimulator on and off and may select programs. The stimulation needs to be individualized. SCEES may function by increasing central excitability involving activation of spared supraspinal pathways to neural networks and modulating spinal reflexes [26]. Further research in optimizing electrode location and stimulation parameters is needed, which may lead to programs for storage and voiding at low pressures. A more developed system may have an effect on other autonomic functions including the cardiovascular system and bowel, Nevertheless, this might as well imply challenges since several programs would co-exist. Currently, there is no experience with long-term SCEES.

Transcutaneous electrical spinal cord stimulation (TESCS) may reduce detrusor overactivity, increase bladder capacity, and lessen detrusor-sphincter-dyssynergia by transforming the automaticity of the spinal neural circuits into a more physiological functioning by activating the spinal micturition centre. Using a non-invasive transcutaneous electrical spinal cord stimulator with electrodes placed over the interspinous ligaments of Th11 and L1 and the iliac crest individualized stimulation parameters were applied [27]. TESCS is non-invasive but requires thorough evaluation and meticulous individualized urodynamic evaluation of the optimal stimulation parameters. It can be utilized in persons with chronic SCI. The initial results of the existing case combined with small studies that can be performed in larger trials may lead to a long-term solution for TESCS as a tool before implanting SCEES. The effects of transcutaneous magnetic spinal cord stimulation on the lower urinary tract were evaluated in a proof-of-concept study in five patients, using a figure-8 coil at vertebra L1 in the midline to allow the magnetic field to be parallel to the spinal cord [28]. Applying magnetic stimulation once a week for 16 weeks, demonstrated an increase in bladder capacity and a decrease in number of self-catheterizations. Yet, the stimulation must be individualized and repeated weekly to maintain this effect [28]. As anticipated for electrical stimulation, magnetic stimulation may facilitate the coordination of the activity in the spinal micturition circuits, but with a lower risk of painful stimulation [28].

In all mentioned spinal cord stimulations, hardly any case reports or small case series exist, pointing out that further studies are required before these techniques can be used in clinical practice (Table 15.1).

**Table 15.1** Different stimulation sites in detrusor overactivity in different neurological diseases

| detrusor overactivity | | multiple sclerosis | traumatic brain injury | incomplete tetraplegia | stroke |
|---|---|---|---|---|---|
| | rectal/vaginal | ✓ | ✓ | | ✓ |
| | genital | ✓ | | ✓ | ✓ |
| | sacral | ✓ | ✓ | ✓ | ✓ |
| | N.tibialis | ✓ | ✓ | ✓ | ✓ |

## 15.6 Perspective

Non-invasive neuromodulatory therapies are available for patients with underlying neurological disorders. In patients with neurogenic overactive bladder (OAB), this therapy can be an option. Due to the non-invasive character, it may serve as an alternative to medical treatment in a well-defined group of patients without risk factors for renal damage. Nevertheless, the evidence for non-invasive neuromodulation in patients with neurogenic lower urinary tract dysfunction is low. There is a lack of prospective, sham-controlled trials. Especially stimulation parameters, duration, and intensity are based on expert experience. Therefore, this therapy should be further elucidated by clinical trials.

Neuromodulation for the treatment of neurogenic lower urinary tract dysfunction (NLUTD) in patients with SCI is developing rapidly. For a long period of time, the treatment of NLUTD was based on the prevention of secondary complications. Oral medication, onabotulinum toxin detrusor injections and bladder augmentation are all qualified to treat NLUTD, but they are not able to restore both storage and voiding function. The sacral deafferentation and anterior root stimulation lead to safe detrusor storage pressures, voluntary voiding in physiologic intervals and continence in patients with complete SCI. This resembles the natural bladder cycle more closely than any other procedure, yet this process is invasive and irreversible. Current research aims at overcoming these obstacles by using external devices. Although these treatments are at an experimental stage, they carry the potential to become common options in the future. In addition, neuromodulation may even be suited to prevent NLUTD instead of only treating it, which will significantly improve the quality of life of the affected persons (Table 15.2).

▶ The treatment of a neurogenic lower urinary tract dysfunction due to a spinal cord injury is complex, challenging, and crucial. The aim is to preserve kidney function, continence, and to improve patient's quality of life. Especially for tibial nerve neuromodulation in MS patients, there are initial data sets that prove its effectiveness. As FES is usually well tolerated, it is a therapy option for selected patients with neurogenic lower urinary tract dysfunction with no immediate risk for the upper urinary tract.

**Table 15.2** Recommended stimulation parameters for electrical stimulation at different stimulation sites

| | | frequency (Hz) | pulse width (µs) | duration/ session (min) | sessions per week | total period (weeks) |
|---|---|---|---|---|---|---|
| stimulation parameters | rectal/ vaginal | 5-20 | 200-400 | 20 | 7 | 8 |
| | genital | 5-20 | 200-400 | 20 | 7 | 8 |
| | sacral | 5-20 | 200-400 | 20 | 7 | 8 |
| | N.tibialis | 5-20 | 200-400 | 20 | 7 | 8 |

# References


1. Blok BF, Holstege G. The central nervous system control of micturition in cats and humans. Behav Brain Res. 1998;92:119–25.
2. Holstege G, Mouton LJ. Central nervous system control of micturition. Int Rev Neurobiol. 2003;56:123–45.
3. Panicker JN, Fowler CJ, Kessler TM. Lower urinary tract dysfunction in the neurological patient: clinical assessment and management. Lancet Neurol. 2015;14:720–32.
4. Pannek J, Wöllner J. Management of urinary tract infections in patients with neurogenic bladder: challenges and solutions. Res Rep Urol. 2017;9:121–7.
5. Nosseir M, Hinkel A, Pannek J. Clinical usefulness of urodynamic assessment for maintenance of bladder function in patients with spinal cord injury. Neurourol Urodyn. 2007;26:228–33.
6. Schurch B, Reilly I, Reitz A, Curt A. Electrophysiological recordings during the peripheral nerve evaluation (PNE) test in complete spinal cord injury patients. World J Urol. 2003;20:319–22.
7. Katona F. Stages of vegatative afferentation in reorganization of bladder control during intravesical electrotherapy. Urol Int. 1975;30:192–203.
8. Lombardi G, Celso M, Mencarini M, Nelli F, Del Popolo G. Clinical efficacy of intravesical electrostimulation on incomplete spinal cord patients suffering from chronic neurogenic non-obstructive retention: a 15-year single centre retrospective study. Spinal Cord. 2013;51:232–7.
9. Lindström S, Fall M, Carlsson CA, Erlandson BE. The neurophysiological basis of bladder inhibition in response to intravaginal electrical stimulation. J Urol. 1983;129:405–10.
10. Aristizábal Agudelo JM, Salinas Casado J, Fuertes ME, et al. Urodynamic results of the treatment of urinary incontinence with peripheral electric stimulation. Arch Esp Urol. 1996;49:836–42.
11. Pannek J, Janek S, Noldus J. Neurogenic or idiopathic detrusor overactivity after failed antimuscarinic treatment: clinical value of external temporary electrostimulation. [Article in German]. Urologe A. 2010;49:530–5.
12. Primus G, Kramer G. Maximal external electrical stimulation for treatment of neurogenic or non-neurogenic urgency and/or urge incontinence. Neurourol Urodyn. 1996;15:187–94.
13. Bourbeau DJ, Creasey GH, Sidik S, Brose SW, Gustafson KJ. Genital nerve stimulation increases bladder capacity after SCI: A meta-analysis. J Spinal Cord Med. 2018;41:426–34.
14. Hansen J, Media S, Nøhr M, Biering-Sørensen F, Sinkjaer T, Rijkhoff NJM. Treatment of neurogenic detrusor overactivity in spinal cord injured patients by conditional electrical stimulation. J Urol. 2005;173:2035–9.
15. Lee YH, Kim SH, Kim JM, Im HT, Choi IS, Lee KW. The effect of semiconditional dorsal penile nerve electrical stimulation on capacity and compliance of the bladder with deformity in spinal cord injury patients: a pilot study. Spinal Cord. 2012;50:289–93.
16. Doherty SP, Vanhoestenberghe A, Duffell LD, Hamid R, Knight SL. Ambulatory urodynamic monitoring assessment of dorsal genital nerve stimulation for suppression of involuntary detrusor contractions following spinal cord injury: a pilot study. Spinal Cord Ser Cases. 2020;6:30.
17. Dalmose AL, Rijkhoff NJ, Kirkeby HJ, Nohr M, Sinkjaer T, Djurhuus JC. Conditional stimulation of the dorsal penile/clitoral nerve may increase cystometric capacity in patients with spinal cord injury. Neurourol Urodyn. 2003;22:130–7.
18. Slovak M, Christopher R, Chapple A, Barkera AT. Non-invasive transcutaneous electrical

stimulation in the treatment of overactive bladder. Asian J Urol. 2015;2(2):92–101.

19. Janssen DA, Martens FM, de Wall LL, van Breda HM, Heesakkers JP. Clinical utility of neurostimulation devices in the treatment of overactive bladder: current perspectives. Med Devices (Auckl). 2017;10:109–22.

20. Andersen K, Kobberø H, Pedersen TB, Poulsen MH. Percutaneous tibial nerve stimulation for idiopathic and neurogenic overactive bladder dysfunction: a four-year follow-up single-centre experience. Scand J Urol. 2021;55:169–76.

21. Kabay S, Kabay SC, Yucel M, Ozden H, Yilmaz Z, Aras O, Aras B. The clinical and urodynamic results of a 3-month percutaneous posterior tibial nerve stimulation treatment in patients with multiple sclerosis-related neurogenic bladder dysfunction. Neurourol Urodyn. 2009;28:964–8.

22. Zecca C, Digesu GA, Robshaw P, Singh A, Elneil S, Gobbi C. Maintenance percutaneous posterior nerve stimulation for refractory lower urinary tract symptoms in patients with multiple sclerosis: an open label, multicenter, prospective study. J Urol. 2014;191:697–702.

23. Welk B, McKibbon M. A randomized, controlled trial of transcutaneous tibial nerve stimulation to treat overactive bladder and neurogenic bladder patients. Can Urol Assoc J. 2020;14:E297–303.

24. Stampas A, Korupolu R, Zhu L, Smith CP, Gustafson K. Safety, feasibility, and efficacy of transcutaneous tibial nerve stimulation in acute spinal cord injury neurogenic bladder: a randomized control pilot trial. Neuromodulation. 2019;22:716–22.

25. Birkhäuser V, Liechti MD, Anderson CE, Bachmann LM, Baumann S, Baumberger M, Birder LA, Botter SM, Büeler S, Cruz CD, David G, Freund P, Friedl S, Gross O, Hund-Georgiadis M, Husmann K, Jordan X, Koschorke M, Leitner L, Luca E, Mehnert U, Möhr S, Mohammadzada F, Monastyrskaya K, Pfender N, Pohl D, Sadri H, Sartori AM, Schubert M, Sprengel K, Stalder SA, Stoyanov J, Stress C, Tatu A, Tawadros C, van der Lely S, Wöllner J, Zubler V, Curt A, Pannek J, Brinkhof MWG, Kessler TM. TASCI-transcutaneous tibial nerve stimulation in patients with acute spinal cord injury to prevent neurogenic detrusor overactivity: protocol for a nationwide, randomised, sham-controlled, double-blind clinical trial. BMJ Open. 2020;10:e039164.

26. Herrity AN, Williams CS, Angeli CA, Harkema SJ, Hubscher CH. Lumbosacral spinal cord epidural stimulation improves voiding function after human spinal cord injury. Sci Rep. 2018;8:8688.

27. Kreydin E, Zhong H, Latack K, Ye S, Edgerton VR, Gad P. Transcutaneous electrical spinal cord neuromodulator (TESCoN) improves symptoms of overactive bladder. Front Syst Neurosci. 2020;14:1.

28. Niu T, Bennett CJ, Keller TL, Leiter JC, Lu DC. A proof-of-concept study of transcutaneous magnetic spinal cord stimulation for neurogenic bladder. Sci Rep. 2018;8:12549.

# 16

Birgit Tevnan

The use of functional electrical stimulation (FES) in home-based therapy represents just one expansion of the field of action for therapists. New and user-friendly devices support therapy in the home environment through simple applications. Especially in neurorehabilitation, the focus should be on increasing the training frequency as well as a high self-efficacy expectation. Enabling evidence-based self-directed training in the form of FES pursues this goal.

For the transfer of FES into home-based therapy and self-directed training, certain supporting factors and barriers can be defined. Therapists can play an important role by introducing and guiding new therapy approaches. The collaborative effort of a therapist-patient team, including caregivers and relatives can promote self-efficacy for all individuals involved. Each patient should be allowed to contribute to their own recovery independently, without a therapist and outside of therapy hours. The potential of individualized self-directed training will be illustrated by a patient example.

B. Tevnan (✉)
Kepler University Hospital, Neuromed Campus, Linz, Austria
e-mail: therapie@tevnan.io

## 16.1 Introduction

Neurological rehabilitation is a complex and time-consuming challenge. Competent care and therapy are required far beyond the acute phase. At best, the rehabilitation takes place in an interdisciplinary setting with a focus on the patient's highest level of function beyond the inpatient phase. The application of Functional Electrical Stimulation (FES) in home-based therapy expands the therapeutic field of action. Modern and user-friendly electrical stimulation devices support therapy in a home environment through their simple use. Especially in neurorehabilitation, the focus is on increasing the training frequency as well as a high self-efficacy expectation. Enabling evidence-based self-directed training in the form of FES pursues this goal. For the transfer of FES into home-based therapy and self-directed training, certain supporting factors and barriers can be defined. Therapists can play an important reinforcing role in this regard. Current evidence in the neurological field supports home-based therapy even in the chronic phase [1, 2]. A home-based therapy option, in combination with technological developments, allows complex applications and treatment techniques to be delivered outside the inpatient setting. Many therapeutic skills allow for a broad range of services beyond the clinical setting. Good education and ongoing training are a requirement for this. The FES has enormous potential for application in home-based therapy. Integrated into a holistic therapy concept, FES in home-based therapy can be an important therapeutic approach in neurological rehabilitation. However, obstacles and difficulties will occur from time to time especially when applying new methods and technologies in practice. The aim of this chapter is to clarify assumed obstacles, show potentials, and strengthen the new fields of application.

### 16.1.1 Relevance of Self-Training as Home-Based Therapy in Neurorehabilitation (Evidence)

Due to the complexity of acquired brain injuries, treatment can often take months or even years. Long-term impairment and consequently, long-term therapies, accompany many patients throughout their daily lives. Home exercise programs, home visits, and therapy in the home environment have a positive influence on the progress of therapy after an impairment to the central and peripheral nervous system. Guidelines such as those of the German Society for Neurology (DGN) make recommendations for therapy duration and intensity. In the case of the chronic progression of sensorimotor disorders, especially with existing deficits and existing potential for improvement, the DGN advocates the continuation of therapies. Intensive interval therapy in blocks with planned breaks is only one therapy option in the chronic phase [1, 3]. After the inpatient rehabilitation phase, outpatient therapy is very often reduced to weekly occupational therapy as well as physiotherapy. This results in a drastic reduction of active therapies. However, interventions of up to 3 h daily are recommended even in a chronic stage (>6 months) [4]. This intensity cannot be covered by therapist-supported time alone. For significant improvements, especially regarding sensorimotor deficits, both a high therapy frequency and many high-quality repetitions are necessary. This can only be ensured through self-directed training, in the home environment [4]. A home exercise program similar to the programs in the inpatient setting can produce the same results if properly imple-

mented. Advantages of such therapy interventions would be a lower financial cost, the possibility of home-based care, and an opportunity for integration into the family environment [5]. For moderately to severely affected patients with acquired brain injury, a caregiver-assisted exercise program is an additional option. Improvement or maintenance of motor function can be supported by such interventions. In many cases, a lower level of psychological strain among relatives as well as a higher self-efficacy expectation among patients can be shown. Setting meaningful goals together can positively influence both the patient's and the caregiver's quality of life [6, 7].

### 16.1.2 Expected Benefit of FES in Home-Based Therapy (Evidence)

The use of FES after acquired brain injury is recommended in clinical trials. The question is: To what extent can this evidence be transferred to home-based therapy? As early as 2005, researchers described the efficacy of FES in home-based therapy. In particular, they emphasized the potential of FES in the preparation of active training and other active therapy methods [8]. A systematic review [9] concluded that self-directed training can improve arm function after stroke, and using FES in this regard may result in benefits for patients. Recent randomized controlled trials show that purposeful activity-based electrical stimulation therapy can be a useful home-based rehabilitation program for promoting hand use [10]. Daily use of FES after a central neurological disorder of the upper extremity is particularly effective in wrist and finger extension and shoulder flexion. Triggered stimulation, as well as sensory feedback, are mentioned as determining factors for a successful therapeutic application. Simple stimulation applications using self-adhesive electrodes and portable electrical stimulation devices can enable therapy in a home setting. However, daily FES therapy requires self-directed performance carried out independently of the therapist [11]. In combination with task-oriented training, distal arm and hand function, in particular, can be targeted. In both acute and chronic phases, FES offers potential in therapy [12]. In the EU-RISE project, FES investment techniques were developed as possible home-based therapy after impairment to the "Lower Motor Neuron" (LMN). Studies showed the relevance and potential to counteract atrophy in a targeted manner. Prevention of pressure sores due to increased cushioning function of the quadriceps femoris muscle and the ischiocrural musculature is mentioned as one of the significant results. Long-term therapy in the home-based setting using FES thus represents a reasonable option for the treatment of a denervated muscle (Chap. 8) [13].

## 16.2 Requirement Profiles

### 16.2.1 Requirement Profile of a Medical Device or Electrical Stimulation Device

Regardless of the evidence and benefits, the actual use of technical medical devices is strongly linked to their "usability" or user-friendliness. A Europe-wide standard for usability has been initiated specifically for the development of medical devices (IEC62366-1) [14]. Therapy time for chronic diseases such as stroke is very precious and often limited. Due to this fact, therapists should carefully consider whether the effort of an application is worth the expected benefit.

In general, the following concrete application factors for technical devices emerge:

- Easy to use,
- Low training effort,
- Low costs.

These requirements also apply to medical devices. Their use should be as simple and intuitive as possible. Practical experience shows that small obstacles are often only tolerated when a maximum result is achieved. If a problem arises directly during an application, a large number of therapists tend to change the type of intervention. Finally, therapy time should actually be used for therapy.

In the case of electrical stimulation devices, other technical requirements can be added:

A maximum of safety is the minimum requirement for any application. Furthermore, specific requirements such as easy adjustability, as well as easy adaptation of current intensity and amplitude, for maximum effect can be mentioned [15]. In addition to these criteria, however, there is also the question of availability and cost. Since many medical cost bearers cover rental costs for certain periods of time, electrical stimulation devices are also available as rental devices. The current market offers a wide variety of products however, these differ considerably in terms of their possibilities and areas of application. The product to be used should be based on the needs of the patient.

Rental and purchase: Distribution channels for electrical stimulation devices vary widely. Accessories such as self-adhesive electrodes are usually included and can be reordered. Various manufacturers also offer rental devices or lease-purchase options.

▶ Intensive research into products with regard to their therapeutic possibilities and quality will pay off for therapists and patients. In the case of consumables such as self-adhesive electrodes, there are significant differences in quality. Cheap is not always the best choice.

### 16.2.2 Requirement Profile of the Therapist

The free choice of therapeutic tools allows therapists a degree of creativity within the therapeutic intervention. With sufficient training and evidence-based practice, therapy can thus be designed effectively. Implementing technical innovations and current research findings in therapy is a challenge in the often-busy workday of a therapist. A certain amount of self-interest and motivation is required here but it is often rewarded by therapy success. The literature recommends reusable training materials in the form of videos or portfolios for training [16]. An increasing number of medical device manufacturers offer in-house and external training seminars, on-site support and webinars, among other services. The initial therapy and device training with the patient should ideally be carried out by the supervising therapist. This is the quickest way to clarify uncertainties and avoid faulty installations. Knowledge of the product including a device briefing in line with regulations, such as the European Medical Device Regulation (MDR) and the ability to carry out qualified patient training, is required in this regard.

▶ Qualified companies offer job-specific training for medical personnel, in some cases free of charge.

### 16.2.3 Requirement Profile of the Patient

In the case of central neurological impairment patterns such as the condition after stroke or other acquired brain injuries, there may be cognitive limitations in addition to motor deficits. Spatial-constructive deficits or attention disorders can complicate the independent use of electrical stimulation devices in home-based therapy. Nonetheless, a supportive social environment, self-interest on the part of the patient and step-by-step instructions are often enough to make home-based therapy and self-directed training possible (Fig. 16.2). A "locked" patient mode that can be set on modern electrical stimulation devices enables simplified and safe handling. By means of a preselection menu, the patient can then select only from the programs that are actually necessary for him. Programs can continue to be adjusted, locked and unlocked using the therapist mode. Independent use can be promoted through various training methods and reusable training material such as instructions on application techniques and video recordings [17]. With therapy provided only once or twice a week, self-directed training should be diligently carried out by the patient and if necessary, with the patient's caregiver. Self-motivation can be an essential requirement for the patient and crucial for the actual use of the device. Consistent daily self-directed training according to therapeutic guidelines can produce relevant improvements even years after an event [18].

▶ The time available for initial training is very important. It is essential that the patient should not be overwhelmed during this process. Additional or more complex electrode applications and programs can often be taught more effectively after an initial acclimation period.

### 16.2.4 Requirement Profile of the Caregiver

A therapist-patient team is ideally complemented by family members or caregivers. A more realistic goal setting and better long-term outcomes could be enabled though including family and caregivers [19]. For the efficient use of FES in home-based therapy, they should already be integrated during the planning phase. The helping hand of a caregiver is useful in many cases, especially for more complex upper extremity applications.

Therefore, the introduction and implementation of a self-directed training and exercise plan can sometimes depend on the caregivers' time, availability and confidence. This collaborative effort can promote self-efficacy expectations for all individuals involved [5]. The positive attitude of all involved toward the electrical stimulation device and its function can be essential to its use. The caregiver can directly support and encourage the patient's motivation and drive. Caregiver-mediated exercise can be an option for patients with limited functions or cognitive impairments [20]. General uncertainty or over-burdening of relatives due to a lack of training or education, on the other hand, can stand in the way of home use.

### 16.3 How to Compose a Home-Based Exercise Program

A home-based exercise program is designed to support the patient in performing self-directed training. With a maximum of 2–3 h of motor therapy per week, it is the patient's responsibility to supplement the time between therapy sessions. This should be done in a targeted manner and

**Table 16.1** Evidence-based supporting factors for the use of home-based exercise programs

| support factors for home-based exercise programs | reference |
| --- | --- |
| involving caregivers into home-based exercise programs as positive reinforcers of self-motivation and self-management | Warner et al. 2015, Korpershoek et al. 2011, Platz et al. 2020 |
| logbooks and treatment plans as a self-monitoring tool for patients and to visualize the achieved performance | Oussedik et al. 2019, Oussedik et al 2017 |
| well-being and psychological gain as a motivator | Poltawski et al. 2015 |
| challenging but adjusted level of exercises as a motivator | Poltawski et al. 2015 |
| promoting self-management by involving the patient in goal setting, home-based exercise program planning, and choice of interventions | Parke et al. 2015 |

with as much active training as possible. Putting together a home-based exercise program is often a challenging task for the therapist. Inactivity of patients after a stroke as well as the sometimes considerably limited perseverance in carrying out home-based exercise programs can be obstacles in the home application. At best, a home-based exercise program is developed together with the patient and relatives during a therapy session. The content should be meaningful and ideally, linked to pre-agreed patient goals [21, 22]. Several factors are known to promote an active home exercise program. The targeted use of the promotion factors described in Table 16.1 can positively influence the actual implementation of a home-based exercise program.

## 16.4    Observations in Practice

FES in home-based therapy is a useful and feasible addition to conventional therapy in neurorehabilitation. Early contact with FES in an inpatient setting leads to a more positive acceptance of FES in home-based therapy. The patient has the opportunity to experience the application of FES in therapy and can recognize its effect and potential at an early stage. This simplifies the transfer to the patient's everyday life. The adherence of neurological patients in home-based therapy and self-directed training proves to be a great challenge. Finding out appropriate ways to promote and incorporate self-directed training can help patients in the long term [21, 23].

### 16.4.1 Potential Obstacles

Recurring negative patterns and further obstacles often come into play in the neurological field. Some are known and are described below. Stumbling blocks and obstacles in therapy can be challenging. A safe environment should therefore be provided to enable the patient to learn and grow.

- *Fatigue:* rapid fatigue and long recovery periods. Up to 70% of all post-stroke patients live with this symptom. Lack of strength and fatigue can severely limit self-directed training as well as the quality of life. Learning self-awareness and time and energy management can be helpful in this regard [24].
- *Depression:* About one-third of all post-stroke patients are affected by depression. Depression has a direct impact on the outcome and participation in rehabilitation [25].

- *Lack of understanding of basic tasks*: In addition to potential cognitive deficits, simply "not understanding" can also be a limitation in performance. Explanations and clear definitions of what is meant could be enough to solve many misunderstandings. Knowing the "how" and "why" also makes it easier to carry on and practice on a daily basis.

## 16.4.2 Self-Management and Self-Initiative

Assuming personal responsibility in general as well as for everyday tasks is difficult for many patients with central neurological impairment [26]. Overcoming this challenge by conducting home-based therapy and self-directed training promotes self-efficacy expectations and self-motivation [19]. As a new role option, personal initiative can be encouraged by gradually taking ownership of the device. Patients with low motor ability also describe FES with EMG triggering as an opportunity for early active training. Each patient should be allowed to contribute to their own recovery independently, without a therapist, and outside of therapy hours. Experienced patients, together with therapists, often become the "experts" for their own most suitable application techniques and parameter settings.

## 16.4.3 General Recommendations for Practical Application

The following factors can promote FES in home-based therapy. Their reinforcement may be relevant for the implementation of home-based exercise programs.

- *Supportive environment*: Committed relatives and therapists can create a supportive environment. Enabling factors such as the "home setting" and providing assistive devices can also be beneficial in the process.
- *Motivation*: It can be a major driver for the implementation of home-based therapy and self-directed training. In the short term, exter-

nal motivation can be supportive, but for long-term perseverance, motivation must be provided by the patient autonomously [27].

- *Openness to new things:* Medical devices with electrode cables and current applications are new territory for many patients. However, brief explanations and experimentation often arouse curiosity. Especially in the chronic phase, a new therapy approach can also mean new motivation.
- *Suitable medical equipment:* Research on FES in general and the current state-of-the-art medical devices is highly recommended. There are various products on the market for both stimulation devices and electrodes. Financial support from health insurance can be a relevant factor for many patients.
- *Proper education:* Training, webinars, and educational exchanges are offered by high-quality manufacturers or distributors. Innovative manufacturers offer certification courses, webinars, online training as well as peer exchange groups. Ongoing information flow and exchange provide new ideas and constant training.

## 16.5 A Case Study of Home-Based Therapy

This section uses a patient example to illustrate practical application possibilities and supporting factors. Personal information was altered to prevent patient recognition.

Anamnesis: Mr. B. is 67 years old. He suffered a left medial cerebral artery infarction 10 months ago. Initial main symptomatology was a hypotonic hemiparesis on the right side and expressive aphasia. Prior to his illness, Mr. B was an active member of society. Recently retired, he enjoyed spending time with his wife and children. Using his private and professional network, he started an association for hobby technicians in his home community shortly after his retirement. He lives with his wife in a first-floor apartment that was furnished and equipped to meet the needs of senior citizens. After 12 weeks of care in an acute hospital as well as 4 weeks of neurological rehabilitation, Mr. B. could be discharged to his home environment.

The initial contact at the first home-based therapy visit showed the following picture:

Initial hemiparesis on the right improved with functional gain primarily on the lower extremity with decreased selectivity. Global activation distally at the upper extremity was already observable in the first weeks after the event. A proximal hypotonic upper extremity with a subluxation in the right glenohumeral joint (GH-joint) as well as the general onset of tone increase of the flexors distal with pushing movements in the near peripersonal space was the highest activity level possible after preparation. Meaningful daily use of the upper right extremity was not possible according to Mr. B. Walking ability for short distances with a walking stick on the left side as well as climbing stairs to his own apartment under supervision was the highest activity level of the lower extremity directly after rehabilitation. Minimal deficits of higher cognitive functions and expressive aphasia recovered almost completely. With a Barthel index of 80 points, Mr. B required little assistance with personal hygiene, dressing, and meal preparation. Low resilience as well as an increased need for rest changed the couple's daily routine. Mr. B. organized physiotherapy and occupational therapy in the form of weekly home visits directly after the inpatient rehabilitation. While in the acute hospital, Mr. B. was able to gain experience with EMG-triggered FES for the treatment of the upper extremity. After his stay in the neurological rehabilitation center, Mr. B. initiated a request for a 12-week loan of an EMG-triggered multichannel electrical stimulation device. During a therapeutic contact, the actual need could be evaluated. At the initial assessment, before the start of the intervention, scores were 23/66 on the Fugl-Meyer assessment (upper extremity), 60/100 on the Motricity Index (upper extremity) and 48/100 (lower extremity), 87/100 on the Trunk Control Test, and 14/14 on the Berg Balance Scale (7-item BBS-3P). On the modified Ashworth scale (mAS), wrist and finger flexors were assessed with mAS 2 and m. triceps with mAS 1. Sensitivity testing showed decreased surface sensitivity and proprioception with decreased localization of stimuli and directions of upper extremity movement.

As an additional limitation, Mr. B. described shoulder pain and pain in the right deltoid region of up to 5/10 on the visual analog scale (VAS), occasionally also at rest. Muscles power grading according to Medical Research Council (MRC) of the upper extremity in functional groups:

- GH-joint: abduction (ABD) grade 2+/5, adduction (ADD) grade 2/5, flexion grade 3/5ə, extension grade 2/5.
- Elbow: extension grade 2/5, flexion −3/5.
- Wrist: extension grade 1/5, flexion grade −2/5.
- Finger: extension grade −2/5, flexion grade −3/5 with strongly reduced selectivity.

## 16.5.1 Therapeutic Goal Setting

Mr. B's main goal was to be able to use his upper right extremity in activities relevant to his daily life. Additional short-term goals relevant to everyday use were defined together with Mr. B. as follows:

- Reduction of shoulder pain during activity and at rest to VAS 2/10.
- Integration of the right upper extremity into everyday life by independently positioning the arm in the field of vision.
- Increased sensitivity and tone regulation of the flexor chain of the upper right extremity through perceptual enhancement.
- Improved function and strength in the upper right extremity.
- Development of an active hand in the form of assistive object fixation with the right hand.

## 16.5.2 Initial Training

After checking for contraindications and receiving approval of cost coverage by the health insurance company, the intervention was started about 7 months after the stroke. On the first day of the rental period, Mr. B was tested using recommended assessments (Winstein et al. 2016). As agreed in advance, Mr. B. and his wife participated in the device training. The training programs chosen were cyclic FES in dorsal extension and finger extension and EMG-triggered wrist and finger extension. Several strategies were used to reinforce the content of the training:

- Photo documentation and transcript by the spouse in her own words.
- Step-by-step instructions of each program with photos of the equipment (Fig. 16.2.)
- Logbook for documentation of actual applications by the patient.

### 16.5.3 Implementation

Mr. B. showed great motivation over the application period of 12 weeks. The FES was applied 5–7 times a week with the different application techniques. Additional programs were added 4 weeks after the initial training and the parameter settings were adjusted accordingly over the course of the training. In addition to active programs with EMG triggering, cyclic programs and sensitive-afferent stimulations with a conductive glove ("mesh glove") were used to promote perception and sensitivity (Fig. 16.1). By applying the electrode volar or dorsal to the forearm in combination with the "mesh-glove", sensory stimulation could be provided in addition to functional training. As described in Chap. 9, the use of sensitive afferent electrical stimulation in the distal area of the upper and lower extremities was particularly useful for deficits in sensory perception. Decreased sensitivity, as well as reduced cortical representation, could be promoted in combination with the "mesh-glove."

Mr. B. predominantly preferred the following applications:

- EMG-triggered FES of triceps and deltoid muscles in combination with arm function training with a roller in the closed chain.
- EMG-triggered FES during wrist as well as finger extension with movement observation.
- Sensitive-afferent electrical stimulation with a "mesh-glove."

As a relevant factor, due to the increased tone of the wrist and finger flexors, a slow rise and fall of the current intensity at each stimulation was shown to be useful. By using a rise and fall time of more than 3 s, an increase in tone triggered by the stimulation could be avoided. This had a positive effect on the increased flexor tone, especially at the beginning of the exercises. With a treatment duration of 15–20 min, a tonus reduction of wrist and finger flexors could be measured from mAS 2 to mAS 1 immediately after treatment. This was possible by a symptom-related functional parameter adjustment (Chap. 6). Complementary to home application, FES could also be used in weekly therapy for more complex applications. Over time, it became apparent that the initial support of the spouse could be reduced to "passing of the electrodes" after the first training phase. Before long, home-based therapy and individual training were called "his personal training time."

### 16.5.4 Evaluation

After regular weekly occupational and physical therapy and accompanied FES, the following changes were evident:

At the interim assessment after 12 weeks, 28/66 points could be achieved in the Fugl-Meyer Assessment (upper extremity), 71/100 in the

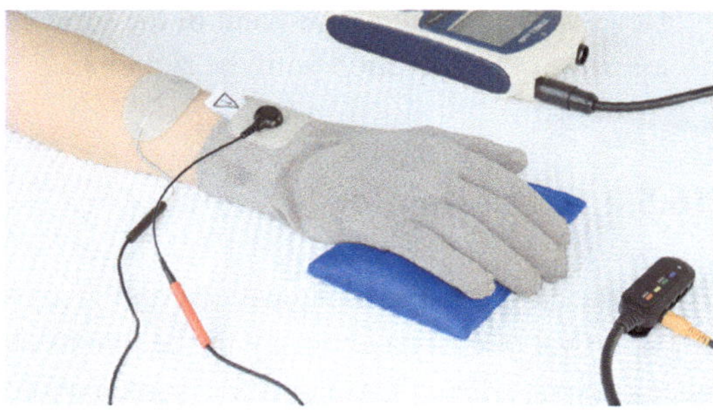

**Fig. 16.1** "Mesh-glove"—sensitive-afferent stimulation with a conductive glove to promote perception

Motricity Index (upper extremity) as well as 70/100 (lower extremity) and 100/100 points in the Trunk Control Test. Wrist and finger flexors and the triceps muscle were assessed with mAS 1. As a subjective improvement, Mr. B. described an increased control over the basic tension of the hand. This was particularly noticeable with reduced visual acuity, such as when putting on a glove. Sensitivity testing also showed progress in the area of distal localization of stimuli, in differential response to sharp and blunt stimuli and in distinguishing temperature differences. This improvement was noted by Mr. B in terms of reduced risk of injury from perceived stimuli. Proprioception of the upper right extremity also visibly improved. Joint positions in the shoulder and elbow could be perceived with certainty. Joint positions in the hand and finger joints could be correctly determined 3/4 of the time.

Muscles power grading (Grade; according to MRC) of the upper extremity in functional groups:

- GHG: ABD Grade 2+/5, ADD Grade 2/5, flexion Grade −3/5, extension Grade 2+/5.
- Elbow: extension Grade 3+/5, flexion 3/5.
- Wrist: extension Grade −3/5, flexion Grade 3/5.
- Finger: extension Grade −3/5, flexion Grade −4/5 with initiating selectivity.

The most noticeable improvement for Mr. B in the area of strength and voluntary movement was the full active extension of the elbow and the significantly increased ability to switch between agonists and antagonists. This was mainly reflected in a meaningful improved selective control. During the joint evaluation of the agreed goals, the shoulder pain was judged to be no longer noticeable. Mr. B. described his right hand as an associated body part and placed it spontaneously and actively in his field of vision. The first functional use of the right hand, in the form of fixing objects, was achieved. In addition, Mr. B. indicated a feeling of control over the hand, especially the distally targeted active relaxation and tone regulation. The training protocol was well received by Mr. B. and his spouse, who supplemented it with personal notes. Together, they were both able to develop a routine in application techniques and strategies during the 12-week loan period. Short videos, repetition of the contact points in therapy, and the possibility of consultation in the accompanying therapy were emphasized as helpful. As a result of the functional improvements and the positive response, Mr. B. and his spouse applied to extend the rental period of the device for another 12 weeks.

**Summary**
FES in home-based therapy and individual training offers the opportunity for evidence-based training at home. With the transfer to a home setting, active training can be offered at an early stage outside of the accompanied therapy time. Direct feedback used as a motivational factor in therapy can promote perseverance in home-based therapy and individual training. Taking responsibility for one's own therapy can additionally promote self-efficacy expectations and personal responsibility [28]. The temporary therapy option through rental equipment makes it possible to use FES as an affordable addition to conventional occupational and physical therapy. The basic requirement for its use is the training competency and experience of the therapist. Furthermore, the patient's self-motivation as well as supporting caregivers are crucial (Fig. 16.2).

# INSTRUCTIONS ELECTRICAL STIMULATION FOR HOME-BASED EXERCISE PROGRAM

## functional electrical stimulation - "wrist & finger extension" program

**program selection:**

hand active (saved)

**material:**

5 self-adhesive electrodes, 3 electrode cables (orange, yellow, white), main cable, towel roll

**starting position:**

sitting, with eye contact to the hand, the hand should lie comfortably without slipping, wrist slightly bent

**procedure:**

- switch on the device
- select program „hand active" (saved)
- set threshold for EMG trigger
- "relax and contract" confirm each time
- "start" and individually set current (mA) for channel 1 (orange) and channel 2 (yellow)
- start the program by pressing the "enter button" (under the rotary knob)

**electrode position:**

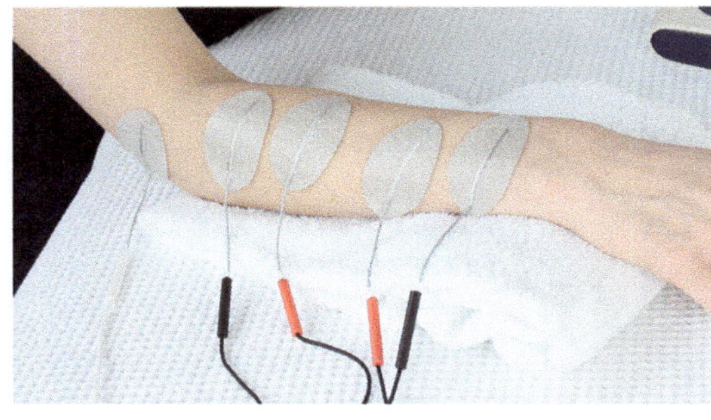

**rear electrodes:**
towards the elbow (channel 1) stick the electrode across the muscle belly in the rear third of the forearm

**front electrodes:**
towards the hand (channel 2) stick the electrodes across the forearm near the wrist in the direction of the little finger

**5th electrode** with white cable: attach to the elbow

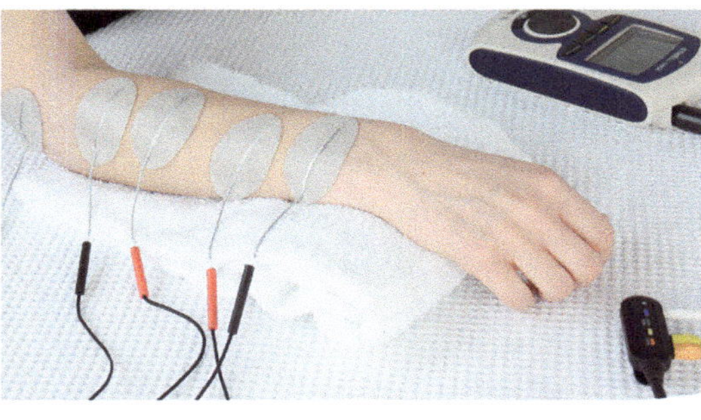

**approx. 18 mA:**
the wrist should be raised
(rear electrodes)

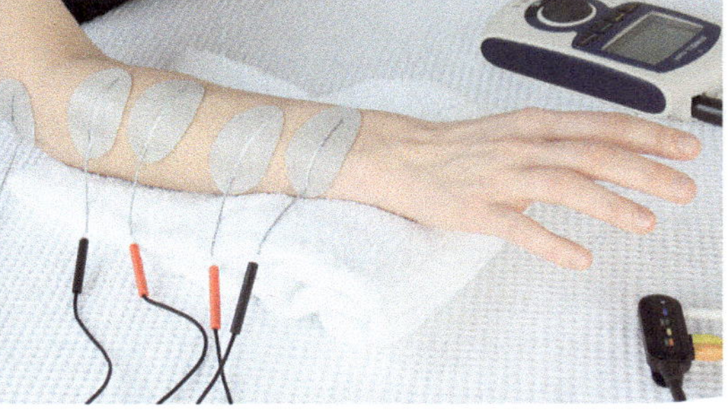

**approx. 24 mA:**
the fingers should extend
(front electrodes)

**The movement sequence should be started by the upward movement of the right wrist.**

**Fig. 16.2** Instructions—exemplary personalized patient instructions to support correct home-based use as reusable training material

## References


1. Nelles G. Rehabilitation von sensomotorischen Störungen. In: Diener P, Berlit D, Elger G, et al., editors. Leitlinien für Diagnostik und Ther der Neurol. Stuttgart: Georg Thieme Verlag; 2018. p. 1–45. http://www.thieme-connect.de/products/ebooks/abstract/10.1055/b-0034-18891.

2. Coupar F, Pollock A, Legg LA, Sackley C, van Vliet P. Home-based therapy programmes for upper limb functional recovery following stroke. In: Coupar F, editor. Cochrane Database of Systematic Reviews. Chichester: John Wiley & Sons, Ltd; 2012. p. 1465–858. http://doi.wiley.com/10.1002/14651858.CD006755.

3. Hsieh Y-W, Chang K-C, Hung J-W, Wu C-Y, Fu M-H, Chen C-C. Effects of home-based versus clinic-based rehabilitation combining mirror therapy and task-specific training for patients with stroke: a randomized crossover trial. Arch Phys Med Rehabil. 2018;99:2399–407.

4. Schneider EJ, Lannin NA, Ada L, Schmidt J. Increasing the amount of usual rehabilitation improves activity after stroke: a systematic review. J Physiother. 2016;62:182–7. https://doi.org/10.1016/j.jphys.2016.08.006.

5. Winstein CJ, Stein J, Arena R, Bates B, Cherney LR, Cramer SC, et al. Guidelines for adult stroke rehabilitation and recovery. Stroke. 2016;47:e98–169. https://www.ahajournals.org/doi/10.1161/STR.0000000000000098

6. Vloothuis JDM, Mulder M, Veerbeek JM, Konijnenbelt M, Visser-Meily JMA, Ket JCF, Kwakkel G, van Wegen EE. Caregiver-mediated exercises for improving outcomes after stroke. Cochrane Database Syst Rev. 2016;12:1–117.

7. Korpershoek C, van der Bijl J, Hafsteinsdóttir TB. Self-efficacy and its influence on recovery of patients with stroke: a systematic review. J Adv Nurs. 2011;67:1876–94. http://doi.wiley.com/10.1111/j.1365-2648.2011.05659.x

8. Gabr U, Levine P, Page SJ. Home-based electromyography-triggered stimulation in chronic stroke. Clin Rehabil. 2005;19:737–45. http://journals.sagepub.com/doi/10.1191/0269215505cr909oa

9. Da-Silva RH, Moore SA, Price CI. Self-directed therapy programmes for arm rehabilitation after stroke: a systematic review. Clin Rehabil. 2018;32:1022–36. http://journals.sagepub.com/doi/10.1177/0269215518775170

10. Minami S, Fykumoto Y, Kobayashi R, Aoki H, Aoyama T. Effect of home-based rehabilitation of purposeful activity-based electrical stimulation therapy for chronic stroke survivors: a crossover randomized controlled trial. Restor Neurol Neurosci. 2021;1–8

11. Hara Y, Ogawa S, Tsujiuchi K, Muraoka Y. A home-based rehabilitation program for the hemiplegic upper extremity by power-assisted functional electrical stimulation. Disabil Rehabil. 2008;30:296–304. http://www.tandfonline.com/doi/full/10.1080/09638280701265539

12. Alona G, Sunnerhagen KS, Geurts ACH, Ohry A. A home-based, self-administered stimulation program to improve selected hand functions of chronic stroke. NeuroRehabilitation. 2003;18:215–25.

13. Kern H, Gargiulo P, Pond A, Albertin G, Marcante A, Carraro U. To reverse atrophy of human muscles in complete SCI lower motor neuron denervation by home-based functional electrical stimulation. Adv Exp Med Biol. 2018;1088:585–91.

14. Fischer H, Endmann A, Reitz T, Gruchmann T. Der usability engineering Prozess für Medizinprodukte nach IEC. Mensch und Computer – Usability Prof Berlin; 2015;172–83.

15. Willand MP, de Bruin H. Design and testing of an instrumentation system to reduce stimulus pulse amplitude requirements during FES. 2008 30th Annual International Conference of the IEEE Engineering in Medicine and Biology Society. IEEE; 2008. p. 2764–7. http://ieeexplore.ieee.org/document/4649775/

16. Ferguson M, Brandreth M, Brassington W, Leighton P, Wharrad H. A randomized controlled trial to evaluate the benefits of a multimedia educational program for first-time hearing aid users. Ear Hear. 2016;37:123–36. http://content.wkhealth.com/linkback/openurl?sid=WKPTLP:landingpage&an=00003446-201603000-00001

17. King TL, Kho EKY, Tiong YH, Julaihi SNB. Comparison of effectiveness and time-efficiency between multimedia and conventional counselling on metered-dose inhaler technique education. Singap Med J. 2015;56:103–8.

18. Bustamante A, García-Berrocoso T, Rodriguez N, Llombart V, Ribó M, Molina C, et al. Ischemic stroke outcome: a review of the influence of post-stroke complications within the different scenarios of stroke care. Eur J Intern Med. 2016;29:9–21. https://www.sciencedirect.com/science/article/pii/S0953620515004288

19. Warner G, Packer T, Villeneuve M, Audulv A, Versnel J. A systematic review of the effectiveness of stroke self-management programs for improving function and participation outcomes: self-management programs for stroke survivors. Disabil Rehabil. 2015;37:2141–63. http://www.tandfonline.com/doi/full/10.3109/09638288.2014.996674

20. Platz T, Roschka S. S3-Leitlinie "Rehabilitative Therapie bei Armparese nach Schlaganfall" der DGNR – Langversion; 2020. https://www.awmf.org/uploads/tx_szleitlinien/080-0011_S3_Rehabilitative_Therapie_bei_Armparese_nach_Schlaganfall_2020-07.pdf. Accessed 07.06.2021.

21. Miller KK, Porter RE, DeBaun-Sprague E, Van Puymbroeck M, Schmid AA. Exercise after stroke: patient adherence and beliefs after discharge from rehabilitation. Top Stroke Rehabil. 2017;24:142–8. https://www.tandfonline.com/doi/full/10.1080/10749357.2016.1200292

22. Rand D, Eng JJ, Tang P-F, Jeng J-S, Hung C. How active are people with stroke? Stroke. 2009;40:163–8. https://

www.ahajournals.org/doi/10.1161/STROKEAHA.
108.523621

23. Oussedik E, Foy CG, Masicampo EJ, Kammrath LK, Anderson RE, Feldman SR. Accountability: a missing construct in models of adherence behavior and in clinical practice. Patient Prefer Adherence. 2017;11:1285–94. https://www.dovepress.com/accountability-a-missing-construct-in-models-of-adherence-behavior-and-peer-reviewed-article-PPA

24. Nadarajah M, Goh H-T. Post-stroke fatigue: a review on prevalence, correlates, measurement, and management. Top Stroke Rehabil. 2015;22:208–20. http://www.tandfonline.com/doi/full/10.1179/1074935714Z.0000000015

25. Jyotirekha D, Rajanikant GK. Post stroke depression: the sequelae of cerebral stroke. Neurosci Biobehav Rev. 2018;90:104–14. https://linkinghub.elsevier.com/retrieve/pii/S0149763417302130

26. Parke HL, Epiphaniou E, Pearce G, Taylor SJC, Sheikh A, Griffiths CJ, et al. Self-management support interventions for stroke survivors: a systematic meta-review. PLoS One. 2015;10:1–23.

27. Poltawski L, Boddy K, Forster A, Goodwin VA, Pavey AC, Dean S. Motivators for uptake and maintenance of exercise: perceptions of long-term stroke survivors and implications for design of exercise programmes. Disabil Rehabil. 2015;37:795–801. http://www.tandfonline.com/doi/full/10.3109/09638288.2014.946154

28. Oussedik E, Cline A, Su JJ, Masicampo E, Kammrath LK, Ip E, et al. Accountability in patient adherence. Patient Prefer Adherence. 2019;13:1511–7. https://www.dovepress.com/accountability-in-patient-adherence-peer-reviewed-article-PPA

Thomas Schick

In a systematic search for literature on Functional Electrical Stimulation (FES), including EMG-FES, one is confronted with a very large number of studies with a wide variety of questions. These studies describe the use of FES in a wide variety of clinical pictures and a wide variety of applications. For simplification and to improve the clarity of reading this book chapter, the term FES will be used exclusively, even if the authors of the primary literature sometimes use the term neuromuscular electrical stimulation (NMES) or even just electrical stimulation (ES).

## 17.1 FES in Stroke Rehabilitation at the Structural and Functional Level

Due to a large number of high-quality randomized controlled trials (RCT) on FES, there are numerous systematic reviews with meta-analyses on scientific questions, especially on stroke rehabilitation. In many studies, subjects are predominantly examined at the structural and functional level and corresponding assessments are used.

In 2019, a meta-analysis on post-stroke care [1] was published with a focus on wrist and hand movement recovery. The authors concluded that EMG-FES is effective in chronic stroke patients and produces robust short-term effects on upper extremity functions. The authors included 26 studies with a total of 782 patients. More than 50% of the studies were of high quality.

In the same year, another meta-analysis [2] by Taiwanese researchers analyzed the effectiveness of restoring arm-hand function in stroke patients. They included 48 RCTs with a total number of 1712 patients and concluded that electrical simulation therapy (cyclic-, EMG-triggered-, sensory stimulation) can effectively improve arm function in stroke patients.

One year earlier, based on literature published over a 10-year period and an included European consensus process, a systematic review [3] recommended the use of FES in stroke patients to improve upper extremity strength and function.

The American Heart Association (AHA) and American Stroke Association (ASA) published a guideline for healthcare stakeholders on stroke rehabilitation for adults [4]. The use of FES is appropriate for patients with minimal voluntary movement or shoulder subluxation. The use of FES for short-term improvement of spasticity would also be appropriate. The rationale refers to the highest level of evidence "A" of class IIa and IIb.

To improve the function and motor impairments of the wrist and forearm muscles, FES should be considered in rehabilitation after stroke in the early and chronic phase due to the existing

T. Schick (✉)
MED-EL, Department Neurorehabilitation
STIWELL, Innsbruck, Austria
e-mail: schick@neuro-reha.info



T. Schick (ed.), *Functional Electrical Stimulation in Neurorehabilitation*,
https://doi.org/10.1007/978-3-030-90123-3_17

high level of evidence "A." This conclusion was reached by a Canadian researcher group [5] in their practice recommendation for stroke rehabilitation (Table 17.1).

A frequently observed problem in stroke rehabilitation is shoulder joint subluxation. A result of the systematic review and meta-analysis [6] on this issue showed that there was a significant difference in the intervention groups in which FES was applied early after stroke to reduce shoulder joint subluxation. The authors concluded that FES can prevent or reduce shoulder joint subluxation in the early phase after a stroke.

A systematic review with a meta-analysis [7] was conducted to answer the question of whether FES should be used for spasticity control in stroke rehabilitation. The authors included 29 RCTs with 940 stroke patients and described in their conclusion that FES should also be considered in combination with other treatment modalities as a treatment option to reduce spasticity and to increase the range of motion after stroke.

**Table 17.1** Guidelines for upper extremity evidence in FES after stroke or cervical spinal cord lesion in rehabilitation and their recommendations

| method | author | year | title | recommendation |
|---|---|---|---|---|
| guideline | Küçükdeveci et al. | 2018 | evidence-based position paper on physical and rehabilitation medicine professional practice for persons with stroke | "It is recommended that electrical stimulation to wrist, forearm and shoulder muscles are considered to improve strength and improve upper limb function." |
| guideline | Winstein et al. | 2016 | guidelines for adult stroke rehabilitation and recovery | "NMES should be considered for individuals with minimal volitional movement within the first few months after stroke or for individuals with shoulder subluxation." |
| guideline | Hebert et al. | 2016 | stroke rehabilitation practice guideline | "FES targeted at the wrist and forearm muscles should be considered to reduce motor impairment and improve function." |
| guideline | Deutsch-sprachige Medizini-sche Gesell-schaft für Para-plegiologie e.V. | 2020 | improvement of the functional capacity of the upper extremities in cervical spinal paralysis. | "Electrical stimulation leads to improvements in muscle physiology and structure. Current evidence shows efficacy in subgroups e.g., improved hand function in chronic incomplete tetraplegia, combined strength training after botulinum toxin injection, or during reconstructive surgery of the upper extremity." |

EMG-triggered multichannel electrical stimulation (EMG-MES) is now receiving considerable attention in neurorehabilitation due to the possibility of combining it with a task-oriented approach. A study currently in the publication phase [8] investigated the effects on the upper extremities after stroke and addresses the question whether EMG-multichannel electrical stimulation (EMG-MES) is superior to pure cyclic ES. The results of this pilot study suggest that this may be the case. A study in 9 chronic stroke patients investigated the cortical effects using fMRI after EMG-MES [9]. Here, an improved arm function (Fugl-Meyer Assessment) and an increased cortical activation on the affected hemisphere of the brain were observed after 8 weeks by task-oriented training in connection with the use of EMG-MES.

EMG-MES combined with the established therapy concept such as mirror therapy (ST) (Sect. 14.2) was also investigated. In a multicenter RCT [10], the severity-dependent use of bilateral EMG-MES in combination with ST has been investigated in post-acute stroke patients. Compared to the comparison group without mirror therapy, the severely affected patients benefited significantly in terms of motor function in the intervention group, as measured by the Fugl-Meyer assessment.

The effectiveness of combining FES with botulinum toxin A (BoNT-A) (Sect. 14.3) was the subject of an early double-blind, placebo-controlled clinical study in 1998 [11]. The authors checked muscle tone using Ashworth scaling before, and 2, 6, and 12 weeks after the BoNT-A injection. In addition, the intervention group received electrical stimulation of the affected muscle for 30 min each for 3 days. The authors concluded that the effect of BoNT-A injection significantly increased by electrical stimulation.

A modern therapeutic approach of combining BoNT-A with EMG-FES and task-oriented therapy in stroke patients with upper limb spasticity was chosen by a Japanese researcher group [12].

Here, the focus was not on spastic muscle stimulation but on the ability to perform goal-directed hand functions after BoNT-A injection. Muscle tone measured by Ashworth scaling, grip function measured by the box-and-block test, and grip strength improved significantly 10 days after BoNT-A injection. The authors concluded that task-oriented training with EMG-FES after botulinum toxin injection effectively reduces spasticity and improves upper extremity function after stroke.

## 17.2 FES in Stroke Rehabilitation at Activity Level

In the previous section, the focus of the scientific literature was on structural and functional deficits after stroke. The following studies refer to the activity level.

Can FES effectively induce positive changes for the activities of daily living (ADL)? A group of researchers [13] investigated this question. They found 20 studies, of which 3 studies reported effects of FES on ADL, 2 months after stroke. In conclusion, the authors emphasized that FES is a promising component of future stroke rehabilitation. In this review, significant effects of FES were found which positively affected ADL within 2 months after stroke.

A systematic review and meta-analysis [14] included 19 studies with activity level effects. They compared the FES therapy group with control groups treated with either placebo stimulation, no training at all, or upper extremity training alone after stroke. The authors concluded that FES resulted in a moderate improvement of activities compared with no intervention or training alone.

An improvement of arm-hand activities using FES has already been described in a previous review and meta-analysis [15]. 25 RCTs on EMG-FES were included, in which the interventions led to significant, homogeneous positive effects on hand activities of the paretic arm, but also on motor functions.

## 17.3 FES After Stroke in Home-Based Therapy

In addition to the clinical use of FES in inpatient and outpatient rehabilitation, another important area is home-based therapy with suitable electrical stimulation devices. Especially in stroke rehabilitation, active rehabilitation at home can be effectively designed by FES, already achieved motor functions can be stabilized or further improved.

A group of researchers investigated whether EMG-FES can be used effectively at home in chronic stroke patients in a randomized controlled trial [16]. The chronic stroke patients underwent an 8-week home therapy program with EMG-FES, followed by an 8-week home therapy program without EMG-FES in the so-called cross-over design. Thus, both groups each completed an 8-week EMG-FES phase. The authors concluded that after the respective 8-week EMG-FES home-based therapy program, the subjects showed only a moderate reduction in damage as measured by the Fugl-Meyer assessment, but a significant increase in active wrist extension above 20 degrees.

Other researchers were able to confirm these results in another RCT [17]. They had 20 chronic stroke patients in the experimental group, for which the event occurred more than 1 year ago. They underwent a total of thirty 60-min EMG-FES sessions at home and compared the results over a period of 5 months. Patients in the EMG-FES group showed significant improvements compared to the control group in active range of motion, modified Ashworth scaling, and hand function tests and were able to fully re-involve their hand in activities of daily living after 5 months.

A systematic review [18] analyzed self-directed therapy programs after stroke. The effects of the individual procedures and the timing of the interventions differed. Stroke patients benefited in particular also from electrical stimulation procedures (Table 17.2).

**Summary**

FES is successfully used in stroke rehabilitation for patients with structural, functional and activity deficits in early and chronic phases. It should also be considered for home-based therapy.

## 17.4 FES for the Treatment of Multiple Sclerosis (MS)

In a retrospective cohort study, a US research group [19] investigated the effects of FES-assisted cycling in activity-based rehabilitation of MS patients with different courses. In particular, patients with primary chronic progressive MS experienced significant improvements in motor tests as a result of FES. The authors concluded that FES as a component of activity-based rehabilitation can maintain or improve various neurological functions.

A systematic review on the effects of FES on foot lift weakness in people with MS [20] included 8 studies addressing this question; 7 studies demonstrated significant positive effects on health-related quality of life. The authors concluded that the review provides preliminary evidence that FES has positive effects on quality of life for people with MS.

**Summary**

Evidence supports the successful use of FES in people with MS. FES can favorably influence motor function and quality of life.

## 17.5 FES in the Field of Neuropediatrics

Is FES applicable and useful in children with a wide range of neurological deficits? The following reviews have investigated this question.

**Table 17.2** Overview of systematic reviews and meta-analyses on FES after stroke with the original title and conclusion of the scientific papers

| method | author | year | title | goal | RCT | n= | conclusion |
|---|---|---|---|---|---|---|---|
| systematic review and meta-analysis | Yang et al. | 2019 | effectiveness of electrical stimulation therapy in improving arm function after stroke | investigation of effectiveness of ES in arm function recovery after stroke. | 48 | 1712 | Electrical stimulation therapy can effectively improve the arm function in stroke patients. |
| systematic review and meta-analysis | Monte-Silva et al. | 2019 | electromyogram-related neuromuscular electrical stimulation for restoring wrist and hand movement in poststroke hemiplegia | functional and structural level EMG-triggered FES | 26 | 782 | "EMG-NMES is effective in the short term in improving UL impairment in individuals with chronic stroke." |
| systematic review | Da Silva et al. | 2018 | self-directed therapy programmes for arm rehabilitation after stroke | functional and structural level home based therapy | 11 | 94 | "Self-directed interventions can enhance arm recovery after stroke, but the effect varies according to the approach used and the timing. There were benefits identified from self-directed … electrical stimulation." |
| systematic review and meta-analysis | Eraifej et al. | 2017 | effectiveness of upper limb functional electrical stimulation after stroke for the improvement of activities of daily living and motor function | activity level FES | 20 | 67 | "FES is a promising therapy which could play a part in future stroke rehabilitation. This review found a statistically significant benefit from FES applied within 2 months after stroke on the primary outcome of ADL." |
| systematic review and meta-analysis | Howlett et al. | 2015 | functional electrical stimulation improves activity after stroke | activity level FES | 18 | 485 | "FES appears to moderately improve activity compared with both no intervention and training alone. These findings suggest that FES should be used in stroke rehabilitation to improve the ability to perform activities." |
| systematic review and meta-analysis | Vafadar et al. | 2015 | effectiveness of functional electrical stimulation in improving clinical outcomes in the upper arm following stroke | functional and structural level shoulder subluxation | 10 | 213 | "FES can be used to prevent or reduce shoulder subluxation early after stroke." |
| systematic review and meta-analysis | Stein et al. | 2015 | effects of electrical stimulation in spastic muscles after stroke | functional and structural level spasticity | 29 | 940 | "NMES combined with other intervention modalities can be considered as a treatment option that provides improvements in spasticity and range of motion in patients after stroke." |
| systematic review and meta-analysis | Veerbeek et al. | 2014 | What Is the evidence for physical therapy poststroke? | functional, structural and activity level | 25 | 492 | "Wrist and finger extensors. The meta-analyses resulted in significant homogeneous positive summary effect sizes for motor function of the paretic arm (synergy) and arm-hand activities. A significant effect was found for the active range of motion." |

A group of researchers [21] investigated the effects of FES on activity abilities of children with infantile cerebral palsy (ICP). Of the 5 RCTs included, 3 reported statistically significant group differences in favor of FES compared to groups without FES. The authors concluded that the available evidence suggests that the use of FES in children shows a stronger effect than no FES and is comparable to the effects of activity training.

The US authors of a systematic review [22] with 37 included studies make differentiated statements. They found that in most studies including children with ICP, FES has positive effects on passive range of motion (PROM), upper extremity functions, sitting stability, walking speed, and foot lift function during walking. Similarly, bone density was positively affected using FES in combination with ergometry. Furthermore, FES can have a positive effect on bladder and digestive tract management. In conclusion, it was described that FES is safe and well tolerated by children with various impairments. The authors further suggest that this therapy should be used more widely in pediatrics.

The effects of FES in supporting foot-lifting function in the swing-leg phase of walking were investigated by a group of researchers [23]. The authors found that there is strong evidence for improved foot lifting function in the swing and initial contact phases of walking. FES resulted in increased walking speed and increased stride length.

An important question in child therapy is the minimum age of the children to be treated. Most studies included children starting from the age of 4 years. A case study [24] describes the safe and appropriate use of FES for upper extremity improvement in a 2-year-old child with hemiplegia.

**Summary**
FES is well suited for the treatment of neurologically induced motor deficits in early childhood. Moreover, it is safe and well tolerated by children.

## 17.6 FES in Incomplete Cervical Spinal Cord Injury

In the past, there has been a significant increase in research interest on FES in the area of tetraplegia. In 2020, a German S2e guideline [25] on upper extremity rehabilitation in tetraplegia has been published (Table 17.1). The aim is to improve the quality of treatment for those affected. The importance of FES as a pre- and postoperative treatment for tendon reconstruction of the arm or hand in tetraplegics after a cervical spinal cord syndrome has already been successfully demonstrated [26]. The importance of choosing the right therapeutic intervention rather than intensity alone in incomplete tetraplegia (C3–C7) was found by a Canadian research group [27] in an interesting retrospective analysis. Subjects received either occupational therapy with a total of 45 h (group 1), 80 h (group 2), or 80 h of FES for hand function in addition to occupational therapy (intervention group). The best and significant functional results were seen in the intervention group with combined FES and occupational therapy, as measured by the Functional Independence Measure (FIM) and the Spinal Cord Independence Measure (SCIM).

In a previous RCT [28], patients who received regular intensive FES for hand function showed better functional outcomes after discharge from rehabilitation. This is also true for long-term observations.

**Summary**
FES can improve upper extremity function after incomplete central cord syndrome.

## 17.7 FES in Lower Motor Neuron Syndrome (LMNS)

The treatment of the consequences of damage to a peripheral nerve or the LMN has been the subject of intense scientific research for several years. Based on current literature and experience, it can be strongly assumed that the targeted use of FES not only preserves musculature in its structure and extent, but also supports nerve regeneration.

For example, researchers [29] wrote that FES and exercise therapy are promising treatments for peripheral nerve lesions and have great potential for translation into clinical practice. They additionally noted that FES promotes nerve regeneration after delayed nerve repair in humans and in animal studies with rats.

In an exciting review [30], the authors conclude, based on the existing literature, that low-frequency ES can effectively promote axonal regeneration immediately after surgery. Promising evidence of maximizing functional recovery in various types of peripheral nerve injuries has been obtained with electrical stimulation.

In an extensive EU-funded research project (RISE-project) dealing with LMNS [31] [32], chronically denervated patients after paraplegic lesion were investigated. Using intensive home-based FES therapy with long pulses and high intensity, the lower extremities were stimulated for 2 years and studied under a wide variety of aspects. Out of 25 patients, 20 were stimulated with an intensity of 5 treatments per week for the required 2 years. The observation showed a significant increase in the cross-sectional area of the quadriceps muscle (+35%) and in the diameter of the quadriceps muscle fibers (+75%). Furthermore, denervation-induced skin atrophy was counteracted where an increase in epidermis was recorded. In addition to cosmetic effects due to the decrease in muscle atrophy, the cushion effects of the thigh muscles to prevent pressure ulceration when sitting for several hours should be emphasized.

In summary, based on the available studies in the field of treatment of denervated musculature in LMNS, the use of FES can also be justified in home-based therapy under expert medical-therapeutic supervision with suitable electrical stimulation devices.

**Summary**
Based on evidence it can be said that FES both supports nerve regeneration and counteracts muscle atrophy in peripheral nerve damage for denervated muscles.

## References

1. Monte-Silva K, et al. Electromyogram-related neuromuscular electrical stimulation for restoring wrist and hand movement in poststroke hemiplegia: a systematic review and meta-analysis. Neurorehabil Neural Repair. 2019;33(2):96–111.
2. Yang J-D, et al. Effectiveness of electrical stimulation therapy in improving arm function after stroke: a systematic review and a meta-analysis of randomised controlled trials. Clin Rehabil. 2019;33(8):1286–97.
3. Küçükdeveci AA, et al. Evidence-based position paper on physical and rehabilitation medicine professional practice for persons with stroke. The European PRM position (UEMS PRM Section). Eur J Phys Rehabil Med. 2018;54(6):957–70.
4. Winstein CJ, et al. Guidelines for adult stroke rehabilitation and recovery: a guideline for healthcare professionals from the American Heart Association/American Stroke Association. Stroke. 2016;47(6):e98–169.
5. Hebert D, et al. Canadian stroke best practice recommendations: stroke rehabilitation practice guidelines, update 2015. Int J Stroke. 2016;11(4):459–84.
6. Vafadar AK, Côté JN, Archambault PS. Effectiveness of functional electrical stimulation in improving clinical outcomes in the upper arm following stroke: a systematic review and meta-analysis. Biomed Res Int. 2015;729768:1–14.
7. Stein C, et al. Effects of electrical stimulation in spastic muscles after stroke: systematic review and meta-analysis of randomized controlled trials. Stroke. 2015;46(8):2197–205.
8. Fheodoroff K, et al. Efficacy of four-channel functional electrical stimulation on moderate arm paresis in subacute stroke patients- results from a pilot randomised controlled study. WCNR Congress. WFNR – Motor control (kinesiology, spasticity, etc.) ePoster ID P0306; 2020.
9. von Lewinski F, et al. Efficacy of EMG-triggered electrical arm stimulation in chronic hemiparetic stroke patients. Restor Neurol Neurosci. 2009;27(3):189–97. https://doi.org/10.3233/RNN-2009-0469.
10. Schick T, et al. Synergy effects of combined multichannel EMG-triggered electrical stimulation and

mirror therapy in subacute stroke patients with severe or very severe arm/hand paresis. Restor Neurol Neurosci. 2017;35(3):319–32.

11. Hesse S, et al. Botulinum toxin type A and short-term electrical stimulation in the treatment of upper limb flexor spasticity after stroke: a randomized, double-blind, placebo-controlled trial. Clin Rehabil. 1998;12(5):381–8.

12. Tsuchiya M, Morita A, Hara Y. Effect of dual therapy with botulinum toxin a injection and electromyography-controlled functional electrical stimulation on active function in the spastic paretic hand. J Nippon Med Sch. 2016;83(1):15–23.

13. Eraifej J, et al. Effectiveness of upper limb functional electrical stimulation after stroke forthe improvement of activities of daily living and motor function: a systematic review and meta-analysis. Syst Rev. 2017;6(1):40.

14. Howlett OA, et al. Functional electrical stimulation improves activity after stroke: a systematic review with meta-analysis. Arch Phys Med Rehabil. 2015;96(5):934–43.

15. Veerbeck JM, et al. What is the evidence for physical therapy poststroke? A systematic review and meta-analysis. PLoS One. 2014;9(2)

16. Gabr U, Levine P, Page SJ. Home-based electromyography-triggered stimulation in chronic stroke, RCT. Clin Rahabil. 2005;19(7):737–45.

17. Hara Y, et al. A home-based rehabilitation program for the hemiplegic upper extremity by power-assisted functional electrical stimulation. Disabil Rehabil. 2008;30(4):296–304.

18. Da-Silva RH, Moore SA, Price CI. Self-directed therapy programmes for arm rehabilitation after stroke: a systematic review. Clin Rehabil. 2018;32(8):1022–36.

19. Hammond ER, et al. Functional electrical stimulation as a component of activity-based restorative therapy may preserve function in persons with multiple sclerosis. J Spinal Cord Med. 2015;38(1):68–75.

20. Miller Renfrew L, et al. Evaluating the effect of functional electrical stimulation used for foot drop on aspects of health-related quality of life in people with multiple sclerosis: a systematic review. Int J MS Care. 2019;21(4):173–82.

21. Chiu HC, Ada L. Effect of functional electrical stimulation on activity in children with cerebral palsy: a systematic review. Pediatr Phys Ther Fall. 2014;26(3):283–8.

22. Bosques G, et al. Does therapeutic electrical stimulation improve function in children with disabilities? A comprehensive literature review. J Pediatr Rehabil Med. 2016;9(2):83–99.

23. Mooney JA, Rose J. A scoping review of neuromuscular electrical stimulation to improve gait in cerebral palsy: the arc of progress and future strategies. Front Neurol. 2019;10:887.

24. Musselman KE, et al. The feasibility of functional electrical stimulation toimprove upper extremity function in a two-year-old child with perinatal stroke: a case report. Phys Occup Ther Pediatr. 2018;38(1):97–112.

25. Deutschsprachige Medizinische Gesellschaft für Paraplegiologie e.V. S2e-Leitlinie "Verbesserung der Funktionsfähigkeit der oberen Extremitäten bei zervikaler Querschnittlähmung". AWMF-Register-Nr. 179–013. 2020. [Zitat vom: 06. April 2021.] https://www.awmf.org/uploads/tx_szleitlinien/179-0131_S2e_Verbesserung-der-Funktionsfaehigkeit-der-oberen-Extremitaeten-bei-zervikaler-Querschnittlaehmung_2020-10.pdf.

26. Bersch I, Friden J. Role of functional electrical stimulation in tetraplegia hand surgery. Arch Phys Med Rehabil. 2016;97(6 Suppl):154–9.

27. Kapadia NM, Bagher S, Popovic MR. Influence of different rehabilitation therapy models on patient outcomes: hand function therapy in individuals with incomplete SCI. J Spinal Cord Med. 2014;37(6):734–43.

28. Kapadia NM, et al. Functional electrical stimulation therapy for grasping in traumatic incomplete spinal cord injury: randomized control trial. Artif Organs. 2011;35(3):212–6.

29. Gordon T, English AW. Strategies to promote peripheral nerve regeneration: electrical stimulation and/or exercise. Eur J Neurosci. 2016;43(3):336–50.

30. Willand MP, et al. Electrical stimulation to promote peripheral nerve regeneration. Neurorehabil Neural Repair. 2016;30(5):490–6.

31. Kern H, et al. Home-based functional electrical stimulation rescues permanently denervated muscles in paraplegic patients with complete lower motor neuron lesion. Neurorehabil Neural Repair. 2010;24(8):709–21.

32. Kern H, et al. To reverse atrophy of human muscles in complete SCI lower motor neuron denervation by home-based functional electrical stimulation. Adv Exp Med Biol. 2018;1088:585–91.

# Absolute and Relative Contraindications



Winfried Mayr

## 18.1 Introduction

Functional electrical stimulation (FES) via skin-attached electrodes relies on relatively simple technical tools, which, only in combination with comprehensive understanding of clinical and physiological operation principles, become an important and powerful therapy option for a wide range of applications.

As the human organism is an electrolytic medium and electrical stimulation relies on impulse fields, that are induced via electrical current flow through electrode-skin-contacts, it is essential to comply with basic technical provisions and limitations for avoiding irreversible electrochemical processes and potential biological tissue damage. In addition, a number of health-related risk conditions need to be co-considered for a decision, if a planned intervention can be administered, requires adaptations, or even needs to be suspended due to intolerable risks [1]. After a thorough initial evaluation regular update assessments are recommended along longer application periods, as on one hand relevant border conditions can change over time, on the other hand in rare cases also negative reactions to the stimulation could appear and need to be detected as early as possible upon occurrence of first adverse signs.

General recommendations for identifying and handling contraindications are difficult, due to an enormous diversity in available devices and electrodes. Even though manufacturers usually provide lists of counterindications and their handling, that had been verified for certification, compliance with those can only cover part of factual risks. Also, electrical parameters and application protocols play an important role in specific risk assessments.

E.g., afferent nerve stimulation with intensity near the sensory threshold can be applied safely, if a passive metal implant is situated close to the surface electrodes. Neuromuscular or direct muscular stimulation with the same electrode configuration can be associated with a considerable risk for implant corrosion and tissue damage. Other concerns, like presence of active implants, intolerance against electrode materials, etc. would equally be relevant for all three modalities. Reality is more diverse than any accurately assembled list. It remains in the responsibility of physicians and therapists to identify additional individual risk factors, rate them, give personalized recommendations and carefully supervise the course of application.

Also, there is to be distinguished between primary assessments ahead a first application and later check-ups, in case of later observed salience. It is necessary to address unexpected observations in follow-up consultations, but also advice patients to stop application, in case of introspection of unusual symptoms or new health conditions, and ask back for qualified opinion and advice.

W. Mayr (✉)
Medical University of Vienna, Vienna, Austria
e-mail: winfried.mayr@meduniwien.ac.at


T. Schick (ed.), *Functional Electrical Stimulation in Neurorehabilitation*,
https://doi.org/10.1007/978-3-030-90123-3_18

As a general rule it is strongly recommended for the work with patients with manifest physical or mental health conditions – critical examples are increased thrombosis- or bleeding risk or epilepsy, or pregnancy – to contact involved clinical specialist and discuss if and how safe application is possible and under what precautions (Table 18.1). Possibilities to apply FES in patients with different forms and development stages of epilepsy require in any case consultations with the caring clinical specialists and strictly controlled conditions for the application with individually necessary safety measures. Generally, compliance with any recommendations by the manufacturer has to be taken seriously, which are obligatory parts of medical product documentation and are validated in specific risk assessment procedures in the product certification. Also, those can be relevant already with begin of an intended treatment or relevant later in case of changes in boarder conditions.

## 18.2 Skin Reaction

Manufacturers are obliged to guarantee that only validated biomaterials are used for contact surfaces and as contact media (e.g., electrode gel). Usually applied impulse currents are charge-balanced without direct current (DC) components. In addition, material and surface-specific charge injection limits per pulse phase must not be exceeded under any operational conditions. Under these precautions, stimulation can usually be applied safely to the intact skin surface. Still, in a minority of patients a slow conditioning phase can get necessary, where the skin can adapt to contact with electrode material, gel and current flow without pronounced irritation, in very rare cases also allergic reactions can occur. Therefore, it is essential to keep an eye on the skin condition after removal of electrodes, in particular at the beginning of a treatment series, but also regularly in long-term applications. Redness that declines within roughly 30 min and appears less pronouncedly with repeated application can be seen as uncritical and suggests stimulation-induced increased skin perfusion. If stronger and persisting alterations are noticed, the intervention needs to be stopped for medical investigation. It is important to explain these necessities to patients in preparation of home-based application and remind them from time to time on a regular basis.

Open wounds are taboo for applying FES for both initiating a session and continuing with series of session. Otherwise, there is a pronounced risk for compromising wound healing or infecting the wound via electrode placement. There are FES systems specifically dedicated to foster wound healing, but these rely on special stimulation systems and application procedures. For other therapeutic applications, it is strongly recommended to await wound healing before initiation or proceeding with application sessions. Should a wound have been caused by the FES, e.g., through locally excessive current density, it is mandatory to identify the exact history and develop provisions for reliably avoiding risks of reoccurrence [2].

## 18.3 Passive Implants

Special attention is required regarding passive metal implants. As FES is an important and versatile tool for movement rehabilitation, often after surgical osteosynthesis or joint replacement, there is increased probability for presence of metal components in or near the therapeutic target area. But metal parts can also be remains from older surgery, forgotten or at least with reduced awareness of type and location by the patient. Such passive metal implants can cause serious problems as they have far better electrical conductivity in comparison to surrounding tissue externally applied electrical current concentrates to pathways with lowest electrical resistance. Embedded metal components develop anodic and cathodic surface areas when current flows through and, like in electrodes in general, electrochemical processes can develop on these active interface surfaces with adjacent electrolytic conductors, like biological tissue. This can result in metal corrosion, electrochemical tissue damage, and migration of corrosion products (foreign body particles) into the biological tissue.

Unfortunately, these facts are often underestimated by manufacturers, statements seeing this interaction as more or less problem-free need to be critically scrutinized for individual application scenarios. The acute impact of short duration neural stimuli maybe so small that it becomes obvious only after longer repeated application, but immediate high risk can be associated with

**Table 18.1**  Checklist for handling relevant contraindications for application of FES

| verification before and during treatment period | | action |
| --- | --- | --- |
| manifest underlying physical or mental disease | ✓ | consult attending physician |
| pregnancy | ✓ | consult attending physician |
| contra-indication according to manufacturer documents | ✓ | absolute compliance – in doubt contact manufacturer |
| acute signs of skin disease or allergy visible | ✓ | no treatment before verification of reason and risk |
| wounds or scars in electrode application area | ✓ | no treatment before verification of reason and risk |
| metal implants in or near the anatomical treatment area | ✓ | verification of exact type and position<br>evaluation of treatment options without electrical field induction in the implant<br>exception: sensory nerve stimulation, not exceeding threshold intensity, generally uncritical |
| presence of active implants (even in distant anatomical regions) | ✓ | verification of exact type and position<br>strict compliance with manufacturer's warnings, ev. consultation of manufacturer, by no means: unauthorized testing |

application with long-duration impulses for direct activation of denervated muscles. Relatively uncritical is application of short duration pulses with threshold intensity for afferent nerve stimulation, as the current intensity is low enough to just reach neural skin sensors, and deeper lying metal components are not exposed to critical electrical field strength—but in any case, the specific configuration needs to be rated.

Therefore, in patients with obvious recent traumatic injuries, but also in persons where indicators for older injuries are suspected, it is of utmost importance to ask for type and anatomical position of implants and preferably for provision confirming medical documents. As soon as implants are verified special care must be taken to keep them securely outside applied electrical field ranges. Usually this can be accomplished by creative placement of electrode configurations, if this turns out to be impossible there is no other choice than omitting FES treatment in the respective body area till the implant gets surgically removed.

Similar considerations are necessary for tattoos in the treatment area, as tattoo colors often rely on metal particles for colourfastness, or metal piercings. In both cases electrochemical interaction with biological tissue can occur as soon as stimulation current is applied, which can result in metal corrosion and tissue damage. Therefore, electrode configurations need to reliably spare those danger zones. Of course, also temporary removal of piercings solves the problem.

## 18.4　Active Implants

A very complex situation occurs, if active implants like cardiac pacer, cardioverter, implants for pain treatment or neuromodulation, or drug administration pumps are present. As such implants usually are encapsulated in a metal shell there are similar risks for electro corrosion and tissue damage like described above for passive metal implants. In addition, risks for electrical malfunction and damage in the electronic circuitry need to be taken into account. Test with frequently implanted actual cardiac pacer models has given evidence that risks for harming the electronics have become very low, as manufacturers have implemented effective protection circuits against potentially dangerous excessive voltage at output terminals of the implant. Consequently, it has become more likely that the electrical field induction, associated with the stimulation, causes malfunction by false interpretation of stimulation artifacts as a valid bio-signal, most commonly an ECG. Modern pacers have sophisticated algorithms implanted to minimize such risks. So usually signals with high amplitude than expected are disregarded, which could, e.g., emerge from stimulation via surface electrodes that are placed close to implanted recording electrodes. The popular assumption, to expect less risk of pacemaker malfunction if just pacer and treatment site are far enough apart, does not hold, in contrary, the resulting small size artifacts are more likely misinterpreted as bio-signal.

Literature on this important topic is in principle available, but published results can hardly be generalized beyond the described specific test setup. Reasons are diversity of pacers, operation modes, and frequent model updates on one hand and patient-related factors like physiognomy, implant position, and indication related setup on the other hand. Studies are only valid for exact conditions; transfer of conclusions is only possible with great caution [3, 4].

In particular critical are cardioverter implants, implanted defibrillators with automated arrhythmia detection. If the monitored ECG gets contaminated by stimulation artifacts it can come to unnecessary delivery of an electrical shock, which is not only highly irritating and painful for the patient, but also substantially reduces implant lifetime due to drain of a considerable amount of energy from the battery. Usually implant manufacturers refuse clearance for use of electrotherapy, generally or at least with limitation to switched off state. It remains more or less impossible to find generally valid criteria for predicting safe operation conditions with all diversity of individual anatomy and locations of implant components. Therefore, utmost care and careful monitoring are required if there are reasons for applying FES despite the increased risk situation. In any case this should not be undertaken without consultation of the manufacturer for acquiring at least a conditional clearance [5, 6].

Meticulous initial assessments and regular re-evaluation are mandatory conditions for ensuring best possible patient safety.

## 18.5　Conclusion

In an overall view, the vast majority of FES applications can be regarded as safe and effective. Nevertheless, it is necessary to keep critical awareness for potential risk factors to be assessed before intervention and monitored along application series. If specific precautions are to be met also measures for ensuring patient compliance are essential. Most crucial conditions for self-responsible home-based application are informed patients and a sustainable confidence base, and a low-threshold option for consulting the therapist in case of worrisome observations.

# References

1. ELECTROPHYSICAL AGENTS - contraindications and precautions: an evidence-based approach to clinical decision making in physical therapy. Physiother Can. 2010;62(5):1–80. https://doi.org/10.3138/ptc.62.5. Epub 2011 Jan 5. PMID: 21886384; PMCID: PMC3031347

2. Fary RE, Briffa NK. Monophasic electrical stimulation produces high rates of adverse skin reactions in healthy subjects. Physiother Theory Pract. 2011;27(3):246–51. https://doi.org/10.3109/09593985.2010.487926.

3. Egger F, Hofer C, Hammerle FP, Löfler S, Nürnberg M, Fiedler L, Kriz R, Kern H, Huber K. Influence of electrical stimulation therapy on permanent pacemaker function. Wien Klin Wochenschr. 2019;131(13-14):313–20. https://doi.org/10.1007/s00508-019-1494-5. Epub 2019 Apr 25

4. Crevenna R, Mayr W, Keilani M, Pleiner J, Nuhr M, Quittan M, Pacher R, Fialka-Moser V, Wolzt M. Safety of a combined strength and endurance training using neuromuscular electrical stimulation of thigh muscles in patients with heart failure and bipolar sensing cardiac pacemakers. Wien Klin Wochenschr. 2003;115(19-20):710–4.

5. Badger J, Taylor P, Swain I. The safety of electrical stimulation in patients with pacemakers and implantable cardioverter defibrillators: a systematic review. J Rehabil Assist Technol Eng. 2017; https://doi.org/10.1177/2055668317745498.

6. Kamiya K, Satoh A, Niwano S, Tanaka S, Miida K, Hamazaki N, Maekawa E, Matsuzawa R, Nozaki K, Masuda T, Ako J. Safety of neuromuscular electrical stimulation in patients implanted with cardioverter defibrillators. J Electrocardiol. 2016;49(1):99–101, ISSN 0022-0736. https://doi.org/10.1016/j.jelectrocard.2015.11.006.

# Index

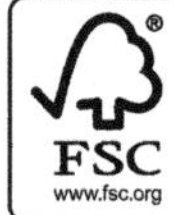